541 - 115128

W9-BZV-295

A TIME OF SCANDAL

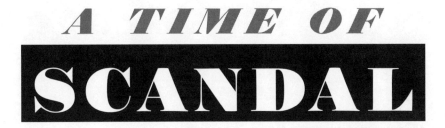

A TIME OF
SCANDAL

CHARLES R. FORBES
WARREN G. HARDING

AND THE MAKING OF THE
VETERANS BUREAU

ROSEMARY STEVENS

JOHNS HOPKINS UNIVERSITY PRESS
BALTIMORE

9 8 7 6 5 4 3 2 1

Johns Hopkins University Press
2715 North Charles Street
Baltimore, Maryland 21218-4363
www.press.jhu.edu

Library of Congress Cataloging-in-Publication Data
Names: Stevens, Rosemary, 1935– author.
Title: A time of scandal : Charles R. Forbes, Warren G. Harding, and the
    making of the Veterans Bureau / Rosemary Stevens.
Description: Baltimore, Maryland : Johns Hopkins University Press, 2016. |
    Includes bibliographical references and index.
Identifiers: LCCN 2016010032 | ISBN 9781421421308 (hardcover : alk. paper) |
    ISBN 1421421305 (hardcover : alk. paper) | ISBN 9781421421315 (electronic)
    | ISBN 1421421313 (electronic)
Subjects: LCSH: Forbes, Charles R., 1878–1952. | Harding, Warren G. (Warren
    Gamaliel), 1865–1923—Friends and associates. | Scandals—United
    States—History—20th century. | United States—Politics and
    government—1921–1923. | Forbes, Charles R., 1878–1952—Trials,
    litigation, etc. | United States. Veterans Bureau.
Classification: LCC E785 .S74 2016 | DDC 973.91/4092—dc23
    LC record available at https://lccn.loc.gov/2016010032

A catalog record for this book is available from the British Library.

*Special discounts are available for bulk purchases of this book. For more
information, please contact Special Sales at 410-516-6936 or specialsales
@press.jhu.edu.*

Johns Hopkins University Press uses environmentally friendly book materials,
including recycled text paper that is composed of at least 30 percent post-
consumer waste, whenever possible.

CONTENTS

....

Illustrations follow pages 94 and 179

PREFACE

....

This is a story of a boy who came to America with his family in the 1880s, lived through various up-and-down adventures, served heroically in World War I, became a prominent government official, and was then the center of a major national scandal—one of a cascade of political scandals in the mid-1920s. The man was Charles R. Forbes, the scandal was the Veterans Bureau scandal, and the "scandal time" the administration of two US presidents. Because the substance of the scandals occurred during Warren G. Harding's administration, they have come down in history as the "Harding scandals." However, their exposure as full-fledged scandals occurred during the administration of Harding's successor, Calvin Coolidge. Together, the two presidencies ran from March 1921 into 1929.

The Veterans Bureau scandal broke as front-page national news in late 1923, soon after Harding's unexpected death. On its heels came the oil scandal, known as Teapot Dome, and while the first two were in play the US Department of Justice was investigated. Three men were at the center of these major scandals: Charles R. Forbes (whom Harding had appointed as the founding director of the new US Veterans Bureau), Albert B. Fall (Harding's secretary of the interior), and Harry M. Daugherty (Harding's attorney general), respectively. The three acquired a lasting label as members of Harding's Ohio Gang, who went to Washington to loot the federal treasury. When hearings on the Veterans Bureau and Teapot Dome ran at the same time in the same Senate office building, visitors to Washington could choose which drama to attend. Allegations became sensations as colorful witnesses described (in the Forbes case) bribes, plots, missing documents, excessive drinking, jumping into a pool fully dressed, greed, revelry run amok. The scandals were moral tales and public spectacles, good stories that took on a life of their own. So good that, until now, the facts of the Veterans Bureau scandal were neglected and Forbes's culpability unexplored.

Colonel Forbes was convicted in federal court for conspiring with others to defraud the federal government by rigging government contracts to build hospitals for military veterans of World War I. He was branded as a criminal, shamed as a disgrace, and served time in the federal penitentiary at Leavenworth. In the public narratives of the scandals in the 1920s and afterward, Albert Fall was a man tempted and overcome by greed, but Forbes was worse than this. Here was a man willing to cheat sick and wounded American warriors out of the services they deserved. He was both a criminal and a pariah.

The personal story of Charles R. Forbes would be worth retelling as a narrative arc of rise and fall; though in life, as we'll see, he thrust aside his painful experiences in the 1920s and lived on to enjoy his grandchildren outside of public view. Of more importance to *A Time of Scandal*, Forbes's experiences thread through and illuminate significant movements and themes in political life in the 1920s. As founding director of the organization now known as the US Department of Veterans Affairs, he is a necessary part of the history of veterans' services in the United States. As creator of the federal system of veterans hospitals that exists to this day, he is part of the history of American hospitals and health care. He participated in efforts to bring business efficiency to government in the Harding administration, and, when he was no longer in office, he was a major character in the drama of the Harding scandals as they played out in the Coolidge years.

The Harding scandals were significant in presenting Coolidge as morally and administratively superior to Harding and the hotbed of scandal attributed to him. Revelations of scandalous behavior by government officials stimulated reforms in executive agencies, including those run by Secretaries Fall and Daugherty, and Director Forbes. As Republicans, Progressives, and Democrats, for different reasons, rallied around the cause of vilifying Harding and his administration, Forbes served as a villain in a historical narrative of the Veterans Bureau scandal that has remained unchallenged until this book.

The disparity between the casual descriptions of Forbes in the historical literature (and in popular fiction, too, as we'll see) and the official dimensions of his job irked me for years, while I was working on other projects. The two views did not seem to fit together. In the literature, Forbes appeared as a character in an American folktale or gangster movie rather than a high-level bureaucrat with oversight of one of the largest budgets in the federal government. The literary character called Charles or "Charlie" Forbes was a stereotyped crony of dubious reputation and hazy background, bandying jokes and brandishing a whiskey glass, whose narrative role was to support negative depictions of Warren Harding. More recent revisionist accounts of Harding have shown Harding as a stronger man and a more skilled politician than formerly depicted but left the secondary characters unrevised. Strings of adjectives have commonly attended Forbes's description: loud, sexual (imbued with animal vitality), coarse, free-spending, heavy drinking (during Prohibition), amoral, back-slapping, rough, poker-playing, picaresque, crooked, a good-time Charlie. In 2010, a popular television series began, set in the 1920s, with a gangster character called "Nucky" Thompson at its center. The series, *Boardwalk Empire*, referred to Forbes as a well-known crook.

Descriptions of Forbes also offered contradictory messages. If, as in one variant, he was a high-living predatory fool, how did he manage to avoid detection of his crimes between 1921 and 1923? He must have been smart. If he managed to steal some $200 million or $225 million (upward of $2.8 billion in twenty-first-century terms) during his eighteen-month tenure at the Veterans Bureau, as often alleged, he must have had confederates within the bureaucracy. No associates were identified. No one in the Veterans Bureau called him a crook when the Senate investigated him after he had left office and employees were free to speak without worrying about their jobs. Did Forbes have direct access to large amounts of cash? (No, he did not.) Stories about a foolish, stumbling leader surrounded by an immoral crop of cronies are ancient and satisfying, but the character of Forbes depicted in stories about Harding does not survive the light of day. Was he framed, as he insisted, and thus a scapegoat or a dupe? Was he a figure of self-aggrandizement? A crafty operator? Was he a hard-working government official struggling to establish a complex bureaucracy in the midst of political intrigue? Or something else? I needed to conduct substantial research before any conclusions could be reached: research into his life, character, and work before the scandal cast its long shadow; into his experiences in the Harding bureaucracy; and into what happened afterward. The questions were simple: Who was Forbes? What did he do?

His responsible position during the Harding administration needs emphasis. Forbes's first task (described in chapter 4) was to take three distinct occupational groups, each from a government office with an established organizational culture, and fuse them together into a supposedly ideal, smooth-running system. At the same time, he had to reorganize, coordinate, and redistribute their services to clients (four to five million military veterans of World War I) from the Atlantic to the Pacific Oceans and from the Canadian border to Mexico. A second part of his mandate came in 1922, when he inherited an unsatisfactory collection of government hospitals, cobbled together by the US Public Health Service from inadequate resources. Some of them were little better than wooden shacks, many in inconvenient locations. He also inherited some huge, disorganized army surplus depots, which were to cause him further trouble.

By the fall of 1921, when Forbes became director of the US Veterans Bureau, most of the military veterans who returned from France with physical injuries and amputations had received treatment in military hospitals or, after discharge, in public or private general hospitals or rehabilitation centers in the United States. In contrast, an increasing number of veterans sought long-term treatment, predominantly for mental illness and tuberculosis, and there were not enough acceptable facilities for them. It was politically and morally unacceptable for returning veterans to be placed in the typical state mental asylum of the day or to end up in chains. Effective medications for mood control lay far in the future. Facilities must be planned to keep unruly patients from harming themselves and others and from self-medicating on street drugs and alcohol (which could be especially dangerous when tampered with by bootleggers). One reported case at the Bronx Veterans Hospital, an expensively converted building without adequate protections, included a patient who returned from carousing in town, was too drunk to recognize anyone, and had to be strapped down. Another was a patient severely bruised who was returned to the hospital by six New York police officers; it took six to bring him in. He had served in France for eighteen months, he said, six months under fire. A shell explosion had hurled him in the air; he had become very "nervous," applied for hospitalization after military discharge, and was the sole support of his mother.

Tuberculosis patients also required special facilities. Again, there were no effective pharmaceuticals, no guarantee of cure. Bed rest, fresh air, and nourishing food were primary treatments. Again, patients were tempted to elope. However good the scenery, it was boring to have to rest for weeks on end, not knowing what the result would be. There was value in placing a new hospital in a peaceful campus with buildings for staff, therapies, and support services that were not easy to leave without outside help. Forbes moved into an expensive hospital building program, funded by Congress, which was bound to be political (where to locate sites) and controversial (in terms of costs).

The combination of the tasks Forbes faced was a massive undertaking. The Veterans Bureau reported a staff of 30,000 during Forbes's tenure and accounted for approximately a fifth of the federal budget, with most of that flowing through in monetary payments to war veterans and their families. Services for the health and welfare of veterans during his tenure became an essential part of the history of US health and welfare policy and of the history of American hospitals (both fields of my earlier research). More broadly, what Forbes did and didn't do—both as public official and private citizen—is important to include in the history of the Harding administration. As it turned out, the Veterans Bureau was his flagship program.

Previous accounts of Forbes are almost universally based on the published transcript of a Senate investigation that was designed to bring Forbes down and achieved this goal. In its way, as we'll see, the investigation was a tour de force. Documenting Forbes's life and work outside of the hearings and related newspaper coverage, required information from a wide range of sources, and some are unfortunately missing. Mrs. Harding destroyed numerous files after her husband's death in August 1923. The government prosecutor for Forbes's trial looked unsuccessfully for a large file of letters and memos between Harding and Forbes, which reportedly included criticisms of Forbes made to the president personally and which could have provided helpful insights about Harding's evolving views of Forbes. Forbes took his personal papers with him when he left the Veterans Bureau, but these and other papers he said he had kept, including letters from Harding and other members of his administration, did not survive Forbes's death. As a result, the personal story of Harding and Forbes in Washington remains thinner than one would wish.

Other characters and sources allow Forbes's story to be told with greater richness than expected. Besides surviving Harding records, these include the papers of significant figures, military and civilian personnel records, records of the Veterans Bureau and Department of Justice (including the FBI), congressional and court records, prison records, and more. These records are supplemented by documents and other treasures kept by Forbes family members, who have helped bring this story to life.

A Time of Scandal covers a broad swath of American life, a large cast of characters, hubris, deception and self-righteousness on various fronts, outrageous claims, love and laughter, gain and loss, and many unexpected wrinkles.

CAST OF CHARACTERS

Charles Robert "Bob" Forbes, b. 1877, an immigrant seeking his place in the world.

> Sarah "Sadie" Mabel Markham, his first wife, m. 1898, later worked as a "forelady" (foreman) in a shoe manufactory. Two children, Mildred and Russell.

> Kate Marcia McGogy Goodwin, his second wife, m. 1909, writer. Daughter Marcia "Awa."

> Katherine Bulkeley Tullidge Mortimer, his third wife, m. 1925, former lab technician; later a federal civil servant. No children.

> Marie Forbes Judkins, his older sister, a professional nurse.

Warren Gamaliel Harding, Republican, of Ohio, b. 1865, president of the United States 1921–1923.

> Florence Kling Harding, his wife, the First Lady.

> Carolyn Harding Votaw, his younger sister, social worker, liaison between the Public Health Service and the Veterans Bureau. Married to Heber Herbert Votaw, superintendent of prisons in the Harding administration.

OTHER NOTABLE CHARACTERS

Gaspare J. "Mike" Allegra, an undercover federal agent for prohibition cases in New York who was assigned to guard/protect Elias H. Mortimer when he became a government informer.

Davis G. Arnold, lawyer, major in World War I, engaged in postwar relief work in Constantinople before returning to civilian life. Acted as chief of staff for General John F. O'Ryan in the Senate investigation of the Veterans Bureau, which focused on Forbes.

James W. Black, a successful businessman from St. Louis, Missouri, who was cited as one of five coconspirators in the Forbes case but died before the hearings and trial took place.

Joel T. Boone, marine surgeon in World War I, younger medical associate of Dr. Charles E. Sawyer at the White House, who went on to a distinguished career but is notable here for recording conversations in his journal.

William J. Burns, former Secret Service agent who founded a well-publicized detective agency, which continued while he was director of the Bureau of Investigation (FBI) at the Department of Justice, 1921–1924. Fired for questionable practices by Attorney General Harlan Fiske Stone and succeeded by J. Edgar Hoover.

George A. Carpenter, Judge, US District Court, Northern District of Illinois (Chicago), presiding judge at the trial of Forbes and his accused coconspirator John W. Thompson in 1924–1925.

Calvin Coolidge, Harding's vice president who became the thirtieth US president on Harding's death in August 1923, won the presidential election in 1924 and declined to run in 1928. The Harding scandals erupted during his administration.

Charles F. Cramer, former lawyer to California oil corporations, general counsel of the Veterans Bureau, and chief of its large legal division, involved in a dubious contract for a hospital site near Livermore, California, cited as one of Forbes's coconspirators, died by suicide in 1923.
　　Lila Davis Cramer, his wife and widow, strong-minded socialite.

John W. H. Crim, hard-driving prosecutor against corruption, including bootlegging, conspiracies, and other crimes; in the Criminal Division of the Department of Justice, 1921–1923, then chief prosecutor for Forbes's trial as special assistant to the attorney general (first, AG Harry M. Daugherty, then AG Harlan Fiske Stone).

Harry M. Daugherty, corporate lawyer in Ohio, Warren Harding's political associate and campaign manager, attorney general, 1921–1924. Daugherty made himself a target for criticism by making some weak appointments, letting his associate, Jesse "Jess" W. Smith, have a desk in the department and conduct business there, and engaging in suspected practices, but though investigated and tried, he escaped the fate of others in the Harding scandals by avoiding conviction and imprisonment.

Charles Gates Dawes, Chicago banker and stalwart Republican, colorful and outspoken. World War I general who organized supplies for the military in Europe in coordination with US allies. Chair of the "Dawes committee" that recommended an independent Veterans Bureau. Created the Bureau of the Budget in 1921 and served as Calvin Coolidge's vice president, 1925–1929.

James S. Easby-Smith of Washington, lawyer, Georgetown University teacher, author, classicist, developed and ran the Selective Service System as a colonel in the office of the Judge Advocate General in World War I, represented the American Legion in pushing for effective veterans' benefits before the Veterans Bureau was established. Became Forbes's dedicated lawyer and friend.

Albert B. Fall, lawyer and US senator from New Mexico, who got to know Harding when both served in the US Senate. Harding's secretary of the interior, where he became embroiled in the oil politics of Teapot Dome. Convicted of bribery for leasing federal lands to oil companies in exchange for loans and eventually spent nine months in prison.

Adolphus E. Graupner, San Francisco lawyer and American Legion committee member, who worked closely with the Senate committee investigating Forbes, particularly on the Livermore case in which Cramer was involved.

Frank T. Hines, a businessman with considerable military experience. World War I general who organized the complicated US military embarkation process. Succeeded Forbes as director of the US Veterans Bureau in 1923, with the goal of raising morale and managing a gigantic business enterprise.

Herbert C. Hoover, engineer and classicist, known for his organizational skills. Secretary of commerce under Presidents Harding and Coolidge. Elected as the thirty-first US president in 1928.

J. Edgar Hoover (no relation to Herbert Hoover), a young lawyer, deputy to the freewheeling William J. Burns, "the Great Detective," who ran the Bureau of Investigation (FBI) under Attorney General Daugherty. Attorney General Stone appointed Hoover as FBI director in 1924.

William Henry "Will" Irwin, a skilled journalist who turned his attention from journalism to fiction after reporting on the horrors of World War I. Commissioned to write a series of articles on the Forbes case drawn from testimony at the Senate hearings and meetings with Mortimer. He had a major influence on the dramatic narrative of the Veterans Bureau scandal.

John Wesley Langley, longtime Republican congressman from Kentucky and sponsor of two major bills, the first and second Langley Acts for the construction of federal veterans hospitals. An overly trusting friend of Elias Mortimer, as a result of which he was sentenced to prison on a prohibition charge.

Andrew W. Mellon, multimillionaire from Pittsburgh, Harding's secretary of the treasury, who continued in that position under Presidents Coolidge and Hoover. Forbes initially worked in the Treasury Department, where two of the three components of the combined Veterans Bureau were located. Mellon originally liked him, but that sentiment did not last.

John B. Milliken, a civil servant who accompanied Forbes on his ill-fated western trip in 1922 and tried to warn him of the danger he was in.

Elias Harvey "Mort" Mortimer from Minnesota, Washington bootlegger, fixer, and confidence man, married to the upscale Katherine Tullidge. Both were Forbes's friends for much of 1922. When Forbes broke with him, Mortimer became a self-confessed coconspirator (to commit fraud against the federal government), gained government protection, and was the chief prosecution witness at Forbes's trial.

Tasker Lowndes Oddie, Republican US senator, former silver prospector and governor of Nevada, member of the Senate Committee on Investigation of the Veterans Bureau.

John Francis O'Ryan, New York lawyer famed for his extraordinary leadership of the New York National Guard, World War I fighting general, counsel and director of the investigation, and impresario of the hearings for the Senate Committee on Investigation of the Veterans Bureau. A major force.

David Aiken Reed of Pittsburgh, Republican, lawyer, chair of the Senate Committee on Investigation of the Veterans Bureau, associated with the interests of Andrew Mellon, critical of Forbes's performance.

Charles E. Sawyer, prominent homeopathic physician and sanitarium owner from Marion, Ohio, White House physician in the Harding administration with additional, partly ambiguous responsibilities for health and welfare policy.

Merle L. Sweet, from North Dakota, Forbes's able executive secretary at the Veterans Bureau and lifelong friend.

George Bowler Tullidge, highly regarded, well-connected Philadelphia physician.
    Katherine O'Donnell Tullidge, his wife, a leader in public-spirited women's social clubs. Both testified for Forbes at his trial.
    Edward Kilbourne Tullidge, their son, a physician with a wayward, checkered career.
    George Bowler Tullidge, Jr., whom Forbes hired for questionably high pay at the Veterans Bureau.
    Katherine Bulkeley Tullidge, their daughter, who married Elias Mortimer in 1919, sued him for divorce for cruelty and abuse, and subsequently married Forbes.

David Ignatius Walsh, Democrat, lawyer, and social reformer, US senator, former governor of Massachusetts, member of the Senate Committee on Investigation of the Veterans Bureau.

Mabel Walker Willebrandt, assistant attorney general, tough-minded lawyer in charge of prohibition cases in the Department of Justice, for whom Elias Mortimer was a valuable informer and to whom he reported.

James M. Williams, ran a dairy business in Philadelphia.
    Margaret O'Donnell Williams, his wife. Mrs. Williams was Katherine O'Donnell Tullidge's sister (and Katherine Mortimer's aunt). Both were ardent Mortimer supporters.

PART

I

AMERICAN DREAMS

HIDDEN STORIES, FATEFUL MEETINGS

Warren G. Harding and Charles R. Forbes met each other for the first time 5,000 miles away from Washington, DC—in the United States Territory of Hawaii, a cluster of islands in the midst of the Pacific. World War I, known as the "World War" or the "Great War" in the 1920s, raged in Europe, but America was still at peace. On February 3, 1915, forty-nine-year-old Harding, a newly elected US senator (Republican, Ohio), arrived in Honolulu after a storm-tossed six-day voyage from San Francisco. He was accompanied by his wife, Florence Kling Harding, who was recuperating from illness; her doctor Charles E. Sawyer; and his wife. Sawyer was a national advocate for homeopathic medicine and the owner-operator of a successful sanitarium in Marion, Ohio, Harding's hometown. The senator-elect was six feet tall, strapping in appearance, and noted for his good looks. His US passport, issued back in 1899, described his face nicely: "full," with a large mouth, strong chin, high forehead, and gray eyes, and—the pièce de résistance—a "Roman" nose. His hair, once dark, had turned gray by his forties and was on its way to the distinguished-looking white he sported in the 1920s.[1]

Forbes was a prominent official in the territorial administration, working directly for the governor. He was not on the dock to welcome the visitors, as sometimes claimed. The Harding party was welcomed by a trio of representatives: Captain James Dougherty, a senior aide to the governor, representing the territorial government; the secretary of the Chamber of Commerce on behalf of Hawaiian business, which was dominated by powerful Republican sugar planters; and a representative of the fraternal Order of Moose. Local members of the order had been assured from the mainland that Harding was a "good Moose," who deserved the courtesy of a formal greeting. Every US legislator visiting Hawaii was a target to be courted, even one newly minted. The territory had a significant American military presence and was dependent on federal funding for civilian projects, including harbors, roads, and public buildings. A large, invited delegation of US congressmen and their families was expected in the spring, their costs borne by the territory. Among them Republican senator Reed Smoot of Utah and Republican representative John Wesley Langley of Kentucky, each of whom would play a part in Forbes's Washington career. Forbes and writer Jack London, who was on an extended visit to Hawaii with his wife Charmian London, were to serve as resident experts for that group. Harding's visit was of minor importance in comparison.

Senator-elect Harding was heralded by the local press as a "dyed-in-the-wool protectionist" who had assured the sugar industry of his support. After years of running a small-town newspaper and participating in Republican politics in Ohio and on the national scene, he was well aware of underlying business agendas. When he left Hawaii after an event-packed, eleven-day stay, he declared that the Hawaii Territory should become a state and that he would be Hawaii's friend when he took his Senate seat: "They say that under the protective tariff people get rich. What if they do?"[2]

Charles R. Forbes worked for the governor of Hawaii, Lucius B. Pinkham, as superintendent (chief officer) of public works and chair of the Harbor Commission. He was an attractive, capable man in his late thirties, the age of Harding's youngest siblings; the youngest, Carolyn, was to become Forbes's friend and a colleague at the Veterans Bureau. As superintendent and commissioner, Forbes was responsible for topographic and hydrographic surveys across the Hawaiian Islands, waterworks and sewers, public buildings, artesian water investigations, harbor improvements, sidewalks, roads, and many other related public functions. Harbor Commission reports were filled with discussions of piers, wharves, landings, waterfront parks, the coastline, and marine railroads across the islands. Controversy could arise on any of these projects, ranging from differences of opinion about which firm would receive a contract, to battles over the rights of landowners, to disputes over how tax funds should be spent. Forbes had the decisive, can-do personality Harding appreciated. During the visit, the two men bonded as friends.

The machinery for official guests swung into gear. Governor Pinkham asked Forbes to see that the senator-elect was "properly entertained." Harding's name was added to previously scheduled events, including a fifty-man dinner of the Bar Association and the governor's welcoming dinner for visiting leaders of the Philippine Constabulary Band. He toured coastal defenses under military escort, visited submarines and three coastal artillery forts, and reviewed troops under the eyes of curious tourists at a fourth fort. The high spot was an excursion to the Big Island of Hawaii to explore the world-famous Mauna Loa volcano at Harding's request. Forbes wrote later that he and Harding talked about God's work while sitting on the crater's rim, "looking down into the seething mass of molten lava." Forbes wife, Kate Marcia Forbes, was in the process of publishing a small book—she called it a booklet—on the Kilauea volcano, for which she had spent time with scientists at the Hawaiian Volcano observatory and researched the Hawaiian legend of Pele, the fire goddess. Her publisher, the *Honolulu Star-Bulletin*, praised Kate Forbes for her "fine and sympathetic pen," and printed four editions. Jack London called it a "notable piece of work." The Hardings were in good hands for learning about the Hawaiian Islands.[3]

Back on Oahu local residents organized a series of small dinners, including one at the Forbes house where Harding read to the company from Kate Forbes's lyrically written book and in a complimentary, jesting spirit, offered her a "life position" on his newspaper, the *Marion Star*. The governor and other leading island figures graced the visitors' farewell dinner at the Commercial Club. The Harding visit was a success. In July, Harding wrote Forbes, "Every few days I have pleasant day-dreams amid pleasant recollections of Honolulu and the Hawaiian islands."[4]

Forbes did not participate in all of the events on the Harding trip. Besides his regular workload, he was working on two significant projects. The first was creating detailed plans for Governor Pinkham's proposal to drain and backfill the foul swamps called the "duck pond district" behind Waikiki Beach, for reasons of both public health and tourism. The second project helped the nationally renowned volcano scientist Thomas A. Jaggar, Jr., chair of the Geology Department at MIT and head of the Volcano Observatory, and newspaper publisher/tourism booster Lorrin A. Thurston, to draft a viable proposal to present to Congress to create a national park around the volcanoes on the Big Island. Forbes had spent weeks making practical plans for the reclamation of the Waikiki swamps and explaining his plan to the governor, the board of health, the Promotion [Hawaiian tourist and business] Committee, the Chamber of Commerce, and his colleagues on the Harbor Commission. He sent his official letter with the plan for the "Waikiki sanitation project" to Governor Pinkham a few weeks before Harding's visit. Though nothing was to be effected until the 1920s, the planned Ala Wai Canal, the ocean boulevard, and the rise of hotels and shops were eventually achieved at Waikiki, as anyone visiting Honolulu can see. Pinkham rightly gets the credit, but Forbes played an early part in this development.

The volcano park also came to pass, via a bill (H.R. 9525) drafted by Jaggar and Forbes, with strong lobbying by Jaggar in Washington, which was signed into law by President Woodrow Wilson on August 1, 1916. Hawaii's national volcanic park, a natural wonder that was compared with Yellowstone and Yosemite, was the eleventh approved US national park, and the first located in a US territory. Given Forbes's later reputation in historical and popular literature as a self-seeking sycophant, it is worth remarking that he seems neither to have sought nor gained public recognition for the part he played, however small, in these achievements.

Warren Harding accepted Forbes at face value, as did most senior military and corporate leaders in Hawaii, without need for probing into his education, his credentials, or his past experiences. Success in the job was enough. Forbes was generally well regarded. He attacked problems with enthusiasm, had an eye for detail, was good company, and was knowledgeable about construction, from penitentiaries to piers. He was also cagy and on occasion misleading about where he had come from—and modern bureaucracy assumed a documented pedigree: birth, citizenship, schooling, credentials. Critics of Forbes in Hawaii, and later in Washington, unable to figure out who he was in terms of heritage and training, or even his political affiliation, found him baffling, unsettling, or suspiciously evasive. Forbes withheld information or hinted rather than proclaimed. Had he really attended an elite private boarding school in New England? (No.) Forbes added fuel to the fire of doubters by producing fantastical stories about his past with the relish of an old-time raconteur. He was what others have called a fabulist, inventing memories of a past he might have had and perhaps half-believed he had or creating stories that seemed appropriate to the occasion. Where was he born? Why, Scotland, New England, Boston, New York. A report circulating in the 1920s, which must have come from him, claimed that at the age of ten he "shipped before the mast" on a square-rigger from Boston to Freemantle, Australia, under a very severe skipper; that only a few days out he was beaten up by the skipper who was drunk; and that "all through the voyage of 164 days he and the other members of the crew were dominated by an inhuman man and cruel captain." This unlikely if rip-roaring tale was undoubtedly well told, for Forbes was a gripping speaker. He was a "character." Love him or hate him.[5]

Who was this man who was to become the central figure of the Veterans Bureau scandal in the 1920s? Here, for the first time, is a brief review of who he was and what he had done, insofar as they can be drawn from original records, before we return to his friendship with Harding. He had had an unusual, up-and-down life, on the upswing in Hawaii.

The name on his birth certificate was Charles McIlroy Forbes, born in the quiet rural parish of Glenluce in southwest Scotland on February 11, 1877, to a family that lived an apparently ordinary life: father working with horses, mother running the household. Appearances were deceptive. The family was living undercover, maintaining a state of secrecy and vigilance. Four years before young Charles's birth, his father, the secretly married Private Charles McElroy of the Eighth Queen's Royal Irish Hussars, deserted from the British cavalry when he was stationed in Ireland. (The queen was Queen Victoria.) The family was hiding in plain sight under the assumed name of Forbes; hiding, that is, from bounty hunters and others who would turn him in. McElroy's regiment was soon to be deployed to India and Afghanistan. Recapture would mean shame and punishment (though deserters were no longer branded) and return to duty. The family survived under the Forbes name as a closely knit, disciplined unit. The middle name McElroy (or McIlroy), given to both sons, was dropped and not revived in the United States. When the Scotland census was taken in the spring of 1881, the Forbes family lived near Edinburgh with five children, ranging in ages from younger than one to ten; young Charles was number three. In October 1881, mother and children left for the United States, traveling steerage. Father came by an undocumented route. Four-year-old Charles was Charles Robert Forbes, nicknamed Bob. He was a smart, outgoing, curious child, blue eyed with reddish hair and the fair complexion to go with it. Given the need for secrecy about his father, he had to have been schooled not to speak of his family to anyone.[6]

Like many other immigrants off the boat without funds, the seven family members crowded into a dark tenement in the disease-plagued, stench-ridden Lower East Side of New York City. The story is familiar. The former cavalryman labored as a stableman. A new baby was conceived, born, and died. The youngest child who came from Scotland died. But then another baby, Emmeline, was born (out of town) and survived the perils of infancy. In 1886, Forbes senior became a US citizen, declaring he was "English" and leaving out salient information on the form, such as the ship and exact date of his arrival. Nine-year-old Bob and his brother, but not the females, automatically became naturalized citizens. Sometime during his schooling, which graduated students at age fourteen, the family moved to Massachusetts. In Pittsfield, his older brother George became an electrician.

An extraordinary opportunity opened up for Bob. Supported by his enterprising parents (who stated for the record that he was born in New York and thus a citizen by birth), on December 5, 1893, the officially fifteen-year-old Charles Robert Forbes (he was sixteen) enlisted as a "Boy in the United States Marine Corps, US Navy" at the US Marine Rendezvous in New York City. As an apprentice musician, he was to master bugle, fife, and drum at the school of the great US Marine Band in Washington, DC. Here he flourished. The curriculum required musical and general education plus expertise in military drills and lasted six months to a year or more, depending on the student. Forbes graduated in less than seven months. This was his equivalent of high school.

Next came his substitute for college. Rated "Fifer" in June 1894, he gained a plum assignment as marine fifer on the USS *New York*, a sleek, technologically advanced armored cruiser, prepared both for war, if and when it came, and for visiting dignitaries. The navy's report of his first voyage read as follows: "The cruiser returned to West Indian waters for winter exercises and was commended for her aid during a fire that threatened to destroy Port of Spain, Trinidad." Fifer Forbes had no problem with military discipline or tight sleeping quarters. The order of military life suited him. Along the way, he acquired an unshakable American patriotism that lasted through the dark days of the 1920s, dedication to the military, impressive tattoos, and a gold-capped tooth.[7]

Two signal events stand out during his life in the marines, one positive educationally, the other negative and life changing. The first was the ceremonial visit of the USS *New York* to Germany as flagship of the American presence at the opening of the Kiel Canal (which joined the Baltic to the

North Sea) in June 1895. There, in his role as fifer for the marine contingent, he saw international figures at close quarters, including the host, Kaiser Wilhelm II, who came to the ship twice to inspect her engineering systems. More than fifty warships from twelve nations swung at anchor in Kiel Bay; thousands of soldiers and sailors teemed the streets, jostling with residents, diplomats, and tourists. Officers of the *New York* waxed ecstatic on their return to New York City. The celebration was "like somebody's show, the greatest on earth." They had a "glorious and a gorgeous time." For a young American, here for a moment was the center of the universe.[8]

The second event, seven months later, was a naval accident. On a cold January day in 1896, when the *New York* was swinging at tide in port at Hampton Roads and the battalion was returning from landing drill, the boarding ramp slipped, plunging men and musical instruments into the dark waters of the dock. Forbes developed pneumonia complicated by empyema, with both right and left sides of the body involved. He recovered somewhat, substituting drum for the fife he had no breath to play, and might have stayed to complete his term of service, which ran until February 1899. However, in the spring of 1897, there was terrible news from home. His eleven-year-old sister Emmeline had died. He received a furlough to go home. On returning to duty, he was hospitalized at the Boston Navy Yard, where his first pulmonary hemorrhage was recorded. Tuberculosis was most likely an underlying problem. (His service had also endowed him with malaria.) At his request, he obtained a medical discharge with a recognized service-connected disability, on the basis of pulmonary disease contracted on duty on the USS *New York*. First, he went to a hospital in Lenox, Massachusetts, and then to his parents' home in Pittsfield to grieve and convalesce. He was twenty years old and a world traveler. Like many disabled military veterans, before and since, he was without a ready ladder for employment.[9]

The review of his claim for a federal disability pension was painfully slow—a salutary message about the urgency of speedy decision making for a future director of veterans' benefits. Eventually, in mid-March 1898, a board of three surgeons examined him in Pittsfield. In his application, he had described himself as "Charles Robert Forbes, Bugler," suppressing the role of fifer, which was not always greeted with the seriousness it deserved. He was working as a carpenter about a quarter of the time, he said. The doctors observed that his hands were soft, not callused as one would expect, and he looked anemic and poorly nourished. Medical examination sustained his report of four slight hemorrhages, convulsions about once a month, but no chill except for one that was followed by pneumonia. The doctors noted "No evidence of vicious habits," that is, sexually transmitted diseases. More months went by. In August 1898, Forbes reminded the Bureau of Pensions that he had been out of the navy for a year. "Could you please help me out with it," he wrote. "I am under a doctor's care since I left the Navy and all my savings has [sic] gone for doctor's bills." Finally, in a certificate dated February 24, 1899, he received the long-awaited pension: $6 a month, backdated to August 31, 1897, with his disability recorded as "Disease of Lungs result of pneumonia." His malaria was not approved as a service-connected disability.[10]

The logical next step as his health improved would be to take up a formal educational program or apprenticeship, but unfortunately, he was not free to do so. During the first part of his convalescence, he had impregnated Sarah "Sadie" Markham of Pittsfield, and the next step was preordained. Clergyman Hubert S. Johnson of Pittsfield officiated at the marriage of Miss Markham to Charles R. Forbes, Jr., on February 24, 1898. Their daughter Mildred was born in Pittsfield on June 5. Forbes was a twenty-one-year-old unable to work or support a wife and child; Sadie was twenty-three. Soon afterward, the senior Forbes family moved back east, to Somerville, Massachusetts. All three of Forbes junior's surviving siblings lived with their parents when the census was taken in June 1900, contributing to the household budget. Forbes senior (the former cavalryman) had become a golf instructor—golf was all the rage. The Markhams also moved, to Brooklyn, New York. Sadie (but not her husband) was listed as living with them in 1900 under the name, Sadie Markham.[11]

The Spanish-American War came and went. The USS *Maine* exploded in Havana Bay in February 1898, about the time of Forbes's shotgun wedding, precipitating military engagement. The USS *New York* steamed to Cuba without its former fifer, bombarded Spanish defenses, and served as the flagship at the decisive battle of Santiago in July, which destroyed the Spanish fleet. In victory, the *New York* steamed up the Hudson River with the victorious American squadron, accompanied by cannons firing, men in tears, whistles shrieking, and the cheers of triumphant crowds. It had been, remarked Secretary of State John Hay, "a splendid little war." Forbes had missed it. With his health improved, on March 2, 1900, he enlisted in the US Army in Boston, using his parents' address, for a three-year period for service in the US Signal Corps, listing his occupation as electrician and claiming New York as his birthplace. He answered, "Yes," to the question, "I have neither wife nor child." He had his navy pension stopped.

Then, confusingly, on May 11, barely two months after enlistment, he deserted from Fort Myer in Arlington, Virginia. The parallel with his father's earlier military desertion is striking, though what Forbes knew about that at the time is unknown. Unlike his father's case, desertion was not a big deal in the United States in mid-1900. Young Forbes resumed life as a civilian, gained practical work experience, and had an equivocal semblance of a marriage. His second child, Russell Markham Forbes, born in Brooklyn in February 1902, started life with a father who was away working on construction and railroad jobs and then vanished. On April 9, 1904, with the army building up its ranks, Forbes was officially captured by the police chief of Suncook, New Hampshire, taken to Boston, confined for less than a month at Fort Strong, and restored to duty without trial. He returned to the US Signal Corps in good health at the relatively mature age of twenty-seven, leaving wife and children to the care of her parents. Forbes reportedly told his commanding officer that he had started divorce proceedings in March 1904, but as the one who left the marriage, he would have had a weak case. The status of the marriage was left, apparently, unresolved; a question that would come back to haunt him later, after he chose to marry again.[12]

To summarize his mixed career so far: Forbes had served in the US Navy as a teenage marine fifer, acquired hands-on construction experience as a civilian, and resumed military life in the US Signal Corps after a false start four years earlier. He was not engaged, as has sometimes been claimed, in the Spanish-American War (1898–1900), nor did he serve in the Philippines.

The Signal Corps gave him first-rate technical training and experience in the field of modern communications. In 1904, its work encompassed balloons, telegraph, telephone and cable communications, photography, and military meteorology, with exploration of new ways to design, install, and support transmission networks via radio, dirigibles, and airplanes. Forbes flourished, rising rapidly up the ranks to sergeant first class and demonstrating his abilities as a leader and teacher. Postings introduced him to the midwest and west of the United States, and then to Cuba (from October

1906 through January 1907), which the United States was governing on a provisional basis. At Camp Columbia, near Havana, Sergeant Forbes was in charge of the mess hall of Company "I." Toward the end of his stay, he was hospitalized with typhoid fever, attributed to the line of duty, but made a good recovery. He was honorably discharged at Fort Monroe, Virginia, in January 1907 with a character of "Excellent." The following comment was underlined: "Service honest and faithful."[13]

Out of the army, Forbes went first to Omaha, Nebraska, where his parents were then living, and then to Washington State before moving to Hawaii. In Omaha, for a while he ran a business supplying items for construction firms. In 1909, the sudden death of his father from a stroke scattered the surviving members of his birth family. Forbes's mother moved back to Massachusetts to live with her eldest daughter, and soon Forbes abandoned Omaha and moved on. Six months after his father's death, he married Mrs. Kate Marcia (McGogy) Goodwin in Minneapolis—an independent, well-educated, ambitious young woman who had worked as a stenographer at Hayward Brothers Shoes in Omaha and, like Forbes, had been married before. They were a good-looking couple: Kate, petite and dark-haired, blue eyes sparkling in an oval face; Bob, medium height, a large personality, a reddish cast to his brown hair. Both of them held strong opinions. They traveled to the American Northwest.

Then in his early thirties, Forbes joined a major construction firm, the Hurley-Mason Company of Seattle-Tacoma, and worked his way up in the business: "from water-boy to superintendent of construction," was how he put it. His boss, Charles B. Hurley, was a substantial, well-liked older man, active in civic and Republican circles, who had put up major buildings in Tacoma, Spokane, Seattle, and Portland, Oregon. A member of the expanding cadre of college-educated professionals in the United States, Hurley had graduated in civil engineering from the University of Pennsylvania—a pathway closed to men like Forbes who had the talent but not the opportunity and if lucky were trained on the job. The two men became friends.

Forbes took up sailing. On one of his sailing trips in lower Puget Sound, he found a site on Vashon Island on which he and his wife built a house. The state of Washington was to be their state of residence into the 1920s and remained Kate Forbes's home until her death in 1960. It was from there, in 1912, that Mr. and Mrs. Forbes went to Hawaii. The Washington (State)

National Guard, of which Forbes was a member, ordered him to go on behalf of architect A. Walter Spaulding, whose firm had a government contract to work on the construction of the new US Naval Base at Pearl Harbor. The US Congress, whipped up by fear of Japanese naval power, had belatedly provided funds to improve the channel, build a dry dock there, plus machine shops and storehouses, and develop the yard and expected immediate action.[14]

The Pearl Harbor enterprise was huge. It included the largest dredging project for the US Navy up until then (conducted by the Hawaiian Dredging Company) and the challenge of building a dry dock big enough for a modern warship on an unstable sea floor of lava-pocked volcanic rock (the San Francisco Bridge Company). Forbes went to manage the work of the Spaulding Contracting Company for the construction of marine barracks and service buildings. He plunged into his work. Kate Forbes was pregnant. She wrote her sister and brother-in-law in Chicago, on arrival: "Climate perfectly ideal just right," but "lonesome," and "Bob awfully busy." Work at the harbor continued until the devastating collapse of the unfinished dry dock in February 1913, a multi-million-dollar Navy disaster. Water, under enormous pressure, exploded through the pumped-out section. Huge wooden beams that formed the structural skeleton of the dry dock were chopped up, thrown, and scattered like matchsticks. The rebuilt dry dock was not formally opened until 1919. Work stopped pending clean up and reappraisal.[15]

Bob and Kate Forbes stayed on. Honolulu had fine hotels and government buildings, parks and a botanical garden, white houses with verandahs or lanais set among palm trees and hibiscus, and electric streetcars on lava-paved streets. Waikiki Beach was noted for "surf-riding," and festivities abounded. The official (American) tone was upbeat. In 1912, there was allegedly the first "spirited" Fourth of July since US annexation of the islands in 1898. The softness of the air was matched by the rancor of its politics. "Hawaiian political meetings are similar to those everywhere, but with a little local color," wrote an observer in the 1920s: "Leis are put around the necks of perspiring sitters-on-the-platform. Speeches are usually in English, and they may or may not be translated. Perhaps the reason for this is that there are more epithets applicable to political opponents in the English language than in the Hawaiian."[16]

Forbes moved from the military-oriented milieu of Pearl Harbor into this slippery civilian environment. In August 1914, the month World War I began in Europe, Governor Pinkham appointed him to the major jobs of superintendent of public works for the Territory of Hawaii and chair of the three-man Harbor Commission. He had been in these positions for less than six months when the Harding party arrived in Honolulu. Pinkham was a colorful character in his early sixties, eccentric and annoyingly slow of speech but bold and far-sighted about the territory's development, and Forbes was in tune with his initiatives. Neither was much interested in political parties. Pinkham had been reluctantly appointed by President Wilson as a "near Democrat" but held that "the best politics were sound administration." As part of Pinkham's administration, the equally apolitical Forbes was a Democrat by association.[17]

Mr. and Mrs. Forbes had come up in the social world. As members of the upper echelons of Hawaii's multiethnic society, they mingled with deposed royalty, visiting ship-owners and dignitaries, and wealthy sugar planters. Influential businessman Walter F. Dillingham and US General Robert K. Evans organized a flying club in Hawaii in 1916 with Evans as president and Forbes as vice president. Forbes and his wife had a daughter, Marcia, born in Honolulu on November 29, 1912. Governor Pinkham became a close family friend, little Marcia's "Uncle Pink." Bob doted on his new daughter, "Papa Bob's Sunshine," a happy creature. All three family members were to look back on Hawaii as a special period in their lives.[18]

In the first few days of World War I in Europe, the commercial port of Honolulu was crowded with vessels serving both British and German commercial shipping. There was ongoing concern about the possible involvement of Japan. Sugar prices soared. So did the price of rice. Hawaii was a US military asset for both the army and navy, and Honolulu Harbor was important for US defense, particularly while work at Pearl Harbor was on hold. Army engineers improved Honolulu Harbor for military purposes along with building land fortifications.[19]

Rather than attempt to account for his convoluted, messy past by writing a celebratory account of the trials and successes of a once-poor immigrant, Forbes created a biography better suited to his new status. The social and professional register, Men of Hawaii, described him as the son of splendidly named, upper-class-sounding parents, Christina Fordyce (Nicoll) Forbes and Charles Robert Murray Forbes. (He had added the "Fordyce" and the "Murray" for effect. Nicoll was his mother's maiden name.) He edited out his period as a marine fifer, as he did on later occasions as well. His higher education was reportedly at Cooper Institute and Columbia University in New York (where he may have attended a few lectures but was not enrolled for a diploma or a degree). Not all who met him believed his statements; and if one thing was untrue, then others might be too. Ranged beside Forbes's undoubted successes in rumor-prone Hawaii were negative stories that anticipated those he would face in the 1920s: rumors of dubious dealings at work, his political allegiance (Republican or Democrat?), his background and professional expertise. As a military man who had come up through the ranks, he had absorbed messages in the military environment as simple truths: hard work on duty, then relaxed, even raucous fun onshore or in the mess; top-down command-and-control as the administrative method; orders specified and unquestionably obeyed; and acceptance of the unexamined virtues of loyalty, duty, honor, and trust. At work, he was disciplined, focused, detail oriented, expert; off-duty he let loose his exuberant, tale-spinning social presence. A political environment demanded more nuance.

Politics in Hawaii was a blood sport and lack of a clear affiliation as Republican or Democrat a mark of personal weakness. Republicans in the legislature held up his appointment for months after he was on the job and rated a "dynamo of industry," "technically equipped," and a "man of ideas and initiative." US District Judge Horace Worth Vaughan of Honolulu, a former Democratic US congressman from Texarkana, Texas, heard scornful criticism among Democrats that Forbes was claiming to be a loyal Democrat when he was no such thing. When Forbes returned from testifying to Congress (on behalf of Hawaii's development needs) in Washington in 1916, brandishing a medal he had unexpectedly received for serving in the US military in the occupation of Cuba (as indeed he did, in 1906–7), this was too much for Judge Vaughan, who wrote off to Washington for facts. A return memo from the War Department responded to a mysterious question about an Edgar Q. Smith, a man not known in Forbes's history, and stated that neither Forbes nor Smith "were ever in confinement in the Bilibid Prison at Manila." The question was obviously in error. Vaughan was not deterred. Later he launched into wild allegations of criminality, based in part on information he got from the army about Forbes's desertion in 1900, although, as the record showed, Forbes had returned in 1904, completed his term, and been honorably discharged.[20]

Forbes attracted rumors. In some ways, he implicitly asked for them. Seven years after he left the Hawaiian Islands, US Department of Justice agents investigated rumors that he had been involved in scandals in Honolulu between 1914 and 1917. Among them: he had padded a payroll, had something to do with the sale of territory bonds in New York, and generally had a "very shady reputation with people on the inside." In mid-June 1924, Special Agent E. B. Montgomery interviewed members of all the leading firms in San Francisco with close relations with Hawaii or engaged in business there, including sugar and pineapple concerns, the Matson shipping interest, and others. Everyone he interviewed had known Forbes personally or by reputation. Montgomery also spoke with Hawaiian residents who were staying in hotels in San Francisco. None of his informants had ever heard of any scandal "involving [Forbes] personally or officially." As James McCandless, a self-described capitalist (investor) from Honolulu remarked, if there had been a scandal everyone would know of it, because everyone in Honolulu knew everything that was going on. There was some criticism of building a bridge or wharf, but that was because of a mistake in the estimates. However, these informants were in remarkable agreement about Forbes's "hot air" ebullience. He "tooted his horn" so loudly that more was expected of him as superintendent of public works than he could deliver. He would have benefited from a course in etiquette, a subject that was coming into vogue.[21]

The decision of his two colleagues on the Harbor Commission in 1917 to bring in three independent professional engineers to review his plans for concrete piers in Honolulu Harbor—while Forbes (the commission chair) was away on the mainland and without consulting him—brought out another emergent problem: his difficulty in handling confrontation. The case showed a more irascible, overly defensive side of Charles R. Forbes. Rather than see whether a positive outcome could be achieved, he was hostile and antagonistic, refusing to consider anything the engineers said. In response, the engineers wrote a strong letter to the press in which they charged that Forbes, whatever his other qualities might be, was not to be relied on for the "design of engineering." Taken together, these were not good augurs for Forbes's future role as a government official in Washington, DC.[22]

Warren G. Harding took up his role as senator in 1915. Charles R. Forbes stayed in Hawaii until the spring of 1917. They kept in touch by letter and during visits Forbes made to Washington to give testimony for Hawaii, which he did with consummate skill, as the published hearings show. On at least one visit, he stayed with the Hardings as a houseguest: Harding wrote Forbes in July 1915, thanking him for the Kona coffee, and asking him whether he received the bathrobe he had left behind, which Harding had returned by parcel post.

German as well as British ships continued to use Honolulu Harbor until America's entry into the war, though some members of the Hawaiian legislature wanted to banish the Germans to open sea—a kerfuffle rightly quelled by Forbes, his Harbor Commission, and US military officials. "Forbes and Silva Not Yet Decided Whether to Have War or Not," declared the local press in March 1917, making sport of Representative Eugene da Silva of Hilo. On April 6, 1917, the US Congress approved President Wilson's declaration of war.[23]

In May, Forbes informed Harding that he was going to volunteer. He had already passed the examination for admission to the Officer Reserve Corps. Harding wrote a perceptive, affectionate letter back, urging him instead to do valuable work in Hawaii, but added: "I don't suppose anything will hedge you off . . . I know the germ of adventure is in your system, and I don't suppose you will ever get it out unless somebody shoots it out on the western battle front in Europe . . . You will excuse me from writing in this strain. It is not my business to tell you what to do. Under normal circumstances I want to help you to do the thing you most wish to do."[24]

On June 9, Major Charles R. Forbes was called to active duty and ordered to report to the commanding general, Western Department in San Francisco. Mid-level officers with his mix of technological, organizational, and leadership skills were invaluable—hard to find as America joined the Great War. In November, he shipped to France with the Forty-First Division of the American Expeditionary Force. The Forbes family left Hawaii for good. Kate Forbes set up their home on Vashon Island, in Washington State. Forbes returned to the United States in January 1919.

From April 1917 through November 1918, two million young Americans were trained and transported across the Atlantic like interchangeable parts, to face the technological ingenuity of exploding shells packed with shrapnel for maximum effect, the efficiency of machine gun fire, and toxic gases designed by chemists, in the scarred and putrid fields of France. General Hunter Liggett, commander of the Forty-First Division, gave as good a description of the situation as any: "A war began in 1914, of the complex causes of which we Americans knew nothing. We never believed that it could happen; we could not believe that it had happened; the only thing more incredible was that we ever could be drawn into it. Yet the force of circumstances had drawn us in three years later."[25]

At home, the federal government, big business, and volunteers collectively mobilized to win the war, with government agencies in the lead. Among the efforts: creating a citizen army through the action of local draft boards with final selection by national lottery; building huge training and transfer camps (cantonments) in the United States; creating a new system of veterans' benefits and expanding the fledgling Bureau of War Insurance into a federal bureaucracy for managing the system; commandeering transport ships and developing the US Shipping Board and its subsidiary, a government-owned shipbuilding corporation; managing the railroads as a national network for the duration; creating the necessary publicity (propaganda) to fan the flames of patriotism and curtailing freedom of speech; booting up industry for war production on a case-by-case basis through quickly negotiated cost-plus government contracts, which favored large business corporations; and adjusting to the rapid relocations in population that accompanied such changes—African Americans from the south to war jobs in Chicago, Detroit, and other industrial centers; women replacing men and taking on new jobs. Thousands of civilians, men and women, went to Washington to work for hundreds of wartime agencies (2,400 by an official count). Near Union Station, a southern journalist observed, were "rows and rows of wooden dormitories, like cantonments, which housed the thousands of women and girls who had come to Washington to feed tons of paper into the war machine, to run red tape, instead of soapsuds, through their fingers." Not least, in swarmed reporters, lobbyists, publicists, and fixers.[26]

Although almost one of every five US draftees was foreign born, on the home front, immigrants were seen as potential spies. The Department of Justice organized a major national network of private informers that numbered a quarter of a million people by the end of the war. With the flow of immigration stemmed during wartime, the stage was set for restrictive immigration legislation in 1921, which was strengthened in 1924. In Congress, convoluted arguments about the uses and control of oil reserves on certain parcels of federal land, which had engaged oil executives, members of Congress, and others since 1909, gained steam in 1917. Those in the conservationist camp wanted to keep oil in the ground, while others argued for private development via government leases to oil companies for drilling (and profit taking). Senator Albert B. Fall of New Mexico, a known advocate of private enterprise, states' rights, and minimal federal control, supported the complicated leasing bill that was signed by President Wilson in February 1920, which gave the Department of the Interior the authority for making regulations, thereby launching Fall into the scandal called Teapot Dome.[27]

In France, Major, later Lieutenant Colonel Charles R. Forbes served as an exemplary divisional signal officer for the Forty-First (training and replacement) Division of the American Expeditionary Force and then for the Thirty-Third under Major General George Bell, Jr., where he replaced an officer who had been badly wounded. Because of the shortage of competent officers, Forbes performed two jobs simultaneously for the Thirty-Third, taking on direct command of the signal battalion during weeks of military engagement, and fighting with the British on the Somme and in the gas-filled Meuse-Argonne offensive. At the divisional level, his job was to ensure effective communication across the battlefront and back and forth to headquarters. On-the-ground communication depended for the most part on telephone and telegraph lines, though he experimented with air-to-ground radio, taking equipment up on a plane for testing. On the ground, speedy and shrewd decisions were vital as the battlefront shifted. Forbes planned and directed the carrying of wire across trenches, mud, barbed wire, and worse, through noisome swamps and guarded rivers. He put himself in the line of fire as Signal Corps personnel kept communication going through thick and thin. Forbes "understands the signal corps game from start to finish," a colleague wrote. The division's chief of staff General William K. Naylor commended him: "During the operations beginning on the 26th of September and continuing until the armistice the signal liaison of the 33rd Division was as near perfect as I believe it could have been made." The divisional commander, General Bell, described him: "Untiring in his devotion to duty, exposing himself fearlessly to enemy fire in order to supervise signal operations in the forward area this officer contributed largely by the ability of his management, to the successes achieved, particularly during the delicate operations north of Verdun, October 8th to 20th 1918 when this Division was astride the Meuse." Forbes received the Distinguished Service Medal. He had been gassed twice, and like many others, needed dental work, but he had not been physically wounded. Eighteen years later he wrote to his daughter Marcia about Armistice Day, November 11, 1918: "I was in a shell hole and at eleven o'clock when we ceased firing I was in the town of St. [Hilaire]," where battle with the Germans had blown up the waterworks the previous night and Allied soldiers who were wounded left to drown. "What bitter memories are carried back," he wrote, "the memory of that War is still clear and vivid. Sherman was right when he said 'War is Hell.'"[28]

There was shock on both sides when veterans of the war returned home in staged batches during 1919. Those on the receiving end expected ex-soldiers to move beyond their war experiences and merge smoothly back into civilian life, but the country had moved along without them. Writer Mary Roberts Rinehart, who was a war correspondent on the Belgian front, described her reactions on returning to the United States: "I was gazing with a sort of terror at an America I hardly knew, a jazzed America, drinking, dancing, spending; developing a cult of ugliness and calling it modernity, and throwing aside the simplicities and charms of living in pursuit of a new god called Smartness." By returning in 1919 to work for his earlier employer, the Hurley-Mason construction company in the Pacific Northwest, Charles R. Forbes avoided the full combination of absurdity, fear, cynicism, and disbelief that marked political and intellectual circles in Washington, New York, and other major cities—although Washington State had its own postwar alarms, including a mayor of Seattle who trumpeted anti-immigrant phobia across the nation under the banner of Americanism and an armed conflict and lynching in Centralia. Forbes reported three hospital admissions for angina pectoris in 1919–21, with treatment for "nervous breakdown-angina." He recovered and went on.[29]

A worldwide pandemic of influenza had killed American civilians as well as forces in military camps in the United States in 1918, with a further outbreak in France in 1919 among soldiers waiting to return, but was downplayed as if it had not been. Strikes punctuated wartime production. Though at its peak the war effort accounted for almost one-fourth of national income, there had been little planning for the demobilization of industry or resettlement of American labor, now swelling up with gun-trained veterans, or for hospitals to treat the sick. In Washington, scandal mongering and slashing personal criticisms flourished. Congress struggled to regain influence after the wartime shift of authority to the president and wartime agencies. Large business corporations, having benefited from wartime contracts, were compelling targets for charges of fraud.

Points of view had changed as well, sometimes in striking directions. Who would have guessed that automaker Henry Ford—known throughout the industrial world for demonstrating "Fordism," or "scientific management," on the shop floor (mass production) would have sparked the prominent Newberry scandal in the US Senate between 1918 and 1922? Ford was an ardent pacifist who turned over his plant at Highland Park, Michigan, to military production during the war, and then in 1918, at President Wilson's urging, agreed to run for the Senate in Michigan to stop another wealthy businessman, Truman Newberry, from filling the seat as a Republican. Ford won the Democratic primary; Newberry's team spent an unseemly amount of money to win the Republican primary, in which Ford also ran; Newberry won that primary and then the election; Ford demanded a recount (same result) and sued Newberry for campaign-financing violation—at its nastiest, "buying votes." Newberry was prosecuted, convicted, and the case overturned on appeal. President Harding publicly supported him and the Senate grudgingly seated him, but Newberry left the Senate as a symbol of big businessmen who used money to subvert American democracy. *Newberryism* was the shorthand term.[30]

In 1919, Forbes became a vice president of Hurley-Mason in Washington State, managing its construction work in Spokane. Republican presidential candidates for the 1920 election were lining up. Senator Warren G. Harding announced his candidacy on December 16; he wrote Forbes at the Spokane City Club accepting his help. In late December, Forbes informed Harry Daugherty, Harding's campaign manager for the primary, that he had about two hundred volunteers working for him, was about to take "Harding propaganda" to distribute in Idaho, and planned to visit every state delegate from Oregon, Washington, and Idaho to the National Republican Convention, where the presidential nominee would be selected. Daugherty considered Forbes an uncontrollable meddler. Harding's strategy was to seek support wherever he could get it, positioning himself in second place in states he could not win outright. The rival Republican candidate in Washington State, Senator Miles Poindexter of Spokane was ahead but might throw his support behind Harding in subsequent rounds. Forbes was advised not to upset him, but in his enthusiasm, he undoubtedly ruffled some feathers. Kate Forbes also worked for Harding, visiting her mother's home in Indiana to do "some publicity work with the South Bend papers." Forbes visited the Hardings at their home in Marion, Ohio; Harding wrote warmly to him; and Dr. Charles and Mrs. Sawyer, who had been part of the Harding party in Hawaii, maintained overtly friendly relations. Harding reassured Forbes that he did not expect to be the first choice for the Republican nomination in Oregon, but "everything is going along very smoothly and in the most gratifying way." He was right. Warren G. Harding was nominated on the tenth ballot as the Republican Party presidential candidate at the party's convention in June and elected president on November 2, 1920, defeating his Democratic opponent, James M. Cox, by a landslide.[31]

John W. Dean's twenty-first-century assessment of Harding squares with Forbes's experience of his friend: "Harding played politics like he did poker . . . and he seldom lost. . . . The presidency was a high-stakes game and Harding played it with zest, all the while appearing casual and disinterested. . . . He let others mention him as a future leader of the nation, but it is doubtful he told anyone his true thoughts." Exulting in Harding's success, Forbes—now a committed Republican—sent Harding a congratulatory telegram from Spokane, and Harding responded with a letter: "You have been a good scout throughout it all. Indeed, you have been a good friend since that afternoon when we first met at the Beach Hotel and you sized up your wards on a trip to Hilo and the Island of Hawaii. . . . I hope I may have some opportunity of expressing my appreciation." Neither man stopped to think whether Forbes would make a good federal official.[32]

WASHINGTON, DC, MARCH – APRIL 1921

On a beautiful Friday morning, March 4, 1921, two men settled into the back of a luxurious open limousine outside the White House in Washington, DC. Democrat Woodrow Wilson, in his last day in office after eight years as president, sat on the right-hand side, where the stroke-ravaged left side of his face was less visible to spectators; Republican Warren G. Harding, president-elect sat on the left, looking sun-bronzed and healthy from a Florida vacation. The sun shone out of a cloudless sky, but the temperature was a few degrees above freezing. Both men wore winter coats and black silk top hats. The convertible top of the automobile was folded neatly down behind the two riders, framing them like a ceremonial ruff. They were about to demonstrate the peaceful transition of leadership in American democracy—no matter what disruptive currents surged beneath the surface—by riding in procession along Pennsylvania Avenue to the Capitol, where Harding would be sworn in as the twenty-ninth president of the United States and would deliver his inaugural address. The two men barely knew each other except by political reputation, and that was mutually negative.[1]

Woodrow Wilson was a member of a white Anglo-Saxon, Protestant social elite whose members chatted with one another at exclusive New York clubs, weddings, funerals, and college reunions. His face was long, forehead noble, hair smoothly parted; he carried his clothes well. He had been governor of New Jersey before assuming the presidency and president of Princeton before that. He had earned his PhD from Johns Hopkins University, studying congressional government. He had been outmaneuvered and outplayed in negotiations with his more wily and self-interested French and British counterparts (Georges Clemenceau and David Lloyd-George) at the Paris Peace Conference in 1919, but even his most severe critics there admired his aristocratic bearing and "finely cut" head and features. When animated and in good health, Wilson was lively, enthusiastic, charismatic, and playful, a man of keen glance and winning smile. At other times, his seriousness was enhanced by the habitual rimless pince-nez that perched across his nose, substituting for more substantial eyeglasses.[2]

Warren Harding came up in the scrappy, deal-making world of entrepreneurship and practical politics in Republican-proud Ohio, where he published and edited the *Marion Star* and firmed up his political career, serving stints as a state senator and lieutenant governor before becoming a US senator. Harding, with a profile that could be imprinted on a Roman coin, was both complimented and belittled by the oft-quoted comment that (at least) he "looked like a president." He was known for being kind, watching baseball, playing poker and golf; for his open manner, resonant voice, and nonconfrontational disposition. He had found it useful to downplay his abilities. Harding was a skilled practitioner in the arts of persuasion, cooperation, compromise, and conciliation and, when advisable, deflection of attention from the subject at hand. His strategic intelligence, judgment, and people skills tended to be underrated. He ran for election as the Republican candidate for president in 1920 against Democrat James M. Cox in a brilliantly organized campaign and won 60 percent of the popular vote. Broadway star Al Jolson wrote the words and music for the Republican campaign song, "Harding, You're the Man for Us," and organized actors to campaign for Harding, including, among many others, movie stars Lillian Gish, Mary Pickford, and Douglas Fairbanks.[3]

Among other changes, the change in administration was a change in personal styles. Wilson was a Presbyterian, Harding a Baptist from a family that later became Seventh-day Adventists. Harding's sister Carolyn married an Adventist missionary, Heber H. Votaw, whom Harding made superintendent of prisons. Racism figured in both Wilson's and Harding's stories, but for quite different reasons. In 1920, Harding was the target of accusations that he had "Negro blood" through an African American great-grandmother, a politically damaging assertion at the time. Federal agents seized virtually all the copies of the accusing pamphlets, but the issue remained as a potential scandal. (Almost a century later, after speculation that Harding could be celebrated as the first black president of the United States, DNA testing found the rumors to be without foundation.) Wilson showed the D. W. Griffith movie *The Birth of a Nation* (1915), an overtly racist film that included hooded white members of the Ku Klux Klan as heroes and African Americans as villains to an invited audience at the White House and made no critical public comments on it.

Wilson had met and married his second wife while in office. The married Warren Harding had had an affair with a married friend, Carrie Phillips (proved by letters that surfaced in 1973), in his hometown of Marion, Ohio. In 1919, he fathered a love child with Nan Britton, a woman in her early twenties who had had a crush on him since she was fourteen and at school in Marion, where Harding's younger sister Abigail was her teacher. According to Britton, their affair continued while Harding was in the White House. Florence Kling Harding had a son from an earlier relationship and legitimated that relationship by a formal divorce. But these matters were not generally known in 1921. A scandal is only a scandal when made public.[4]

Woodrow Wilson's public image and his recent tragic life formed an essential backdrop to Harding's projected image as he took over. Lacking Senate approval of the League of Nations in 1919, Wilson had decided to get the support of ordinary voters by taking his message out across the nation. Illness defeated him. He could not complete the arduous cross-country train trip he had undertaken and returned to Washington. A major stroke in October 1919 left him incapacitated and confined to the White House. Though his mind was clear and he could walk very slowly with a cane by the time of Harding's inauguration, he was still physically and emotionally impaired. His left arm and leg were weak, and his eyes readily dropped tears. It was this man, not the vigorous leader of earlier years, who rode to the Capitol in March 1921. Helped from his wheelchair at the White House he was lifted into the backseat of the limousine. On request, photographers put down their cameras during these transitions.

Wilson's prewar administration had extended the regulatory role of the federal government through the Federal Reserve Act, the Federal Trade Commission, and the Clayton Anti-Trust Act, and introduced an income tax. He had also segregated federal offices by race (white and black). After he took the United States into World War I in April 1917, Wilson oversaw powerful new federal agencies to mobilize, redirect, and manage resources for war, then brought the nation through war to the Armistice (ceasefire) in November 1918, and on into international discussions for peace. The Treaty of Versailles, formally ending World War I, was signed on June 28, 1919.

The proliferation of executive agencies during the war, following previous expansion in the executive functions of the federal government, was followed again by the dissolution of many but not all of the wartime agencies after the war. Two that continued were the US Shipping Board and its shipbuilding business, which was still gearing up production when armistice was declared; and the Bureau of War Risk Insurance, which managed the postservice benefits of World War I military veterans. Even with what was left, the federal government was a huge, unwieldy collection of centers with specialized missions, some of which duplicated or overlapped with others. The incoming Harding administration was faced with two generic questions on the "administration" part of the Harding agenda: (1) the size and complexity of the executive and (2) its authority versus Congress. The first was represented by proposals for government efficiency, accountability, and reform—an agenda that echoes into the present. The second centered on how Congress would exercise its legislative and investigative roles as a check to a powerful executive.

Observers regarded Harding from a wide variety of perspectives, both before and after the inauguration. It was not that he was a chameleon—his behavior and his policies were quite consistent—rather, he evoked varying responses from different quarters. For the highly educated idealist, Harding was ill-educated and directionless, a small-town American with small-town capabilities and less-than-perfect manners. In contrast, his successful maneuvering to get elected suggested a man who was shrewd and goal directed. Washington social doyenne Alice Roosevelt Longworth famously proclaimed Harding a "slob." The less aristocratically born, wealthy social leader Evalyn Walsh McLean, wearer of the Hope Diamond, disagreed. Her Harding, a loyal friend, was a "stunning man," despite his habit of chewing tobacco, "biting from a plug that he would lend, or borrow," and not caring "if the whole world knew he wore suspenders." The socialist politician Eugene V. Debs was an inmate at the federal penitentiary in Atlanta in March 1921 for promulgating socialist views during the Great War; Wilson had not pardoned him. Harding released him on December 24, together with twenty-three other political prisoners, declaring, "I want him to eat his Christmas dinner with his wife," and invited him to the White House for a chat on December 26.[5]

The opinions of eminent Americans who supported Harding, advised him, and served in his cabinet were positive overall. Multimillionaire Andrew W. Mellon accepted Harding's invitation to become secretary of the treasury; approved of Harding's platform of "normalcy," "honest money," "sound finance," and freeing business from undue regulation; and worked hard to resolve the financial crisis of 1921 as the nation reeled under the impact of the national debt (incurred by the war), the collapse of wartime demand, unacceptably high unemployment, and a chaotic tax structure. Although Mellon was cool toward Harding, whom he would reportedly not have employed in his own business, he enjoyed the trust Harding placed in him. Harding, in turn, considered Mellon inadequate as a politician. Herbert C. Hoover, Harding's secretary of commerce (and a future president), praised Harding for standing up to bankers when he demanded supervision of their foreign loans; standing up to the steel industry when he pressed for the abolition of the twelve-hour day and seven-day week; and vetoing an overly stringent farm bill. Hoover gave Harding a mixed personal review, which included after-the-fact disapproval of Harding's poker-playing "cronies"—a loaded word denoting socially unacceptable acquaintances. But he also recalled: "Harding encouraged me in everything I wanted to do. I never knew him to give a promise he did not keep." Harding's administrative style was to choose people he thought would do a good job and let them get on with it.[6]

Albert D. Lasker, who achieved fame and fortune in the advertising business but took a two-year stint as head of the troubled Shipping Board at Harding's request, considered him "a man of utmost integrity, a man to whom you could unbutton your thoughts and your soul." (Harding told Lasker, "You are the only, single, solitary man I have around me that doesn't want something.") Charles G. Dawes, a successful Chicago banker, was sufficiently impressed by Harding to create (in June 1921) the first federal budget and standardize business methods across federal departments. His assessment of Harding: "Deliberate, when time is not the essence of decision, he has the quality of almost instantaneous action when it is." For Dawes, Harding was the "ideal chief of the business machine of the government." He sought strong, decisive leaders and expected them to exercise initiative, making it clear over his first year in office that his goal was not a weaker government but a better one. The restoration of normalcy in the world "must come through the initiative of the executive branch of Government," he told Congress in December 1921.[7]

Perhaps the best summary of Harding that was made during the time he was president was by well-known Washington journalist Mark Sullivan in July 1922, after plenty of time to observe him. Sullivan remarked on two of Harding's important characteristics: On one hand, he was a "real politician" with a gift for telling stories, creating an atmosphere, and raising a laugh. On the other, he "made the impression of a cool capacity." He needed all the coolness and capacity he could summon. The year 1921 was distinguished by postwar malaise, discontent, disillusion, a "kind of fretful sullenness," the sense of living in a "cock-eyed" world. Drinking and flouting the liquor laws, weak moral character, suspect status as an immigrant or alien, wartime corruption, sexual freedom, greed, lackluster government, and stereotyped messages from the culture at large wove together, fanning fears for the moral fabric of the nation. Woodrow Wilson had won the war; Warren Harding was left with its effects.[8]

Wilson's negative views of Harding stemmed at least in part from Harding's membership on the Senate Foreign Relations Committee, which opposed Wilson's commitment to the new League of Nations, more specifically, American participation in it. For Wilson, the League of Nations was a necessary vehicle for establishing lasting peace; quite simply, it was the right thing to do. For his international efforts, he received the Nobel Peace Prize. However, in the United States, foreign relations meant fostering advantageous trade, not bailing out failing nations. The war had fostered exclusiveness, self-interest, and a narrowly defined "Americanism." The Foreign Relations Committee, chaired by Henry Cabot Lodge, revised Wilson's document to provide safeguards to block perceived threats to American independence, and these "reservations" were a possible vehicle for negotiation, but Wilson would not budge. At a meeting of the committee at the White House in August 1919, Harding asked what Wilson meant when he said that moral claims outranked legal claims with respect to the league and relationships with other nations—not an unfair question, though Wilson thought he had already explained this satisfactorily. Afterward, Wilson described Harding to cabinet member David F. Houston as having "a disturbingly dull mind . . . it seemed impossible to get any explanation to lodge in it." He had not changed his opinion since. Houston, who had studied political science at Harvard, took a similar view of Harding's "mediocre mind and ordinary standards of thinking." In another observation, this time on Harding's style of leading from below through consensus rather than setting directions from above, Wilson asked, "How can he lead when he does not know where he is going?" The idealistic preacher and the practical politician could not (or would not) understand each other. Wilson was a man of his class, working for "the faith in which I was bred and which it is my solemn purpose to stand by until my last fighting day." Harding was a man of his class, too, mobilizing effort in the trenches of politics and seeking divine guidance through the Psalms of David and passages in the Gospels; and "there's still wisdom in the sayings of old Solomon." Warren G. Harding had studied at a small Ohio college. He was not a member of the university-educated upper class.[9]

For journalists and cartoonists writing about a people "tired of men with burning convictions" and "more or less afflicted with moral shellshock," Harding was a gift. Negative views of government or the war had been banned during wartime. Afterward, official Washington offered numerous opportunities to be sardonic, superior, or satirical. Woodrow Wilson aimed to "make the world safe for democracy" but was felled by the forces of democracy at home. Warren Harding rode in under the banner of a "return to normalcy" when there was no such thing. Writers embraced the idea that Americans were living in a fictional world—like characters in a novel or a movie. Senators moved in a "region of fictions," a popular pundit observed: "They represent the Republican party, when there is no Republican party, no union of principles, no stable body of voters, no discipline, no clear social end to be served." The Democrats were no better, a squabbling band of sectional interests. The art of "ballyhoo" (salesmanship or showmanship) was a fruitful theme; particularly, ballyhoo as a distinctive feature of the nation's commercialized national press, fed by ubiquitous press agents. The papers were "an escape, a thrill, an opiate," their stories given "trade-mark identification" to make them similar to the human interest story in a confession magazine. Dramatic stories—murder, adultery, arrests, betrayals—sold newspapers and upped their advertising revenues.[10]

The wartime Committee on Public Information had shown how efficiently public opinion could be developed and manipulated. Its title was a good one for control of news and opinions and firing up patriotism. The committee's expertly managed wartime propaganda machine, based on the latest advertising and communications techniques, drew on talented writers, actors, illustrators, and others. Its campaign to sell war bonds included standardized four-minute pep talks delivered by trained speakers in the nation's ubiquitous movie theaters. Sales messages permeated America's postwar culture of consumerism. Stock characters and emotive themes influenced the public's views. A serious study of public opinion explained that humans view reality in terms of stereotypes, including familiar plots and unifying themes, through stories invented and transmitted in social settings, which become what "everyone" believes. The dismal chaos of the modern world was more manageable when viewed through common prisms. Newspapers, tabloids, plays, movies, and popular songs circulated stereotypes: the romantic hero, the gangster and the mob, the flapper for whom "anything goes," the corrupt government official, the wicked wife, the predatory male driven by sex and the liberation of the "id," the "rough-and-ready hail-fellow-well-met, who is anybody's match at a story-telling contest."[11]

Warren Harding was the "modern type" of what is meant as "typically American"; namely, "the Square head, typical of that American whose artistic taste is the movies, who reads and finds mental satisfaction in the vague inanities of the small town newspaper, . . . who has his car and his bank account and can sell a bill of goods as well as the best of them." Sinclair Lewis published a best-selling novel, *Babbitt* (1922), along these lines. In 1921, F. Scott Fitzgerald worked on a play, *The Vegetable: Or, from President to Postman*, based on stereotypes (the president, the postman, the general, the flapper, the bootlegger). His play opened in Atlantic City on November 19, 1923, but closed almost immediately. The timing was awkward, not long after Harding's unexpected death, and farce was not his métier, but the play includes a very funny spoof of a rambling, "bloviating" Harding speech. Elsewhere, Harding was the "the oldest of stage heroes, Everyman"; his interior secretary Albert B. Fall, was a "stage sheriff of the far West in the movies." Their selves were to vanish behind these alternative realities. That was to be true of Charles R. Forbes, too, when he accepted Harding's gift of a job and came to work in Washington, DC.[12]

Warren Harding arrived in Washington on March 3, the day before the inauguration, in the early afternoon by special train from his hometown of Marion, Ohio, accompanied by supporters and friends. He talked Pennsylvania Railroad officials into speeding up the trip by traveling nonstop between Harrisburg, Pennsylvania, and Baltimore, Maryland (a "first" in the railroad's history), and thus arrived half an hour earlier than expected. He and his wife were met at Union Station by Vice President-Elect Calvin Coolidge and his wife, Grace, and other official greeters, backed up by a cheering crowd. Two hours later, while Harding was engaged in a round of meetings with visitors and newspaper correspondents at the Willard Hotel, a vanload of Harding belongings arrived at the main entrance of the White House while the Wilsons were still in residence. A reporter described these as tagged boxes and bundles, some labeled "President," some "Hon. W.G. Harding," some "President-Elect." They included his golf clubs.

At a meeting with fifty or so reporters, Harding firmed up the image of accessibility and friendliness he hoped to maintain as president, a contrast with Wilson's remoteness. He reminded them that he was "just a newspaperman myself" and asked for their cooperation. He came off well. As one reporter put it, "It is a mighty solemn affair to see the greatest and most powerful government the world has ever known turned over to new untried hands. And it was impossible not to feel a great gratitude that the hands were the big, rough capable hands of this slow, sweet, big Middle Westerner."[13]

There was much to do. The Republican Party was riven with competing constituencies and conflicting views, including those of the crusading "America-first" conservatism of Senator Hiram Johnson of California, the belligerence of Senator William E. Borah of Idaho, and the Progressive outlook of Senator Robert M. "Fighting Bob" La Follette, Sr., of Wisconsin. One of Harding's main tasks was to keep the party together to ensure that needed legislation was actually achieved by a Republican congress and a Republican president. Harding expressed his aspirations for a more peaceful, satisfying life at home, which might be achieved in unexpected ways, and it largely was, eventually, and via rising prosperity—but not until the administration of Calvin Coolidge. In 1921, it was impossible to define as normal a world swept by periodic waves of political hysteria. Attorney General

A. Mitchell Palmer had overseen anticommunist raids and arrests during the Red Scare of 1919, in which vast and evil conspiracies seeking to overthrow the government were conjured, civil liberties dismissed, and Americans were encouraged to spy on their neighbors. Under prohibition enforcement bribes and offers of bribes were commonplace and conspiracy and corruption spread insidiously. "Undesirable aliens" and even native-born Americans (such as socialist leader Eugene Debs, who was born in Indiana) had been imprisoned for the expression of "un-American" ideas.

Two million mostly young Americans who had been drafted and sent to fight in France were home, and they, together with another two million demobilized conscripts who had worked in the United States, competed with other laid-off workers for scarce jobs. Many, if not most, war veterans reintegrated into civilian life quietly and apparently successfully. Men who had been plucked from home and subjected to low-paying jobs and military discipline in the United States were understandably resentful when they saw workers in the private sector get high wages in the war economy. African Americans who had fought for their country faced continuing segregation at home. Needy and disabled veterans were angry and frustrated, even defeated, by the barrier-like red tape of applications between them and the federal benefits to which they were entitled. Bands of veterans suffering from tuberculosis wandered in Arizona and other mountain states looking for somewhere to be treated—high altitudes and dry climates being touted for improved health. Frantic families struggled to cope with a family member who had returned from the war with psychiatric problems, without having to consign him (for veterans were almost always men) to an unacceptable state or local mental asylum. A more general movement, led by the newly formed American Legion, pressed for a special payment to all veterans who served to compensate for wages they had lost by not being able to participate in the civilian war economy. This soldiers' bonus was a controversial political issue inherited by Harding, with huge costs involved if granted, and it would not go away.

Still, the mood was festive in the nation's capital as Harding arrived in town, even though there were fewer out-of-town visitors than there might have been because Harding had firmly squelched efforts by the inauguration committee to create an extravaganza of inaugural balls and over-the-top decorations. Extravagance was not the right message to send. The town looked good. Floodlights illuminated the Capitol's great dome to magnificent effect, signifying the grandeur of official Washington, the authority vested by the Constitution in the US Congress and, not least, the promise of a stabilized new America powered by electricity. Illuminating the eastern sky, in competition to the lighting of the Capitol, a huge electric sign flashed the message, "Jesus, the Light of the World." An on-the-spot reporter for the *Los Angeles Times* observed, "A stranger to our ways might be in doubt whether the impending event [the inauguration] was to be something Scriptural or something political, so equally do the lights shine." It was not clear to anyone what the change of administration would mean. On the east front of the Capitol, shivering sightseers could hear the amazing acoustics of the new "voice magnifier" (loudspeaker system) being tested out for Harding's speech on the morrow—the first inaugural speech to be recorded and transmitted by radio and the first that bystanders could actually hear. On Wilson's inauguration for his second four-year term in March 1917, shadowed by the apparent inevitably of entry into World War I, a stiff wind blew his words away.[14]

Near the Potomac River, the great Lincoln Memorial was in its final stages of construction, with its phalanx of columns, one for each state, and massive statue of a godlike seated Lincoln looking out across the Reflecting Pool toward the Washington Monument. Three presidents, three wars, symbols in history: George Washington and American independence, Abraham Lincoln and the end of the Civil War; Woodrow Wilson and World War I, marking America's involvement in a world war begun by others. And now there was a new president. But these were serious thoughts. This was a time to celebrate.

Visitors who were getting chilled could find a movie as exciting as anything on the political scene—and backed dramatically by live musicians. At Crandall's Metropolitan, F Street at 10th, *The Scoffer* was playing: "Seldom has the screen revealed such a torrent of power as surges through this masterful drama of man's hate against man's fear; woman's perfidy against girl's love, and scoffer's skill against God's might. A burst of vivid realism that mental weaklings will not enjoy." At Loews Columbia, Mae Murray starred in *The Gilded Lily*: "The story of a greater love that arose from the ashes of an unworthy sacrifice." *Officer 666* was at the Rialto, and there was always Charlie Chaplin in *The Kid*, as well as other entertainments. There were no open bars because of the Volstead Act (Prohibition). A week before, in the biggest liquor raid yet in Washington, federal agents made fifty arrests—mostly hotel bellhops trading caramel-doctored alcohol as whiskey. Still, someone might know someone who knew where one could get a drink.[15]

Warren Harding had been busy between the election in November and the inauguration in March. First, a vacation with his wife in Brownsville and Point Isabel, Texas, with a party that included influential Washington socialites Edward "Ned" and Evalyn McLean. Then on to inspect the Panama Canal with two fellow US senators, following concern that the area had inadequate military protection. In Panama City, Harding pledged brotherhood with President Belisario Porras of the Panama Republic and turning his face from Europe declared his hope that the Americas, North, Central, and South, would be united peacefully in cooperation by which he meant through trade. Sailing home via Jamaica, he made similarly friendly comments to the British governor there, Sir Leslie Probyn. On arrival back in the United States at the naval base at Norfolk, Virginia, Harding's welcome included a flight of army planes and seaplanes that accompanied his ship to the dock. A special edition of the *Washington Post* was parachuted down, and aerial photos flown back to the capital. Here were presidential trappings indeed for a man who was still a US senator. But that career was shortly to be ended.[16]

On December 6, 1920, Senator Harding spoke before the Senate for the last time as a senator and asked legislators to clear the legislative books, cooperate with him, be tolerant of one another, and "give the best that is in all of us." Nice sentiments, but too much to expect. He discussed the issues facing the country, receiving applause from both sides of the aisle. He then left for his home in Marion, Ohio, where he conducted a series of interviews and discussions with Republican leaders, potential cabinet members, and, in his words, "the best minds and intellects in this great country." Harding announced his new cabinet on February 21, 1921, but there were still ambassadorships and numerous other appointments to make. According to one report, there were 690,000 individuals on the executive rolls in December 1920, not including the military and judicial and legislative lists. Most positions were under civil service regulation, but 240,000 could be seen as potential patronage appointments for Republicans. Harding would be "the greatest job dispenser in the world."[17]

The Harding cabinet was generally praised as an expert and dedicated group. In the light of what happened later, the two most problematic cabinet appointments were of Harding's political supporter, Ohio corporate lawyer Harry M. Daugherty, appointed as attorney general, and Harding's friend in the Senate, Senator Albert B. Fall, as secretary of the interior. Daugherty, then in his early sixties, garnered suspicion from the beginning. He had managed Harding's successful campaigns for the Senate in 1914 and for the Republican nomination for president in 1920. (The campaign for the presidential election was run by Will Hays.) Broad chested, with a large nose in a plumpish face, sharp eyes, receding hair, and flashing smile, Harry Daugherty was known for his bulldog methods and his skills as a political operator, deal-maker, and schmoozer. When attacked, Daugherty stood his ground and swung back at his opponent.[18]

Albert B. Fall, also in his early sixties, was a more promising appointment. Former President Theodore Roosevelt described him as "the kind of public servant of whom all Americans should feel proud." Herbert Hoover wrote Fall on his resignation from government in March 1923, well before charges of scandal circulated about the leasing of government oil reserves to corporate friends, that the department had "never had so constructive and legal a headship as you gave it." Born in Kentucky, Fall was indelibly linked with New Mexico, where he had been a cowboy, a farmhand, a miner, and a prospector and where he learned to use and carry a gun. He passed the bar exam in New Mexico; developed a law practice based on Mexican ranching, mining, and development; and was elected to the US Senate as a Republican when New Mexico became the forty-seventh state in 1912. Harding recognized him as knowledgeable about Latin America and the American West and as a man with a first-rate personal reputation. With erect posture, gray-brown eyes, a straight nose, and an arrestingly bushy, well-trimmed mustache whose ends curled down each side of his mouth, Secretary Fall had an authoritative western look, which he cultivated by wearing a string tie and wide-brimmed black hat. He could have served as a character in a cowboy movie that starred Tom Mix as noble hero, with Tony his faithful horse.

Secretary of the Navy Edwin Denby was a third cabinet member who ran into trouble later for his role in the Harding administration, specifically, for allowing (or not knowing about) the transfer of what became the infamous government oil leases from the navy to the Interior Department. In 1921, Denby, too, was regarded as a strong leader. Herbert Hoover described him as one of five cabinet members who "stood above the others." Attacks on Denby were "among the cruelties of the times," Hoover wrote; he was driven from the Coolidge cabinet by "political persecution and public hysteria." Unfortunately for themselves, both Fall and Denby were to crumble when subjected to hard-swinging accusations of malfeasance by a Senate investigative committee. Denby resigned. Decisiveness alone was not enough.[19]

Outside of cabinet positions were many who deserved a lesser, but still prominent, recognition: men such as Scott C. Bone, who served as the campaign's director of publicity in New York; E. Mont Reily of Kansas City, whose contribution seems mostly to have been his early and continuing enthusiasm for Harding; and Charles R. Forbes, for whom Harding had a special affection and respect. Harding had observed Forbes's work as chief territorial development officer for the governor of Hawaii, had seen him in Washington when he gave testimony about Hawaii to congressional committees, had been in touch with him during the war and after, and appreciated his work for the primary campaign on the West Coast. He had risen in life by his own efforts—though exactly what those were no one knew. He lacked a pedigree, and that mattered as government was becoming more professionalized and American society more formally stratified by education and social class.

Such was the state of affairs when Harding took a needed vacation, before taking on the weight of the presidency.

Inauguration day came and went. The procession arrived at the Capitol with due pomp—cavalry, army vehicles, motorcycles, marchers, bands. Woodrow Wilson entered the Capitol through a side door to avoid climbing a formidable flight of steps, greeted people, and signed last-minute legislation in the President's Room, next to the Senate chamber. Then, frail and having done his duty, Wilson declined to participate in Harding's inauguration ceremony and was driven to his new home on S Street.

Among the bills Wilson signed on his last day in office was an act for an appropriation of $18.6 million for the construction of federal hospital beds for World War I veterans, a topic that was soon to figure prominently in the life of Charles R. Forbes. However, this 1921 law, the first Langley Act (Public Law 66-284), named after the Congressman John W. Langley whom Forbes had met in Hawaii, was passed long before Forbes became responsible for veterans hospitals. The new treasury secretary, Andrew W. Mellon, implemented the legislation. Because appropriate beds for the treatment of war veterans with tuberculosis were of urgent concern, Mellon sent for an expert in that field from his hometown of Pittsburgh, Dr. William C. White, and the two men added an expert in neuropsychiatry and two others on hospital and medical planning. The "White Committee" was to be an irritant for Forbes, and vice versa, in 1922. But of greater significance in 1921, this last-minute signing of legislation for war veterans signified two major problems for the new administration: first, the lack of a national system of hospital and medical services in the United States, into which war veterans could be absorbed and, second, that nothing much had been done for the provision of services that Congress had guaranteed for its sick and wounded warriors until frustration was evident on all sides.[20]

The Harding inauguration went well. On the platform built for the occasion over the steps of the Capitol's East Portico, the new first lady, Florence Kling Harding, was animated, her glasses glinting in the sun. Harding was an emblem of vigor. United States Chief Justice Edward D. White administered the presidential oath of office. There was a fanfare of trumpets, and the US Marine Band played the national anthem. Then President Warren G. Harding delivered his speech in a strong voice, bareheaded, from time to time pointing upward with his right hand for effect. The loudspeaker system worked.[21]

His words were convoluted, but the message was understood: "When one surveys the world around him after the great storm, noting the marks of destruction and yet rejoicing in the ruggedness of the things which withstood it, if he is an American he breathes the clarified atmosphere with a strange mingling of regret and new hope." He spoke of the war's "delirium of expenditure. . . . Our supreme task is the resumption of our onward, normal way." The themes were as expected: probusiness, administrative efficiency, lower taxes, sound commercial practices, concern for agricultural problems, greater operating freedom for business, American self-reliance in production eased by tariffs on imported goods, in favor of a draft in wartime, and belief in the "God-given destiny of our Republic." Then the drive home to the

White House, surrounded by the famed roan horses and cavalrymen from Fort Myer across the river—to the challenge of the real world.

Los Angeles business leaders read Harding's message as a "Let's Go" signal for commerce, including renewed hopes for the sagging movie industry. There was general optimism elsewhere as well. Secretary of the Treasury Andrew W. Mellon and Herbert Hoover at Commerce would not let the business community down. Secretary of State Charles Evans Hughes, a former governor of New York, Supreme Court Justice, and 1916 presidential candidate, would stay on message. Indeed, Hughes built America's international relations anew after its rejection of the League of Nations covenant, improved relations with Latin America, and directed and set the tone for the 1921–1922 international naval disarmament conference, which agreed to limits on the world's five major naval powers. However, optimism had to be tempered with reality; too much could not be achieved at once.[22]

The opening of the white baseball season in Washington in mid-April, with President Harding throwing out the first ball for the Washington Nationals (a.k.a. Senators), was a festive occasion. The black baseball season, represented by the Washington Braves, began the following week. President and Mrs. Harding were accompanied to the game by Secretary and Mrs. Herbert C. Hoover, Attorney General Harry M. Daugherty, and his associate Jess W. Smith, and Charles R. Forbes. The Senators lost to the Red Sox, 3 to 6. Forbes was a guest that evening at the White House, described by the *Washington Post* as a "long-time friend" of the president and Mrs. Harding, an accurate description. There was no reason for him to be described in any other way in the foreseeable future—unless President Harding maneuvered him into a highly visible, contentious job, and that seemed unlikely as bat struck ball at the start of the baseball season. In a humdrum job, he would just remain a White House friend. Instead, Harding was to push him into the spotlight by force of circumstance and political expediency.[23]

In mid-March, Forbes was mentioned in the newspapers as a possible member of the seven-man US Shipping Board, the organization established for the rapid production of wartime ships. On Armistice Day, only half of the 2,311 ships were completed. The rest were no longer needed, and the board's new mission was liquidation without destroying the shaky domestic shipping industry by swamping the market with low-priced ships. Harding favored the creation of a Merchant Marine, but Congress resisted. Forbes had submitted a formal application for a position on the Shipping Board. His nomination file made a good case for him, and at first, he seemed a likely choice. However, Washington State put up a more favored candidate and in the end California won the West Coast slot—with a man Herbert Hoover called "unscrupulous and untrustworthy." Forbes was reportedly offered a special mission for the Shipping Board in London but turned this down. There was humor in some stories about finding a job for Forbes, and venom. Politics as usual. Rumors from the West Coast claimed he was a carpetbagger who did not actually reside in Washington State. A telegram from Kate Forbes in Forbes's Shipping Board dossier attested that her husband was a resident of King County, Seattle, and had owned the house on Vashon Island for seven years, and a deputy tax assessor on the island affirmed that he had "assessed Colonel Forbes in his own house" in 1919.[24]

Harding mentioned the position of governor of the Territory of Alaska when he informed Forbes of the difficulties in naming him to the Shipping Board. There was, he said, a "very strong contention between the conflicting elements in Alaska over the Governorship." He was thinking of appointing an outsider to restore amity, and Forbes might be that man; "this might afford you a fine opportunity for constructive service and making a brilliant record." As Forbes remembered it, he went to discuss the possibility with the new interior secretary, Albert Fall, who waxed enthusiastic about the possibilities for American business enterprise and pointed out desirable locations for development on a large map of Alaska. That evening Forbes dined with Harding, who raised the possibility of ambassador to Peru, but when he got back to his hotel after midnight, a visiting delegation from Alaska was there to congratulate him on the governorship and to lobby him further. Next morning Harding's secretary, George Christian called to invite Forbes to lunch with Harding and told him that Fall had called with doubts about Forbes's eligibility because he had served in Hawaii in a Democratic administration. Forbes declined the positions in Alaska and Peru and went to New York for a dinner with friends at the Yale Club.[25]

Rather than give up on Forbes on the basis of reasonable offers made and refused, Harding continued in his urge to get his protégé a place, thus offering a window into his tenacious personality and adding a frantic element to the proceedings. By then, it was late April. But, then, unexpectedly, an important job became vacant and needed filling. Harding propelled Forbes into managing the Bureau of War Risk Insurance, the federal agency for monetary payments, insurance, compensation, and disability benefits for World War veterans, working under an assistant secretary of the treasury. Decisions that affected dissatisfied war veterans were politically critical, and there was a need to move fast. Forbes had managerial experience and was a decorated veteran. He was not an unreasonable choice. But, then, after fourteen weeks, Harding was to launch him out on his own as director of a new, independent, consolidated Veterans Bureau, responsible for one of the largest budgets in the federal government. Thus, Forbes was set to become a lightning rod for criticism: first, in April 1921, because of demands on the Bureau of War Risk Insurance to provide timely and more effective services and, then on a larger scale in August, when three feuding government offices were brought together under his direction as the new US Veterans Bureau. In 1924, his name would become vilified, together with those of Interior Secretary Albert B. Fall, Attorney General Harry M. Daugherty, and others, as a corrupt, betraying toady of a weak, blind-sided president.

Late in the evening of the Yale Club dinner, Forbes received a telephone call to return to Washington. Next morning White House physician Dr. Charles E. Sawyer met Forbes off the overnight train at Union Station with the White House car to take him to the president. Besides his clinical role, Sawyer was now Harding's adviser on domestic health and welfare policy. Harding called in Treasury Secretary Andrew W. Mellon, to whom Forbes would report. Forbes was sworn in as director of the Bureau of War Risk Insurance.

THE DREAM OF EFFICIENCY IN GOVERNMENT

On April 27, 1921, Colonel Charles R. Forbes, the new director of the Bureau of War Risk Insurance, became a government insurance and benefits executive with more than four million clients on the books: the men and a few women who served in the military in World War I. The bureau had been set up in the Treasury Department after World War I began in Europe to insure American merchant ships, freights, and cargoes against damage incurred in a hostile environment—a program managed by twenty individuals out of four rooms in the Treasury Department. After the United States entered the war, a new, progressive program of benefits for US servicemen was designed. In a huge, scaled-up effort, the bureau hired thousands of staff—up to 17,000 at one point—to write the necessary rules, regulations, interpretations, and explanations; to design application forms, processes, and files; and to locate, counsel, and ensure compliance from all prospective beneficiaries, wherever they might be. The bureau opened offices in France. Men filled out applications in the trenches. By December 1920, the Bureau of War Risk Insurance had adjudicated more than 430,000 claims for death and disability compensation, with more coming in every month. The good news for Colonel Forbes was that most of the technical aspects of insurance, including eligibility for compensation and compensable benefits, had been dealt with under previous directors. When Forbes told Harding, "I know nothing about insurance," Harding said, rather cryptically, "that was an advantage." The bureau needed someone to improve and expedite existing programs.

Veterans of World War I (then simply known as World War veterans) were also eligible for medical and hospital care and job training. Two other federal agencies were responsible for these services. The US Public Health Service provided medical examinations and hospital care, and an independent Federal Board for Vocational Education managed a countrywide program of job evaluation, vocational education, and placement. Relations among the three groups were strained in 1921. Hapless applicants for benefits struggled to get prompt and helpful attention from different branches of government and find all the records they needed: military and demobilization papers, war risk insurance records, medical information, and job assessment. "Red tape" was a constant refrain. For the administration, the big issues for veterans' benefits in the spring of 1921 were questions of organization and management: how to coordinate services for war veterans at the federal and local level to provide effective services in the field, how to speed up claims, get veterans into jobs, produce more and better hospital beds, and—in a climate of widespread criticism—create a better public image of war risk insurance as a whole.

Forbes's predecessor as director of the Bureau of War Risk Insurance, Richard Cholmeley-Jones, described it as "one of the largest financial institutions the world has ever known." The number of staff was down to 6,000 by the time Forbes arrived, facilitated by efficiency studies and job consolidations. Ninety percent of the workers were women, almost all of them stenographers and clerks. They worked at arrays of desks in an imposing ten-story building on Vermont Avenue that consumed the entire block between H and I Streets, with overflow space in a new annex and other buildings. The executive suite was on the tenth floor. Forbes wrote later that he accepted the director's job "with much misgiving." The pay was reasonable, $7,500 a year, the same salary as a congressman. The responsibility was huge.[1]

Warren Harding entered the presidency with a commitment to improving efficiency in government, making Colonel Forbes, as head of a large unit that was in many ways a "business," part of his larger enterprise to modernize the executive branch of the federal government. Readjustments within existing departments were relatively simple. Efforts to consolidate medical and monetary services for World War I veterans were under way as Forbes arrived on the job, facilitated by the fact that the Public Health Service and the Bureau of War Risk Insurance were both part of the Treasury Department, and both were responsible to the same assistant secretary. However, even here there were professional and cultural barriers and external constituencies that divided the two groups and made transitions difficult. Further coordination of services for veterans with vocational education was problematic, as those were housed in the Federal Board for Vocational Education, a separate agency. Though business methods might form an admirable agenda for improvements in government, intergroup politics intervened at all levels. Then as now, the more comprehensive the plan for reform, in whatever area of government business this might be, the more difficult it was to achieve.

Where should veterans' services be placed, and how should they be organized? During his famous front-porch campaign for the presidency (on Women's Day, October 1, 1920, to be precise), Harding had suggested the establishment of a large new Department of Public Welfare, which would bring together scattered federal government offices relating to "health, education and social justice" and would logically include services to war veterans. "Let's make social justice real and functioning, rather than visionary and inefficient," he proclaimed to the female throng, members of whom were now allowed to vote. Whether or not he expected this to be achieved, Harding supported the creation of a public welfare department throughout his presidency. To act as his representative for advancing the proposal, he requested Congress to confirm the appointment of Dr. Charles E. Sawyer, his old friend from Marion, Ohio, as White House physician with the rank of brigadier general (duly approved), on the understanding that Sawyer would also have authority to survey and report on the consolidation of appropriate federal offices in the welfare field. Sawyer became his point man for advancing legislative proposals for the proposed department, working with Senator William S. Kenyon of Iowa, the progressive Republican who chaired the Senate Committee on Education and Labor. The proposal called for a cabinet-level department with four assistant secretaries, each in charge of a major division: education, public health, social service, and veterans' service. Veterans' benefits would then be recognized formally as similar and parallel to health and social services for other civilians, rather than as distinct, separate, and unique. Three policy questions thus came into play: (1) where veterans' services should be administered within the executive offices of the president; (2) the fate of the welfare department, to be decided by Congress; and (3) Sawyer's incipient role in veterans' affairs as White House adviser on domestic programs, which would become a major source of uncertainty for Forbes.[2]

General Sawyer was a major speaker at Senate hearings on "social welfare" in April 1921 and at joint House and Senate hearings on "public welfare" in May. (Both terms were used.) The goal, he said, was to develop "the highest type of American citizenship," and as a matter of economy and efficiency, this could best be done through bringing diverse federal service agencies together into "one united family." The proposed siblings splintered in opposition, as might have been expected. Educationalists wanted a cabinet department of their own. Health had a bigger case to be independent than did education. Given that women were voters and social welfare was considered a women's issue, assurance was needed that a woman would be the secretary of social welfare (but drawn from which professional division?). Organized labor opposed moving the Children's Bureau and the Women's Bureau out of the Department of Labor. Figures presented by the chief of the Bureau of Efficiency (an agency established in 1916) showed that the proposed Department of Public Welfare would have 37,000 employees, drawn from twelve organizations, with the largest number, 19,000, from the Public Health Service. In contrast, the Bureau of Education had only 256 employees and the Children's Bureau even fewer. Supporters of the Bureau of Education would resist joining any new department, whatever it was called, if it would be numerically swamped by other units. Plans may engage reason but fail against the force of human interests, then as now.

Harding also looked favorably on other efforts to reorganize the executive branch of the federal government. Walter Brown, his appointee on a joint congressional Committee on Reorganization came up with a suggested list of ten executive departments, which included a combined War and Navy Department named Defense [painfully achieved in 1947], renaming the Post Office "Communications," and establishing a new Department of Education and Welfare, which excluded Health. Major change did not come from any of these or other efforts in the 1920s, except in the case of World War veterans, for whom veterans' groups were pushing for an autonomous federal organization.[3]

Besides the political strengths of the various parties involved in all these efforts, veterans had a strong argument for special treatment because of the relative allocation of federal funds in the 1920s. Health, education, and welfare services for the general population were almost entirely paid for by local and state governments. By far, the largest federal expenditures on public or social welfare were for military veterans of World War I and previous wars, including the Civil War. According to one accounting, when the costs of separate outlays for veterans of earlier wars were added in, 97 percent of total net federal social welfare expenditures went for military veterans in fiscal year 1923. The remaining 3 percent covered all other "ordinary social welfare" categories, including services to American Indians, immigration control, and federal prisons, which were the three largest remaining items. (A new model of funding through federal grants to states for maternal and child welfare services, the Sheppard-Towner Act, signed by Harding in 1921, was further down the line).[4]

The amount of money flowing to veterans meant that, in pushing for a new public welfare effort, Charles E. Sawyer, the domestic policy adviser to the president, had a huge interest in veterans' programs. He had never served in the military, but his ability to exert authority was fostered by his appointment as a brigadier general in the Army Medical Corps, called to active duty at the White House. Army Surgeon General Merritte W. Ireland was pleased to accommodate a close confidant of the president by recommending Sawyer to his new rank. Sawyer received offices in the War Department and other accoutrements. The sight of the short, erect Sawyer with his neat white beard, in his first ever military deployment, wearing a general's uniform and perched on the top of a cavalry horse, caused mirth in journalistic circles. But that was to underrate him. Sawyer established a network of individuals and organizational representatives seeking access to the president, while enlarging his acquaintance among influential members of the Washington community.

As Forbes remembered it, Sawyer was his first visitor at the Bureau of War Risk Insurance. "Now let's do some real work," he said. The first thing he wanted to do was "kick out Dr. Haven Emerson," the bureau's eminent, aristocratic, sometimes irascible and condescending medical director, who had allegedly insulted Sawyer and his field of homeopathic medicine. He probably had—this was a man who did not pull his punches. Forbes was wary: "Immediately I sensed a pitfall into which I would inevitably stumble unless I watched my step." Sawyer kept watch on what Forbes was doing through reports from informants within the bureau.[5]

On Forbes's second day on the job, he was called to give an official statement in a House hearing that was from one perspective a piece of the public welfare proposal, but from a second, a rival to it: "consolidation of government agencies for the benefit of disabled ex-service men." This was a major congressional proposal for the establishment of a new, consolidated veterans' bureau, through combining the Bureau of War Risk Insurance with related elements of the Public Health Service and the Federal Board for Vocational Education. (Sawyer expected this to be initially housed within the Treasury Department and then transferred to the Department of Public Welfare on its creation.) Forbes was an old hand at briefing congressional committees from his work for Hawaii and handled himself well. He reminded his hearers, "I just took over the office yesterday," added some anecdotes from his wartime experience, and noted that "at the next hearing, or in a short time, I will be better able to give you some of my own ideas, after consultation with my associates."[6]

The spirit of reform wafted through bureaucratic corridors and crevices as cabinet members prepared to achieve Harding's commitment to the "business organization of government." Among other things, business administration meant standardization of budgeting for federal offices, audit and cost controls, reduction of overlapping functions, and coordination of efforts across departments in areas such as purchasing and construction. Before Harding, there was no single federal budget. Each department prepared its own requests for Congress without overall executive planning and surveillance. There was no center, no single "business." The new Budget and Accounting Act (June 10, 1921) established for the first time a centralized Bureau of the Budget and an independent Office of Comptroller General, a significant achievement for the Harding administration.[7]

From the beginning of Harding's administration, cabinet members were expected to make their departments more efficient: Hays at the Post Office, Weeks at the War Department, Hoover at Commerce, Fall at Interior, among others. Albert B. Fall, having come to the cabinet with strong views about the business (and probusiness) organization of government, pushed the definition of *business organization* to include what he took to be Republican business policy. "There was no shilly-shallying, no indolence about this energetic man," a contemporary observer wrote. "He came to office with his mind made up that the whole conservation policy was a piece of sentimental nonsense." In the spirit of a business entrepreneur, Fall communed with another strong appointee, Secretary Edwin Denby at the Navy Department, which controlled vast in-the-ground government oil reserves (but had no use for unrefined oil), seeking authority for these to be transferred to the Interior Department, which had staff experienced in mining and oil. (In return, the Navy would reportedly get fuel-oil tanks constructed at Pearl Harbor.) Commerce Secretary Herbert Hoover described Denby as one of five cabinet members who "stood above the others." In May 1921, President Harding signed an executive order transferring the navy's oil leases on government land in California and Wyoming to the Interior Department. Later the transfers were to appear nefarious. However, in 1921, it was not clear what limits would, or should, be put on cross-departmental transfers or other actions done in the spirit of a business-and-efficiency-minded federal government.[8]

At the Department of Justice, Attorney General Harry M. Daugherty hired William J. Burns, a famous detective, whom he had known for forty years in Ohio, to head the Bureau of Investigation (the fledgling FBI). Burns was a character, for whom successes were achieved via whatever worked, not excluding burglary, breaking and entering, stalking, harassment, or bribing to get someone's letters or into bank accounts, as Daugherty no doubt knew. Burns kept control of his international private detective agency and felt free to use both public and private agents while he served the Department of Justice. As liquor crimes proliferated as a result of prohibition, the significance of a national police increased. Sometimes it took one crook to nail another. The combination of Burns and his young deputy, J. Edgar Hoover, created an odd amalgam of old and new: on one hand, old-style detective work that might involve criminal acts; on the other, modern information systems. Hoover was a data-and-systems-oriented lawyer who built an extraordinary national identification system, trained agents, and standardized the reports of agents in the field. Fingerprints were being used. Harding had his fingerprints taken. An association dedicated to fingerprinting suggested that everyone's prints be taken and kept at local post offices, to be used for identification by police as necessary. But that was taking efficiency too far.[9]

In this context of reform, efforts were made within the Treasury Department to consolidate medical and insurance services for World War I veterans. A few days before Forbes was appointed, Treasury Secretary Mellon transferred the fourteen district offices the Public Health Service had established across the country (to provide the medical examinations needed for veterans claiming benefits) to the Bureau of War Risk Insurance, in the hope that this would reduce delay in adjudicating claims. This was a significant move toward coordinated services for veterans but still only a partial effort. For the moment, the Public Health Service retained control of veterans' services provided in its own hospitals and dispensaries. Meanwhile, the Bureau of War Risk Insurance assumed responsibility for assigning beneficiaries to hospitals and supervising the care of those receiving treatment under contract with nonfederal hospitals. Forbes had no time to study his new position. When he arrived at his desk on the tenth floor on his first day, 4,000 health service employees were in the process of transferring to his bureau, grudgingly in many cases. Mutual distrust would not suddenly go away. Several hundred physicians were included in the transfer: commissioned Public Health Service officers with salaries and benefits fixed by rank and length of service, which were typically higher than those paid to doctors in the Bureau of War Risk Insurance. The transferred doctors worked "on detail" to the bureau, maintaining their higher status as part of the Public Health Service. Conflicts in organizational allegiance were inevitable, plus doubts and feelings of superiority with respect to Colonel Forbes as a nonphysician—a layman raised up beyond his proper place.

With the new medical responsibilities the Bureau of War Risk Insurance moved toward becoming a comprehensive veterans bureau—and on that topic political momentum was building, spurred on by Congress, the Harding administration, medical experts, the American Legion, and other veterans' organizations. As often in politics, opinion became enshrined in a conveniently reassuring truth, namely that veterans' services were not working well because they were offered in a tragically dysfunctional "system"—a word in vogue among politicians and efficiency engineers. Putting the blame on the system freed Congress and members of the former administration from shouldering blame for shortchanging services promised to World War I veterans, whom Congress had virtually ignored in 1919 and in 1920. In 1921, it was as if an advertising agency flew slogans across the sky: "Organizational Reform! The Answer to Administrative Problems. Change the system and services will improve. Consolidate for efficiency!"

A plan to consolidate veterans' services was drawn up in Harding's first two weeks of office. Harding had the report in hand. The chair of the committee from which it came was General Charles G. Dawes, popularly known as General "Hell 'n' Maria" Dawes for colorfully expressed frustration before a congressional committee. Dawes was a respected Chicago banker who had run the supply service while the American Expeditionary Force was in Europe and liked to get things done. The Dawes committee report made the point explicitly: "The present deplorable failure on the part of the Government to properly care for the disabled veterans is due in large part to an imperfect organization of governmental effort." Dawes wanted someone to cut though bureaucratic inertia, "someone with a meat ax." Red tape must go. His committee met on April 5, 1921, worked through the next day, took testimony from Sawyer (of the White House), Cholmeley-Jones (Forbes's predecessor), Public Health Service and American Legion leaders, and others, and reported out on April 7, three weeks before Forbes joined the Bureau of War Risk Insurance. Forbes had jumped on a rapidly moving train.[10]

The Dawes committee hearings were based on a proposal to place a consolidated veterans bureau in the Treasury Department, where two of the three components were already located. However, Dawes made a significant change when he drafted the committee's recommendations. To give the director of the new bureau the greatest possible freedom to make and execute decisions, as an army general would, freed from the constraints of being a subsection of another department (the Treasury), Dawes recommended that (1) the proposed director would report only to the president and (2) the bureau would be an independent federal organization. His committee members quickly endorsed this tack, and this conclusion was made public and warmly embraced by the American Legion.

Inadvertently, Dawes had undercut the proposal for a department of public welfare. General Sawyer was appalled. Public welfare was supposed to integrate all similar services into one department, for reasons of efficiency. A new federal entity just for veterans would isolate services for World War I veterans into a political and social sphere separated from that of other civilians and might separate them from veterans of other wars as well. Once an independent entity—a veterans bureau—was in place, the inclusion of veterans of future wars into a public welfare department would be politically difficult, if not impossible, to achieve. (Such concerns had merit. When a Department of Health, Education and Welfare was finally achieved in 1953, it did not take over veterans' benefits. To this day, US war veterans are served by a dedicated federal organization, now a cabinet department.)

General Dawes, who liked and respected General Sawyer, tried to backtrack and urge that the proposed location of the bureau be switched back to the Treasury Department under an assistant secretary. The day before Forbes was sworn in Dawes wrote to American Legion leaders, in the hope that they would support the idea of having an assistant secretary in charge of veterans' affairs. The idea of direct report to the president was all his idea, Dawes said. His essential message was "if we really want to help the disabled soldiers, we will not object to a modification like this which is not vital." Too late. Veterans' organizations grabbed onto the prospect of an independent federal agency and did not let go. As debate continued into the summer months, the Dawes committee plan stuck like glue, namely, to transfer the whole of the Bureau of War Risk Insurance, all Public Health Service programs dedicated to veterans, and all vocational rehabilitation services for veterans in the Federal Board for Vocational Education into a new "independent" federal organization. Its managing director would be responsible directly to the president but would not be a cabinet member. The alternative, favored by many, was to locate the combined bureau in the Treasury. Congress would make the decision about placement.[11]

The number of World War veterans needing help was sobering; veterans, their families, survivors, and advocates were socially visible and politically active. More than 53,000 American servicemen had died in battle and more than 63,000 from other causes, including tuberculosis and epidemic influenza, and 204,000 servicemen were wounded without being killed. Coverage for aggravation of preexisting conditions, most notably for the flaring up of tuberculosis and for mental illness, increased the number of beneficiaries seeking inpatient hospital care after discharge. In this war as for later wars, the most lasting medical needs were for chronic diseases. The grief and grievances of ex-servicemen and their families simmered and boiled across the United States. American bodies were still being shipped back from France. More than 5,000 flag-draped coffins stretched across the army pier in Hoboken, New Jersey, in late May 1921, welcomed home in a ceremony attended by President Harding. The last shipment arrived in

August 1922: 1,064 dead men and boys delivered from temporary burial in France, this time with a formal ceremony at the Brooklyn Army Base. Between these dates, on November 11, 1921, Presidents Harding and Wilson joined a solemn procession to Arlington National Cemetery to dedicate a new national monument, the Tomb of the Unknown Soldier, and (on the following day) the landmark international Naval Disarmament Conference began in Washington, opened by Harding with a moving antiwar speech. The families of the dead applied for life insurance and survivor benefits; the sick, maimed, and disabled sought the medical and institutional care to which they were entitled (but which was vaguely defined in the initial legislation); and the unemployed demanded vocational training.[12]

Complaints flooded into the Bureau of War Risk Insurance. Republican Senator John Jacob Rogers of Massachusetts reported early in 1921 that he spent most of his time as a US senator interceding with the three veterans' agencies on behalf of individual constituents. The Bureau of War Risk Insurance received 25,000 letters every day from one source or another, plus telegrams and phone calls. "Some of these letters are very pathetic," Forbes told a congressional committee. He interviewed some of the applicants himself. To help improve access to services, the bureau ran a "clean-up" drive to locate eligible men who had not filed a claim because they were ill-informed, disorganized, illiterate, isolated, mentally ill, in long-term hospital residence, had no fixed abode, or had landed in prison.[13]

In parallel, the American Legion continued to push for a generic soldiers' bonus to be given to all who had served in the ranks, a proposal that Harding, backed by Treasury Secretary Mellon, strongly opposed on budgetary grounds. The goal of the bonus was to adjust the paltry pay received by conscripts by providing a sum of money to help compensate for what they might have earned in wartime jobs at home. World War I veterans were well organized, and their organizations were demanding more. Violence at home was a possibility. Membership in the legion, established in France in 1919, took off under the patriotic banner of "100 Percent Americanism." In 1920, the legion had more than 800,000 members. Disabled American Veterans, founded in 1920 as an activist organization of and for disabled ex-soldiers, was a second influential force. Seventy-five thousand veterans paraded down Fifth Avenue in New York to demand the bonus, watched by 100,000 spectators. Congress favored the proposal. To stand firm and counter claims for the bonus, Harding needed to show that the delivery of government benefits to veterans was effective, generous, and humane, particularly to disabled veterans, who had the strongest case for government beneficence. That load was on Forbes's shoulders.[14]

Colonel Richard G. Cholmeley-Jones, Forbes's predecessor, had served as director for less than two years after accomplishing the mammoth task of establishing a system for selling and managing government-run war risk insurance policies in wartime France. During his time in Washington, the three agencies serving veterans were frequently at loggerheads, and all were roundly criticized by Congress and by veterans' groups. The American Legion, which had had run-ins with Cholmeley-Jones, remembered him as someone who "worked himself into a hospital bed" after his "tremendous, really impossible assignment." Ten months after leaving office he died at the age of thirty-seven. His colleagues believed the job had killed him. When Forbes's life was unraveling in 1923, he remembered a warning he received from Cholmeley-Jones: "Colonel Forbes, you are coming into a job that will bring you only grief and sorrow. I have done everything within my power to build up this institution and make it really worthwhile. It is politically stagnant, and I do not believe that you or any other man will ever be able to put it over." The first difficulty Forbes would face, he said, was the Public Health Service.[15]

Nevertheless, Forbes was a fresh face, someone of apparently unjaded spirits, indeed, of optimism and energy, and his former work experiences served him well: constructing complex building projects and communications systems, enlivening the public works agenda in Hawaii, rallying his troops in the war. Staff members liked him as he walked around the floors appreciating their work and encouraging their efforts. His convivial personality gave the bureau an upbeat tone. He worked well with the assistant secretary of the Treasury, Edward Clifford, to whom he reported. General Sawyer showered praise on both men in a letter to General Dawes: "I have always contended that the only thing that was necessary here was to get the machinery in motion, and these boys have oiled it up, tightened up the bolts and kicked out the nuts and are on the way, much to the gratification and satisfaction of everybody concerned." The president appointed Forbes, wrote Sawyer in another letter, because "he knows him to be a great producer of results. He makes little fuss about what he does. He believes that the thing to do is to deliver directly from the bat, and that is what he is doing every day, much to the satisfaction of everybody concerned." Sawyer was happy to emphasize Forbes's success as a mid-level bureaucrat and an administration team player. Harding was pleased with Forbes's reports. Mark Sullivan, a gifted journalist and contemporary historian, heard from one observer of Harding's during the early months of his administration that "whenever he mentioned Forbes's work he looked pleased; here was one part of his Administration, Harding felt, that was clearly making good."[16]

After barely a month on the job, Forbes wrote General Dawes to give him a progress report on the Bureau of War Risk Insurance. Among the "constructive steps" under way, he reported, were organizational overhauls and coordination between War Risk Insurance and the Public Health Service. Improved procedures for examining and hospitalizing the sick, following the transfer of out-of-hospital medical care to the bureau, were "well under way." Many "delays, misunderstandings, and duplication of effort" had been avoided. Reorganization had already been completed in eight of the fourteen Public Health Service districts. Reorganization in the bureau included the appointment of a planning committee with the goal of efficiency. "Four divisions and thirteen sections of the bureau have been abolished," Forbes wrote, and the personnel of the bureau reduced from 5,768 to 5,264 (the recently added Public Health Service staff not included)—an estimated savings to the government of $654,820 in annual salaries, while achieving improved services. He hoped the bureau's enormous, lagging caseload would be current within the next sixty days. The letter reflects Forbes's leadership style: a mix of rapid action, high goals, effort, and exhortation, with more than a dash of overpromising thrown in. Dawes wrote an encouraging letter back, sensibly cautioning him not to boast: "The mere reading of your letter inspires me with confidence that the Bureau is in the right hands. . . . Keep plugging away and above all avoid early publicity. Do not endanger an anticlimax by allowing your work to be praised by the press too quickly, and, in the long run, you will certainly find a very general and public appreciation of it."[17]

Expecting that a veterans bureau would soon be established under new legislation, the bureau's medical division established a section for district organization with fourteen district offices to supervise medical care, and a hospital section. On August 1, 1921, responsibility for medical treatment in contract hospitals was transferred from the Public Health Service to the bureau. (Public Health Service–owned hospitals for veterans were transferred nine months later.) The bureau was becoming heavily involved in hospital processes and procedures. A new veterans hospital construction program was also (finally) under way under the supervision of the hospital consultants (the White Committee) appointed by Treasury Secretary Mellon.[18]

At the White House, General Sawyer was a thoughtful strategist. He was aware from the time of the Dawes report that a quasi-autonomous veterans bureau, if and when it was established, would be huge, expensive, contentious, and politically visible. If things did not go well, it could turn into a political disaster for the president and for the Republican Party. Sawyer envisaged someone at the helm who was a "master mind" and had a national reputation and experience in "large affairs." This was not a description of Charles R. Forbes. A Republican general would be ideal. Sawyer's candidate was General Charles G. Dawes. "It is your duty to your personal friend, Mr. Harding," Sawyer wrote Dawes. "I know that you will be invited to do it." Dawes's secretary suggested another well-known military leader, Major General Leonard Wood—President McKinley's personal physician, army chief of staff before the war, a leading candidate for the Republican nomination for president in 1920, then governor of the Philippines. Neither man was interested. The job promised to be managerially fractious and personally unrewarding, and men such as Dawes and Wood merited a cabinet position. However, Dawes did agree to work for President Harding for a year (June 1921–June 1922) to develop the nation's first federal budget and a Bureau of the Budget to administer it.

Sawyer developed a good relationship with Dawes. At the end of June 1921, President Harding presided over a large meeting of government officials and bureau chiefs in the auditorium of the Department of the Interior to introduce General Dawes in his new role and highlight the Harding administration's commitment to economy and efficiency in government. Forbes was presumably there as director of the Bureau of War Risk Insurance. (There is no surviving list of attendees.) "There is not a menace in the world to-day like that of growing public indebtedness and mounting public expenditures," Harding said. Dawes was the star of the show. In a rousing one-hour presentation, he sent out clear messages about business efficiency, economy, and the need to coordinate efforts across organizational lines to avoid duplication and reduce waste. As a start, Dawes promised to take a cut in his "own little appropriation" as budget director, and he did. He urged all present to "save all you can" and concluded by asking bureau chiefs to stand if they supported him. "The entire audience arose," the minutes show, followed by the president, Vice President Calvin Coolidge, and the cabinet. Loud applause ensued. At the Bureau of War Risk Insurance, the efficiency message rang loud and clear. Forbes's task was to consolidate administrative functions and to cut staff and budget.[19]

Republican Representative Burton E. Sweet of Iowa, introduced the bill that became the veterans bureau legislation. The Sweet bill, H.R. 6611, passed the House of Representatives on June 10, 1921, and was referred to the Senate. It put the new Veterans Bureau in the Treasury Department, with the director serving as an assistant secretary. As expected, the bureau would be composed of the Bureau of War Risk Insurance, the Rehabilitation Division of the Federal Board for Vocational Education, and related functions of the Public Health Service. There would be a central office in Washington, DC, and up to fourteen regional offices for the combined services, with suboffices as necessary in the larger regions. All of these (and other) provisions were to be carried into the final legislation, except for the bureau's administrative location, an issue still under debate. The Senate Finance Committee referred the Sweet bill to a subcommittee chaired by powerful Republican Senator Reed Smoot of Utah, an apostle of the Church of Latter-day Saints, who was known for his commitment to organizational efficiency. Smoot referred the bill to the Bureau of War Risk Insurance for comment.[20]

With two months' experience under his belt, Colonel Forbes submitted technical amendments. Smoot also talked with Colonel John Thomas Taylor, the legislative representative of the American Legion in Washington, who supported all of the bureau's revisions; the legion had no doubt worked on them. The Senate hearings thus began with the buy-in of the major government agency that would be affected (Forbes's bureau) and the most powerful veterans' lobby. Taylor, a Republican from Pennsylvania, stood out among the army of lobbyists and publicists in Washington in 1921. A legionnaire who knew him described him in action: "Donning his spats, swinging his cane, he would march down Pennsylvania Avenue to the marble halls of

Congress, stalk into committee rooms, present the legion's case for this measure and that. If reporters buttonholed him as he left a closed committee session, asking if a pending bill would pass, he would answer them with due gravity, 'The American Legion favors it. It is inevitable legislation.'" Smoot made it clear that he intended to report to the Senate as soon as possible.[21]

In the first week of July 1921, Smoot opened a substantive hearing on setting up a federal veterans bureau. Colonel Forbes was present. General Sawyer was not. He may simply have assumed that the new bureau would be placed in the Treasury Department, as noted in the bill. Edwin J. Bettelheim, Jr., chair of the national legislative committee of the Veterans of Foreign Wars of the United States, delicately brought up the question of who would be director of the bureau. Smoot asserted that "we agreed . . . the other day" that the director would be the director of the Bureau of War Risk Insurance, "who shall be appointed an Assistant Secretary of the Treasury." Smoot had known Forbes at least casually and by reputation since the two men participated in the impressively staged visit of the congressional delegation to Hawaii in 1915, but more pertinently, Smoot had almost certainly discussed Forbes's possible appointment with President Harding. Massachusetts Democrat Senator David I. Walsh, a strong critic of the management of veterans' services, helped Bettelheim out by seeding doubt: "Your point is that that language makes the present incumbent the Assistant Secretary of the Treasury?" Bettelheim waffled: It was "just an embarrassing situation; that is all." He believed Forbes to be "a very good man" but pointed out that the assistant secretary was not automatically the present director of the War Risk Bureau. However, for Smoot, and presumably the American Legion, Forbes was the sole candidate for the job. One way out of the dilemma of who would be the assistant secretary was to remove the veterans bureau from the Treasury altogether. Legislation evolves in such awkward pirouetting.[22]

Hearings resumed on specific parts of the bill, such as how open ended the rules should be for a veteran to claim aggravation after the war for a premilitary condition, or the status of a stepmother as an eligible dependent, or what happened to her pension when a woman remarried (It ceased: "It has always been that way," Smoot said.). Forbes expressed concern that the Sweet bill was too broad in providing government-paid dental work, allowing dentists to engage in bribes, kickbacks, and self-referrals, and proposed to establish public dental clinics (which he did). But attention finally turned back to the placement and directorship of the new bureau. Smoot asked Forbes the critical question, "What do you think about changing this bill so as to make it a separate bureau and taking it from under the Treasury Department entirely?" This question should have been asked of Andrew W. Mellon or Charles E. Sawyer, not of someone with a clear interest in the outcome, but Smoot was playing Forbes, as well as his committee members. Forbes said first, "I think it is rather late now" but then added that the placement would work if the director had sufficient authority. (He was right. Authority was to be a moot point.) Senators Smoot and Walsh disagreed about the proper location for the bureau; the former was in favor of an independent bureau, the latter for keeping it in the Treasury. Smoot wanted to wipe out "red tape." A further problem he noted was that under this bill vocational training for veterans would be taken from an independent federal board (the Federal Board for Vocational Education) and dropped under an assistant secretary in the Treasury Department. Smoot wondered whether professionals in vocational education might perceive this placement as an insult to their field and as a demotion of their experts. Pressed to answer, Forbes agreed that an independent bureau would be "more advantageous." Smoot concluded it was "the only way to do it." Walsh, ambiguously, said, "That is a very happy thought." Thus, the way was set to report out a bill for an independent veterans bureau whose director would report only to the president. Harding wrote Forbes to make his wishes clear, namely that "when I sign the new Act I shall at the same time send my nomination of a Director to the Senate. I do not mind telling you that I am going to nominate a man named Forbes for this place."[23]

On August 1, 1921, the Senate unanimously passed the Sweet bill as agreed in conference. The next day the House passed it 264 to 4. (The four naysayers were congressmen who opposed the bill for striking out a proposed increase in the fee for paying for attendants for totally blind veterans, so effectively this was unanimous too.) No legislator wanted to be viewed as antiveteran. Harding was vacationing at Mount Prospect, New Hampshire, and could not sign the bill immediately. Vice President Coolidge was in New England, and the Senate president pro tempore was ill in Atlantic City; and so the bill sat unsigned for a few days. President Harding signed the legislation to establish a Veterans Bureau (Public Law 67-47) on August 8, to take effect August 9, 1921. From that day into the twenty-first century, for better or for worse, services to US war veterans were sequestered from those of the general population.[24]

The act created immediate challenges. It abolished the Bureau of War Risk Insurance, but the Veterans Bureau could not be established without someone to direct it; and the appointment of a director required Senate approval. There was no time to consider a candidate other than Forbes, even if anyone wished to do so; but by then, his appointment seemed a done deal, even a simple job upgrade. In the Senate, in the words of the *New York Times*, Reed Smoot "got busy" rallying his troops with such success that Forbes's confirmation was achieved within five hours on August 9, the same day the legislation took effect. All insurance and compensation activities, together with those parts of the Public Health Service that dealt with medical evaluation and medical care for veterans, and the vocational rehabilitation of veterans were absorbed into the new United States Veterans Bureau. (Hospitals and their staffs were to be transferred to the bureau from the Public Health Service in May 1922.) The new, consolidated bureau would organize and provide services to World War veterans across the full spectrum: from insurance benefits and evaluation of disability, through decisions about medical, dental, and hospital care, to job education and training.[25]

On the evening the law went into effect, General Sawyer, still pressing for a department of public welfare, went to dinner with General Dawes, the budget director. The two men had become allies in the cause of government coordination and consolidation. "From his suggestions, I always get ideas and from his sympathy always encouragement," Dawes wrote in his journal. Things were "moving pretty well" at the Bureau of the Budget. He was turning his focus to coordination of activities across the federal government in areas such as purchasing and liquidation. Formally, relations between Dawes, Sawyer, and Forbes were civil. Each worked for the president, reported directly to him, and revered him. Dawes, by far the most renowned of the three, described Harding in glowing terms: He was the "ideal chief of the business machine of the government." And again, "My personal and official association with President Harding is a delight to me. His mind is quick as lightning." Sawyer had an emotional relationship with both Warren and Florence Harding that was deeper and longer than that of Forbes. Florence Harding, in particular, depended on Sawyer for her health. Forbes looked up to Harding as an inspiring older brother or father figure. All three men were part of the presidential circle. In July, Forbes spent a weekend with the Harding party cruising down the Potomac on the presidential yacht, together with Dawes, Sawyer, General John J. Pershing, Attorney General Daugherty, Senator Edge, and Senator and Mrs. Harry S. New.[26]

Harding continued to get a good, if mixed, press. Some praised and some denounced his "gradual drift in the direction of aggressive leadership of the executive field of legislation," as illustrated by his insistence in passing legislation to restore business and economic relations with Colombia (in August 1921) and in preventing the passage of the "bonus bill" for veterans in an effective speech to the Senate. The first opened up Colombia for American investment; the second protected the Harding-Mellon fiscal program.

The day after the Veterans Bureau was established Forbes went with Sawyer and the bureau's legal adviser, Charles F. Cramer, to visit Walter Reed Army Hospital. Colonel Forbes declared to wounded veterans at the hospital's Red Cross Hut that the Veterans Bureau "was established for you and you alone" and promised to give them what they deserved, including "perfectly equipped" hospitals in pleasant settings. He also urged them not to expect too much at once, but this was a message no one wanted to hear. The establishment of this cobbled-together, three-prong bureaucracy was supposed to be an answer, not a further set of problems.[27]

Two days after the bureau's establishment (that is, on August 11, 1921) Charles and Kate Forbes, accompanied by their eight-year-old daughter, Marcia, attended a small dinner of "intimate friends" at the White House to celebrate Dr. Sawyer's sixty-second birthday. Kate Forbes reported the informality of such an occasion: Harding sent for his dog, Laddie Boy, which rushed in "boisterous and happy," begged for food from the table, and was finally called to order by Florence Harding: "Warren, leave that dog alone. Laddie, come here."[28]

Treasury Secretary Mellon wrote Forbes with congratulations and best wishes: "I am sure that you will meet the tasks committed to your care in the same efficient manner that has characterized your work since your appointment as Director of the Bureau of War Risk insurance.... You have my best wishes for great success in this important undertaking and assurance of my hearty cooperation."[29]

Work at the now-defunct Bureau of War Risk Insurance was an invaluable training ground for setting up the Veterans Bureau during the fourteen weeks Forbes served there. He worked hard. When in Washington, he usually arrived in the office at 8 a.m. or earlier and put in a ten- or twelve-hour day, sometimes more. He continued his hands-on leadership style that had worked well for him in the War Risk Bureau. He met staff throughout the organization, inspiring them and familiarizing himself with their work. However, the transition to the new entity, untethered from the Treasury Department, represented an enormous change in scope, scale, and vulnerability. The consolidated Veterans Bureau, launched on the rhetoric of business organization and efficiency, was started with a false assumption. It assumed success would be attained through structural change alone; that is, with the development of a more perfect system, without taking into account the upheavals this would cause or the cultural, political, and personal aspects of change. If reorganization were achieved, then any remaining failures in delivering services, which there were bound to be, would fall squarely on the system's chief executive in the full spotlight of publicity.

The complications of a visible government position were nicely stated by Herbert Hoover before he accepted the job as Harding's secretary of commerce: "I knew that if a man engaged in public life he was bound to create opposition every time he took a stand on a public question; that he was fated to accumulate enemies; that in the United States the laws of libel and slander had little potency, and that the customary form of reply to sober argument was proof of guilt by association or assumption of corrupt motives." Democracies, he averred, were "fickle and heartless."[30]

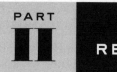

PART

II

REALITY CHECKS

HARDING'S FLAGSHIP PROGRAM
The US Veterans Bureau

Photographs of the swearing-in of Colonel Charles R. Forbes as the first director of the US Veterans Bureau on August 9, 1921, show him in sensible attire for the season—loose, extra-large white trousers (he had put on weight), blazer and tie, with a determined look on his face. The task ahead of him was formidable. Next to him stood Representative Burton Sweet, who initiated the legislation that established the Veterans Bureau, and on Sweet's other side, General Charles E. Sawyer in his role as White House representative, buttoned-up and belt-clasped in his military uniform in the sweltering, un-air-conditioned heat.

The immediate challenge was to integrate three professional cultures—fiscal, medical, and educational—into a consolidated system. Vocational educational services were transferred from the Federal Board for Vocational Education overnight. On August 10, the Veterans Bureau acquired more than 6,000 employees in vocational rehabilitation, responsible for 90,000 men in training in 3,000 schools and colleges across the United States. For both the medical and educational communities, Forbes's appointment as director rammed home a dismal message: the Veterans Bureau was the Bureau of War Risk Insurance under a new name, a victorious beast that was about to swallow them up. Forbes's job was to consolidate services previously given by the three groups into a smoothly running national organization based in Washington; create standardized procedures and oversight mechanisms; decentralize the combined services to fourteen new district offices (plus more than a hundred subdistrict offices) across the United States and install managers in each of these; improve inadequate medical and hospital care, particularly for outpatient specialty services and hospitalization of veterans with mental illness and tuberculosis; shake up vocational education; and get beneficiaries into jobs. This all had to be done at once. Arguably, reforming veterans' services demanded more drastic, destabilizing reforms than any others undertaken by federal agencies in the Harding administration or for that matter in the Coolidge and Hoover administrations that followed.[1]

Congress, having signed off on the legislation as a problem solved, simultaneously increased the demand for services by relaxing the requirement that a strict 10 percent disability rating must be shown for veterans to qualify for medical and related benefits. Under the assumption that soldiers were in good health when they were inducted, the door was opened to claims for all kinds of medical problems as war-related. Section 13 of Public Law 67-47 authorized the bureau to provide hospital, medical, dental, surgical, convalescent treatment, and prosthetic appliances to any veteran who could show a disability or aggravation of a previous condition in the line of duty, if the claim for benefits were made within a year of the legislation—initially by August 9, 1922, later extended, or a year after military discharge if that were later.

The bureau's "clean-up" campaign, which looked for needy veterans who had not applied for benefits, added about 180,000 more ex-servicemen to the rolls. The exact number, 179,868, was provided by the bureau's 300-member logistical support team at headquarters—emblematic of the demands of scientific management and business efficiency. Bureau employees and volunteers helped veterans with their claims, one by one, across the country, assembling the military, discharge, and medical papers necessary to evaluate each case. Forbes's one and only annual report, for fiscal year 1922, was filled with tables and statistics. Almost 31,000 veterans were hospitalized under the bureau's auspices in March 1922, and almost 110,000 beneficiaries were in vocational training programs in April, both, as it turned out, the peak months for these services.[2]

As director, Forbes had three immediate goals: (1) get the bureau's district offices up and running as quickly as possible; (2) take a sharp look at the provision of vocational services, the weakest link in the chain; and (3) provide inspirational leadership, starting at headquarters. On occasion, he came down from the executive suite to interview applicants in the building's new welcoming center. A couple of weeks into his new role a reporter wrote, "Colonel Forbes has the real human touch with the men." He "impresses one with his sincerity, his clear, logical mind, his executive force and directness of thought and action. . . . [He] mingles with the boys, holds conferences with them, getting their stories." As Forbes said: "A sick man is never a contented man ... it is our job to make the men ... as contented as possible."[3]

He kept his executive offices and core staff, and acquired an invaluable secretary who acted as his personal and executive assistant, Mr. Merle LaRue Sweet (no relation of Representative Sweet), an experienced civil servant in his late thirties. Forbes and Sweet formed an appealing physical counterpoint: the midsized, squarish, dynamic, and expansive Colonel Forbes, and the six-foot, lanky, black-haired, pipe-smoking, whimsical Sweet from North Dakota. He traveled with Forbes on many of his official trips, handled his schedule and travel expenses, wrote reports and dictated letters, paid his boss's insurance premiums for him, managed his bank account, and conducted independent site visits. In short, he got to know him well. Sweet liked his job and liked his boss. Both men worked hard and had a sense of the ridiculous. When called as a witness in the Senate investigation of the Veterans Bureau in the fall of 1923, months after Forbes had left government, Sweet testified that he knew nothing about Forbes's engaging in any conspiracy, as then alleged; believed Forbes lived within his government income of $10,000 a year; never saw Forbes take a drink at the Veterans Bureau, and never observed him anywhere under the influence of liquor; and he was uniformly positive about Forbes's work record. "I must confess to a personal regard for Col[onel] Forbes," he added. "I have an affectionate regard for him." He solemnly replied to questioning that yes, he recognized he had a higher loyalty to his country than to the Veterans Bureau and, no, that did not change his views.[4]

The object of the Veterans Bureau, Forbes announced after meeting with President Harding, was to create "a coordinated and an efficient business, conducted as great going concerns are run everywhere else in the land." Veterans would be given the benefit of the doubt in cases in which an individual's eligibility for services was ambiguous: "the presumption is always in favor of the claimants." Action on all claims would be prompt. The new legislation extended Forbes's responsibility for policing the hospitals to which the Bureau sent patients on a contractual basis, even shutting them down when deficient and although the US Public Health Service would not transfer its veterans hospitals for another nine months, this too was anticipated. Forbes made it clear he would not stint: "I intend to have a hospitalization program put into effect that will provide a place in a perfectly equipped institution for every temporarily disabled man or woman desiring treatment, and I intend to have his surroundings such that he will be happy while there." Brave words, with expensive connotations, but they met Harding's need to show optimism and progress in the Veterans Bureau and forestall the passage of the "Soldiers' Bonus."[5]

Forbes faced the enormity of his task with outward equanimity, accepting General Dawes's earlier model of a strong chief executive who wielded a meat-ax and cut red tape. Few stopped to consider the mechanics of his expanding job, its size and changing scope; its organizational, interpersonal, and political pitfalls; and, not least, the ever-present Washington danger of hubris. By the end of June 1922, ten months into his directorship, almost 30,000 individuals were working for the Veterans Bureau. By then, almost half of all bureau employees worked through decentralized districts, with a further third working in Veterans Bureau hospitals. Colonel Forbes was charged to do what Congress had not agreed to do for other civilians; that is, provide a "department of public welfare" for World War I veterans.[6]

An immediate need was for a senior official to oversee the transition of vocational rehabilitation into the organization. In late August 1921, Forbes announced the appointment of Major Arthur Dean, head of the Vocational Training School at Columbia University, as an assistant director of the Veterans Bureau. Dean had spent eight years as director of vocational education in New York City and served as a major in charge of reconstructive work in army hospitals during the war. He was "one of the best informed men in the country," Forbes announced, and "particularly fitted to assist in the mammoth work of rehabilitation of the ex-service man." However, "assist" meant "working under my direction." Once again (as in his spat with consultant engineers in Honolulu), Forbes proved inept in working with civilians in leading professions who had a high opinion of themselves. The day Dean was appointed—and apparently without consulting him—newspapers reported that President Harding and his cabinet had discussed a radical departure from the policies favored by vocational educational specialists, who believed in finding education and job placement for veterans near where they wanted to live. The new plan was to develop a huge residential vocational school at an abandoned army cantonment (in Chillicothe, Ohio) where there were buildings in which trainees and faculty could live and others would be available for workshops and teaching. Forbes suggested there should be four such national centers. He had taught the rudiments of communications technology to raw recruits at special centers in wartime France and knew that education in the trades could be done effectively in this way, at least in the military. Professor Dean must have recognized immediately that he would have little voice in policy making. Worse, he might find himself constrained to carry out policies in his area of professional expertise with which he strongly disagreed.[7]

Forbes's assertive style reverberated through debates about the poor quality of vocational education during the early weeks of his administration. "The men are farmed out in cheap tailoring establishments and mushroom institutions, where the only interest to the proprietors or instructors is the amount of money that can be obtained from the government," he told the press. "It is nothing short of slavery to put men in certain types of these institutions. We want to establish schools so the men will be honestly and properly rehabilitated instead of destroying their morale." He named schools that had submitted vouchers to the government for nonexistent students, closed some New York schools, and was prepared to close the Berkeley Pre-Vocational School in Boston, with 500 trainees, in the face of considerable pressure not to do so. A William Blackburn of Lynn, Massachusetts, aged 72, he reported, had "cost the government $130 a month since July 24, 1919, to teach this man how to write his name," which he could now trace in a "feeble scrawl." Blackburn had reportedly enlisted in the naval reserve and his disability was "indigestion."

By mid-October, Forbes had disallowed training contracts at thirty-two schools (Southern California was the worst area, he said) for reasons ranging from "asininity" (his word) to graft. Universities around the country were looking askance at the projected government training centers. They would not impinge on university-type courses, Forbes assured them: "We will call the schools 'technical training centers,' if they like." However, the Chillicothe experiment was not a success. World War veterans did not want to go to a center far from home, particularly one in which they might be treated as if they were still in the military.

Arthur Dean, for whom this outcome was obvious, was conspicuous by his absence from the public press. Forbes's enthusiasm "ran away with him," the *New York Times* reported; there had been too much "muddling through."

Nonetheless, the vocational education system needed cleaning up. At the district level, as new staffs were assembling and trying to work together, counselors struggled to make sense of the patchwork of placements, apprenticeships, educational offerings, and employers who ranged from excellent to exploitative.[8]

According to Veterans Bureau staff, the Federal Board for Vocational Education had allowed ex-servicemen to enter training in any field they chose, no matter how unrealistic. Here, in paid government-sponsored training, as listed in Forbes's annual report, were aspiring actors and aeronauts, auctioneers and auto painters, bankers and bell boys, candy makers and clergymen, designers, editors and reporters, fingerprint readers, grocers, gunsmiths, hotel managers, industrial art workers, jewelry factory workers, lawyers, lens grinders, musicians, nurses, officials (city, county, state, and federal), piano and organ tuners, real estate agents, stagehands, telegraph operators, warehouse packers, and many others, several hundred categories in all—a mirror of postwar American aspirations. A Veterans Bureau officer lamented: "Men without any background whatsoever have demanded that they be trained for some musical vocation and a large number have insisted on training for the vaudeville stage." Another: "The cultured invariably seem to want rough outdoor life. The illiterate and uncultured often want indoor work. The strong want light work as an objective. The weak often disown their disabilities and want to train for rigid work." The new district managers pressed on as best they could. Forbes lambasted the system at the first annual meeting of district managers in Washington in October, his words reported in the *Washington Post*: "I am only astounded that rehabilitation chiefs would send men to school and shops where the most cursory investigations would have found conditions to be as I have exposed them." He exhorted his new lieutenants into action. The bureau was going to be operated "on sound, modern principles, and every phase of it is going to be clean and above board. . . . I know that with the help of God we can put it over by all working together."[9]

Arthur Dean participated in a major conference on rehabilitation called by Forbes in December 1921, but he was neither the welcoming speaker nor conference chair. Forbes opened the session, stressing the need for the "human touch." Dean lasted in his position as assistant director through mid-January, when Forbes dismissed him. His firing raised hackles on several fronts at once, not least among the vocational education workers who had worked for the Federal Board and now worked for the Veterans Bureau. For Disabled American Veterans, Dean's dismissal was tantamount to a "blow straight to the heart" and was caused because he disagreed with Forbes's "wild-cat scheme" of national training centers. Dean returned home, claiming he was intending to resign anyway, but Forbes "beat me to it." From Columbia University's Faculty Club, he accused the Veterans Bureau of being dominated by the "War Risk Insurance group," lamented the bureau's interference into professional policies, and damned Forbes as an uneducated nonprofessional who had nothing to do with "real" education. Dean added an extraneous social-class critique. Forbes had built "public works," using "'employees' and rough materials" before coming to government, he proclaimed; that is, he had run a construction gang of uneducated migrants or, as Dean put it, "coolie labor." When asked by a reporter, Forbes gave no reason for Dean's leaving: "Just say that Prof. Dean for some time has been under the weather."[10]

Forbes clashed with his medical service chief as well: the eminent Dr. Haven Emerson, detailed to the Veterans Bureau from the US Public Health Service (the man who had insulted General Sawyer). Emerson was a national leader in medicine, hospitals, and public health, who considered himself a consultant with no line responsibilities. Forbes needed a medical workhorse who would deal with the bureau's increasing responsibility for medical services and help develop staff in the Veterans Bureau districts. Each man bristled when annoyed. Each sought victory over compromise. Emerson was an aristocratic superstar who felt no intrinsic loyalty to the bureau and certainly not to Forbes. It would never have occurred to him not to speak his mind. He was famous for his intolerance of "fuzzy-minded nitwits who speak with authority concerning matters they do not understand."[11]

Matters came to a head while Forbes was making his first major trip as director of the US Veterans Bureau to inspect services in the American West in his second month in office (September 1921). In Oakland, California, Forbes was greeted as the hero of the hour. An elaborate ceremony in his honor at Oakland's municipal auditorium included members of the American Legion, the American Red Cross, the Oakland and San Francisco fire department bands, community singing, speeches, vaudeville, syncopated music, and a dance. However, as the *Oakland Tribune* put it, in the modern world of a national press and telegraphic communications, he could not escape "the centers of two storms which have been whirling over the heads of his department." One was the usual flurry of local concern that cropped up everywhere reform was in view; in this case, proposals to abandon the Palo Alto Hospital as a center for veterans and cancel contracts with private hospitals, both of which would mean withdrawing federal money from the area. The second was national news that Haven Emerson had charged the bureau with political patronage and inefficiency—sizzling the wires from coast to coast. Forbes, caught unawares, lashed out. Dr. Leon Fraser, the bureau's executive officer in Washington, sent him news of some unrecorded dereliction of duty by Emerson—though Forbes said later that he had been misinformed. Forbes shot off a cable or telegram (later he could not remember which) to tell Emerson he was dismissed. Emerson's version was that Forbes had accepted his resignation just after he began as director, to take effect September 15.[12]

Emerson's initial tirades predated those of Arthur Dean but continued far beyond them. Like Dean, he saw Forbes through the lens of social and professional class. In his view, the bureau was "being made the football of politics." It was wasting half a million dollars on political patronage, with "plumbers and policemen . . . being substituted for scientific medical men." One version substituted "blacksmiths" for "plumbers," thus casting aspersions on three stalwart occupations. In Emerson's view, the director of the Veterans Bureau was far from being a "professional, with science and ethics at his disposal," or, by analogy, a gentleman, who knew how to behave. Forbes retaliated in a similarly aggressive tone: "I expected some such silly statement from a disgruntled employee whose services have proved unsatisfactory. . . . The facts are that I found the medical division, under his direction, in a chaotic condition. He had 65,000 cases awaiting action and was losing ground every day while sick and destitute men clamored for aid. . . . I intend to keep no employee who obstructs legitimate veterans' claims by incompetence and I would have dismissed Emerson earlier had I had a substitute." Furthermore, he added, "It is too bad Emerson lost his head and his manners." Press coverage was on balance favorable to Forbes. The *Washington Post* called Emerson's remarks "the only pessimistic note heard recently" about veterans' services. The *New York Times* considered the firing of two top figures at the bureau to be appropriate business practice: "Naturally the director prefers lieutenants who are in sympathy with him. . . . He has addressed himself to the solution of the insurance, hospitalization and rehabilitation problems with intelligence, courage and resolution." Nonetheless, the contretemps left ripples of anger in its wake.[13]

Calling Emerson an "employee" was like waving a red rag at a bull. Emerson continued his attack with the thoroughbred scorn of a patrician. He became an implacable enemy, fanning fires of moral outrage about lay interference in medicine into virulent personal criticism. By May 1922, he was explaining in print that he had resigned "because politics interfered with professional efficiency," that under Forbes there was "vacillation" and "interference with professional policies," educational and medical, plus "flagrantly unfit appointments" and "special favors for claimants coming from suitably endorsed sources." Nothing, he wrote, stood in the way of success except the "quality of leadership and direction of the Veterans Bureau." The bureau's real potential as a place where medical professionals would regain their proper standing would not be fulfilled until the president replaced "his political lieutenant from the realms of pioneer power plant construction" with a "real administrator" and established a "regime of competence and merit." If this critique had not struck a chord in various constituencies, it might have been regarded as an entertaining skirmish, which in many ways it was. Public Health Service physicians, working for the bureau and feeling the Forbes machine steamrolling over their prerogatives, were the first and most obviously receptive audience, but anyone with a grievance against the bureau (and there were many, some of whom had been battling with parts of the system for years) formed a large, inchoate second: politicians with a vested interest in the bureau, veterans and their supporters frustrated about the slowness of change, conservatively minded legislators and other citizens who saw their tax dollars flowing excessively into Forbes's domain, community leaders and organizations whose members bewailed lack of services or low standards in existing hospitals and vocational schools, and many others. Emerson made it possible for critics to see Forbes from two dramatically negative perspectives: (1) as the central problem of the Veterans Bureau and (2) as an inappropriately elevated public servant who was ill-prepared, ill-mannered, and possibly unethical. Forbes was a decisive and charismatic leader who could be undiplomatic to the point of hurting himself, as well as others, when maneuvering in the civilian world.[14]

Haven Emerson did not address Forbes's criticism of the medical work done while he was medical adviser to the Bureau of War Risk Insurance, and did not develop a more sympathetic view of Forbes. In an oral history completed in the 1950s, he said simply: "I resigned and Forbes was subsequently sent to jail, to my great delight." Forbes later regretted firing Emerson. "I saw and read a great deal of his work afterwards," he said. But he stuck to his basic point, namely, that Emerson was "a wonderful physician but not a good administrator."[15]

The good news was that he brought in two superb, result-oriented military officers to replace Emerson and Dean. Both were detailed to the bureau from the US Army. Both understood loyalty and chain of command, as did Forbes. The practical and affable Lieutenant Colonel (Dr.) Robert U. Patterson, in his mid-forties, came in to manage the rapidly expanding medical division. Patterson had commanded US Army Base Hospital No. 5 (the Harvard Unit) in France and held the Distinguished Service Medal and the British War Medal. Eventually, he became surgeon general of the army, a major-general, and on retirement a medical school dean (at the Universities of Oklahoma and Maryland, respectively). Colonel Robert I. Rees, also a career army officer, took over the rehabilitation division. Rees had served as an aide to General John J. Pershing in the war with responsibility for educational work in the American Expeditionary Force (AEF). He was a brigadier general when he left the army in 1924 to work in the private sector at AT&T. Rees began to get the vocational system under control. He had no problem shutting down inferior schools or policing the length of vocational training, which was much longer in the United States than in other countries. Up to four years of paid training was allowed, compared with six months in England, and twelve to eighteen months in France. In May 1922, Albert A. Sprague, a Chicago businessman who spent most of his time working for veterans through the American Legion, paid tribute to what Rees had accomplished in only a few weeks. Forbes "turned over to him a disorganized, poorly functioning and a badly overloaded machine. I believe that chaos is being eliminated slowly but surely." However, Sprague warned, the vocational training part of the bureau was the "most difficult and dangerous part . . . where, if there is a big scandal, it is going to break." This comment was prescient in one way (there would later be a scandal) but not in another. The scandal would center on new problems: those of hospital construction and hospital supplies.[16]

While coping with changes in Washington, DC, Forbes and his staff selected managers at top speed to get the district offices off the ground and running. The fourteen districts, each covering services in more than one state, were based on the old Public Health Service districts, repurposed, and expanded to cover the complete span of veterans' services. There were no villains in the culture clashes. It was only human for the former physician manager of a Public Health Service district to feel entitled to the much-larger job—and for physicians to believe the bureau should be medically run. "Colonel Forbes has already replaced the medical men by laymen in Chicago, Dallas, Seattle, Cincinnati, and other cities," reported the journal *The Survey* of the early weeks of Forbes's tenure. The bureau also established 126 suboffices (the law allowed a maximum of 140; Forbes was deliberately saving money here), each of which needed a manager. Then as now, good managers were in short supply.

Six of the district offices had more than a thousand Veterans Bureau employees, working in offices, dispensaries, and vocational schools, not counting hospital staffs. The urgency to get going meant that managers were selected for their availability. There was no time to wait for a "best fit." Some of the prospects were already on the spot working for one or other part of the service. Others were recommended by the American Legion and other veterans' organizations, by the Red Cross, and by congressmen, senators, and local dignitaries, in good faith or as patronage positions. Each manager had to meld together the claims, medical, and vocational training personnel and deal with a vociferous chorus of critical veterans and politicians. When managers failed, they had to be replaced. The physician manager in Philadelphia ran afoul of local critics and was brought back to headquarters; the bureau's executive officer, Major (Dr.) Leon Fraser was moved out of Washington to solve problems at the visibly disorganized district office in New York. Jobs were wearing at all levels. Fraser commented to a friend during his New York experience, "Frankly, I have had rather too long a sojourn with the Bureau."[17]

Forbes relocated District Office 4, which served veterans in Washington, DC, Maryland, Virginia, and West Virginia, to the Arlington building (Veterans Bureau headquarters, where the number of staff was shrinking)—thus saving a substantial amount in rent and showing that local clients were being served. Progress was uneven across the country. The American Legion placed representatives in every district to help in the transitions. The first national meeting of these legion representatives was rowdy with complaints, reported a bureau officer who attended. The second meeting, five months in, was "much more dignified and less caustic"; district managers were at least "trying to handle the work properly." But there was also abundant criticism along lines that would continue to haunt the bureau—"political appointments" in District 1 (Boston); allowing "politics" to enter the district office in District 11; the continuation of "old dissensions and ill-feeling" between the personnel previously employed in the Federal Board for Vocational Education, the Public Health Service, and War Risk Insurance in Districts 2 and 3; closer contact needed between the district and central office in District 5; general issues on competence of staff and low salaries; not enough centers for psychiatric and tuberculosis care in District 10; and a report that "some fifteen hundred men are roaming around Arizona without being properly hospitalized," from District 12. There were no complaints about graft or stealing.[18]

The country was so large and the span of responsibility for disabled veterans so great that at any one time something was bound to be seriously wrong with veterans' services somewhere in the United States. The bureau was newsworthy, and stories about its services and deficiencies were widely disseminated through national news services such as Associated Press and United Press International. Complaints about poor conditions at the Longview Hospital in Cincinnati were headlined in the *Washington Post*: "Charges Insane Yanks Must Sleep on Floor." Denver hospitals, like those in Arizona, were reportedly in crisis, flooded with 7,000 veterans with tuberculosis who had flocked in from other states in the belief that treatment of tuberculosis at high altitude was essential for a cure. Tuberculosis specialists disagreed, but that made little difference.[19]

Forbes pushed ahead. Anticipating the transfer of Public Health Service dispensaries and outpatient clinics for veterans (plus their staff), he approved an ambitious program for establishing federal government clinics in every district and subdistrict along lines that still read as "modern." The largest type, designed for the nation's nineteen largest cities, was a comprehensive multispecialty clinic, which included internal medicine, general surgery, tuberculosis, ophthalmology, ear-nose-throat, orthopedics, physical therapy, dentistry, x-ray, laboratory and pharmacy, with facilities for social service and administration. "Neuropsychiatry," a major diagnostic category for disabled veterans, was not included; there were too few trained psychiatrists, and it was assumed that patients who were severely mentally ill required hospitalization. The bureau operated sixty-three clinics within five months, including all the largest ones, fourteen of them associated with the district centers.

Forbes had expressed his concern about dental price gouging in the private marketplace. After ten months on the job, eighty-seven Veterans Bureau dental clinics had opened. Graduate nurses were assigned to do follow-up work on more than half a million cases in the districts, where they provided medical care, made home visits, conducted school and placement interviews, and dealt with individuals struggling with a wide variety of medical and reentry problems, including the need for "social adjustment." Concurrently, Forbes reorganized the central office into eight divisions (plus some special sections) to support the decentralized system. He brought in an experienced social worker, Albert E. Haas, former national service director of the American Legion to help veterans negotiate with the district services. Haas trained the contact representatives (mainly ex-servicemen), who helped clients present their claims and explained the services made available under the law.[20]

Forbes's official report for the fiscal year ending in June 1922 described the first months as a "trying" period for bureau employees, who were busy standardizing procedures for monetary and medical claims, conducting claims reviews that were already in the pipeline, and transitioning into their new roles. More than 300,000 case files had been sent out from Washington, though there were thousands more to go, and new claims were going directly to the districts. The bureau included a foreign relations subdivision, responsible for thousands of US veterans living in Puerto Rico, Canada, the Philippines, and other countries. Reflecting the segregated federal bureaucracy of the time, there was a "Negro Section," responsible for the needs of black veterans. This was headed by Dr. J. R. A. Crossland, an African American physician from St. Joseph, Missouri, who was a prominent Republican and former US minister to Liberia. He was assisted by an all–African American staff of clerks and stenographers. Crossland's son, Sergeant J. R. A. Crossland, Jr., was killed in action in 1918 and buried at St. Joseph with military honors.[21]

As he had in wartime, Forbes functioned well under stress. After the fracas with Emerson and Dean, he had made excellent leadership appointments. But it was clear that no one could manage the central office, work the Washington political circuit effectively (to make himself known and safeguard his reputation), and be visible in every district on a regular basis as entrepreneur, salesman, and troubleshooter, encouraging workers and adjudicating disputes, though in this latter task he was very effective. Major William F. Deegan, a prominent member of the American Legion in New York, remarked at the end of one long meeting: "There is something about you, Col[onel] Forbes, that when you are away from us, we cuss you and when we are near you, you have the iron hand on us. You have a magnetic personality."[22]

The decentralized services for Veterans Bureau beneficiaries meant that Forbes spent half his time away from Washington. Fortunately, he liked to be on the move. He made efficient use of overnight train travel on comfortable sleepers, took staff with him to write reports, and often reserved a "drawing room" in which to conduct meetings. A typical travel schedule for shorter trips: left Washington, DC, at 12:20 a.m. (i.e., after midnight) for New York City, arrived 6:10 a.m. the same day; left the next day for Boston, overnight arriving 8 a.m. on day 3. Left Boston on day 4 for Washington, DC. The days were spent working with Veterans Bureau clients, staff, and other figures in the districts. For some trips, he used his own automobile—an Aero-Eight manufactured by Cole.[23]

Charles F. Cramer, head of the bureau's 200-man legal division and an acquaintance of the president and Mrs. Harding, was a possible deputy for Charles R. Forbes—at least on paper. Cramer was slim, well turned out, and bespectacled, in his forties, with a high forehead and receding hair, blue eyes set in an oval face, and a damaged arm. He had been general counsel for two oil corporations in California before moving to Washington as the agent of California wartime oil interests, selling aircraft fuel to American allies. When the demand for military aircraft fuel disappeared, he had to fall back on private practice. In 1921, a reasonably paid government job was attractive. Cramer's wife, Lila Davis Cramer, was his most obvious attribute when the two of them were seen together: a twenty-something stunning redhead who stood 6 feet tall in her shoes, with a shrewd mind and the looks of a showgirl. The Cramers married in 1918, when his career was at its height, and made a three-month trip to Europe in 1919 at the invitation of the British government. Lila Cramer played the Washington social game with zest, gave and attended lunches with members of Congress and their wives, had a box at the Washington opera ball, made newsworthy trips to the Adirondacks, and attended the Yale-Harvard boat races with her spouse.[24]

However, Cramer had no particular commitment to the Veterans Bureau. Forbes had known little about him when he recommended him for appointment. Political interests were involved. Cramer had the strong support of the California Republican congressional delegation. Glowing references for him came from the two US senators from California, Hiram W. Johnson and Samuel M. Shortridge, and from Congressman John I. Nolan of California—influential Republicans all. Johnson had sponsored Cramer as a member of the exclusive Metropolitan Club in Washington. Attorney General Daugherty also supported Cramer. Harding's wishes to favor this group were the deciding factors. Mr. and Mrs. Cramer had bought the house at 2314 Wyoming Avenue previously owned by Warren and Florence Harding, and Mrs. Harding relied on Cramer for initiating corrective action in response to letters of complaint from veterans that were received at the White House when Forbes was away. Forbes appointed Cramer as a "special expert," a category falling outside civil service procedures, and awarded him a salary equal to his own as director of the Bureau of War Risk Insurance.[25]

Forbes did not give Cramer broad authority in the bureau. Their personal relationship was strained, particularly after an awkward set of negotiations done by Cramer on Forbes's behalf in the fall of 1921. Forbes learned that Cramer was going to be in Northern California on other business and asked him to scout out sites for a tuberculosis hospital in the region. Senator Hiram Johnson of San Francisco, a demagogue and former governor of California who could arouse public fury at the snap of a finger, was pressing Harding to get a veterans hospital built in Northern California. "Turbulent popular feeling is breath in Johnson's nostrils," was the way one commentator put it. Johnson disliked Harding, and Harding had reason to do him a political favor in exchange for his support. Forbes had no authority to select sites or build hospitals at the time, but he could make suggestions to Treasury Secretary Andrew Mellon for consideration by his consultants on hospitalization (the White Committee). Cramer, eager to please all sides, found the grape-filled Cresta Blanca vineyard at Livermore, secured an option for its purchase at a price far above prevailing prices, and Forbes, or someone for him, signed a letter to the Treasury Department recommending a contract.

Trouble ensued when Treasury officials saw the recommended price—$150,000 (more than $2 million in twenty-first-century terms). Mellon's consultants had already considered the site and rejected it. The situation had become politically embarrassing for Harding. Mellon handed the problem to Colonel Forbes, Cramer's boss. Forbes, the former vice president of a major construction company, had the price brought down to $105,000 (still high) and included in the contract seven to ten additional acres and water rights for the whole property, plus a sixty-foot easement on both sides of the property. With these adjustments, the Treasury acquired the Livermore site, and the consultants put it on their list. Cramer had also arranged to employ a California architect who turned out to be expensive and incompetent. Forbes was not inclined to involve Cramer on projects that fell outside his role in the legal department.[26]

The most obvious individual for Forbes to partner with in Washington was Dr. (and Brigadier General) Charles E. Sawyer, White House physician and Harding adviser. Both men worked directly for Harding, revered him, and supported his policy agenda. Their partnership was a nonstarter. Sawyer saw himself as the overseer of health and welfare policy, had little confidence in Forbes's ability to direct the Veterans Bureau, and disagreed with him on fundamental questions. Notably, Sawyer thought Forbes was too soft toward veterans instead of toughening them up and favored expensive, specialized medical treatments over the milder approaches of Sawyer's homeopathy. Forbes had accepted the idea that he, and he alone, was running a federal business: the US Veterans Bureau. Personal jealousy of each other's involvement with Harding no doubt also played a role. Sawyer kept an eye on what was happening in the Veterans Bureau and talked freely with its staff, as he had with the Bureau of War Risk Insurance. His appointment as White House public welfare adviser provided entrée to government offices as a matter of course. Forbes became frustrated when Sawyer waved a letter in front of him signed by the president and reported what he said were the president's views. Without a federal public welfare department, Sawyer had no other domain in which to exert authority over health and welfare policy, and he was protective of what he saw as Harding's best interests. Sawyer could be difficult. To Forbes, quite simply he was a meddler.

With respect to management style, Forbes followed the Dawes committee report of April 1921, which suggested corporate authority and a military-type command-and-control model for the Veterans Bureau. Eliminating or cutting through red tape was an important part of the mission. However, two months later, General Dawes established the federal Bureau of the Budget, which required new rules in the interest of modernization, not tossing all regulations away. What, exactly, was red tape? The Veterans Bureau was an "independent federal organization," but what did that mean? It was still part of the federal government, which included partially implemented civil service regulations and rules for advertising and bidding on government contracts. Forbes's driving energy and assertive entrepreneurial action in the interest of speed were suited to the initial organizational reforms in the bureau, but in the long term, any director would have to play by civilian, not military rules, and what those rules were was not always clear.

Instead of partnering with Forbes, Sawyer found a new opportunity for exerting influence through Budget Director General Dawes. Dawes was planning federal coordinating boards as part of the administration's efficiency agenda. President Harding signed executive orders for two such boards, a Federal Purchasing Board and a Federal Liquidation Board, in August 1921, just after the Veterans Bureau was created. Sparked by Sawyer's interest in public welfare and backed by Harding, Dawes next had in mind a coordinating board for federal activities for public health, veterans' relief and other activities, including hospitalization, which would necessarily involve the Veterans Bureau. Sawyer was "a man of great ability and common sense," Dawes wrote in his journal, "but he needs an authoritative position to fully control the wasteful duplication in building and the use of facilities now going on." The major federal hospital construction projects were for veterans, and Forbes would be the main target, but the new coordinating board would also include hospital activities of the army, navy, the marine hospitals of the Public Health Service, St. Elizabeths Hospital (a huge federal psychiatric hospital in Washington, DC), the National Home for Disabled Soldiers, and Indian Affairs—each supplying a member of the board. Harding signed an executive order to establish the Federal Board of Hospitalization on November 8, 1921, with Sawyer as its chair and chief coordinator. Thereby, Sawyer assumed titular authority in two major areas: (1) the construction of veterans hospitals and (2) hospital supplies. The stage was set for an open clash between Sawyer as multiagency "coordinator" and Forbes as head of the executive agency with immediate interest in new federal hospitals. Forbes became vice chair of the board.[27]

Harding's first budget message to Congress in December 1921 called for lower federal expenditures in fiscal 1923 than in 1922, a sign of his efficiency agenda. The Bureau of the Budget would be the instrument to impose this policy. Dawes recognized that the destabilizing reorganizations required in the first year or two of the Veterans Bureau required further expenditures during the transition. With costs centralized into one budget, however, for the first time, Americans could see how much was being spent on World War veterans. The approved budget of the new consolidated Veterans Bureau was $510 million (more than $7 billion in twenty-first-century terms). Colonel Forbes was responsible for the expenditure of more than a million dollars a day. A leading senator pointed out that this was "more than the entire expenditure of the whole United States in any year prior to 1897."[28]

How quickly would World War I veterans be recast as an expensive social burden? The magnitude of the administrative machinery to handle their affairs was becoming obvious across the nation, including the establishment of new, multipurpose district offices in major cities. For example, in New York, Veterans Bureau District 2 leased the eighth and tenth floors of the Grand Central Palace building, stretching between Forty-Sixth and Forty-Seventh Streets and Lexington Avenue in Manhattan. "One of the largest and most important leases of the year," reported the *New York Times*. The name of the building suggested excess, though it was simply one of the buildings near the Grand Central railroad station. Forbes explained, to no avail, that the combined rental was less than what had been spent before. The revealed size of the Veterans Bureau raised questions about preferential treatment for disabled veterans compared with ordinary employed and unemployed Americans, who had neither a national health service nor paid vocational training. Rumors of waste and graft in government built on such observations. Members of Congress had little interest in posing philosophical or moral questions of how much the nation *should* spend on its war veterans, and why. Legislators pushed for as much as they could get for the voters in their constituencies. Congress was not designed to be efficient.[29]

As he had been in Hawaii, Forbes's performance was underrated, as were the enormous problems he faced. In his first nine months in office (August 1921–May 1922), he created the Veterans Bureau districts while absorbing additional services into the bureau, forged ahead under pressure, took decisive action whatever the fallout might be, and brushed off hostile criticism, not always with tact or common sense. There were problems across the system, including grumblings from staff moved out from headquarters to other parts of the United States, or moved in reverse to the central office, but the bureau was accepted as a single government entity, here to stay. That was probably all that could be achieved in this time frame. Meanwhile, Forbes had acquired an army of critics.

Naval officer Joel T. Boone, a White House physician who worked with General Sawyer, wrote in his journal of a lovely spring day in 1922: "Rode horseback with Gen'l Sawyer in Potomac Park. . . . Gen'l Sawyer says Colonel Forbes is an autocrat. There is apparently friction." Leading mental health expert Thomas W. Salmon wrote to Colonel Sprague of the American Legion early in April 1922: "A good many rumors reach me regarding Forbes' coming downfall." If that meant getting a superb man in the job, all to the good, but if not, he noted, a change of director could be another blow for disabled veterans. Sprague was of the same mind. There was no point in "trying to cross the stream on another horse," and someone else could delay things further: "Forbes certainly has shown his disposition to work hard, to cooperate and I feel has his heart set on making good."[30]

HIGH STAKES
Controlling Veterans Hospitals

Ideally, in the late spring and summer of 1922, Forbes and his staff would be able to concentrate on improving effectiveness at all levels of the Veterans Bureau after the major disruptions of reorganization, work on continuing problems, reduce the pressures felt by all concerned, and raise morale, but there was no time to slow down and reappraise because yet another set of reforms was under way. New battles loomed; this time over veterans hospitals.

Under a presidential executive order of April 29, 1922, the US Public Health Service transferred fifty-seven veterans hospitals to the US Veterans Bureau, effective two days later. Public Health officials, relieved of the burden of struggling to provide hospitals with inadequate resources and in the face of constant criticism, could surely sigh with relief. Six large tuberculosis hospitals were included in the transfer, and some smaller facilities for neuropsychiatric illnesses, but nine of the hospitals were deteriorating wooden wartime structures built by the army in 1917 to last five years. Public Health Service hospital staffs transferred too, including another batch of commissioned Public Health Service physicians who were seconded on detail. Nine other hospitals, under construction by the Treasury Department under the White Committee, would be transferred to the Veterans Bureau as each was completed. In addition, several disorganized and uncataloged military surplus depots, which had been dumped on the Public Health Service because of their potential use for hospital supplies, were shifted to the Veterans Bureau. On top of his other duties, on May Day 1922, Forbes assumed responsibility for these hospitals, personnel, and supplies, as well as a nascent national hospital system.

A wiser man might have resigned at this point, declared victory in organizing the Veterans Bureau, and left hospital management to the next incumbent. Counting his tenure at the War Risk Insurance Bureau, Forbes had been working nonstop for a year. His health was threatened and his marriage at a point of crisis. Forbes, however, considered control of designated hospitals for veterans an intrinsic and continuing part of his mission. He tried to explain the importance of his sense of mission to his wife, no doubt on more than one occasion, in terms of "inborn impulses that I possess," that is, as stemming from his intrinsic personality rather than from Washington-derived hubris or promises he had made or being on a treadmill. No one's ambitions or ideals were greater than his, he wrote on one occasion, and their fulfilment was the greatest purpose of his life. He stayed.[1]

The Veterans Bureau was already responsible for decisions about whether beneficiaries should be hospitalized and where they should be treated. The bureau also contracted with existing nonfederal hospitals (private, state, and local government) to provide hospitalization for veterans, for which those hospitals were reimbursed, and shut down unsatisfactory facilities. Before May 1922, however, the bureau had to rely on hospitals run by others, which ranged from excellent to terrible. In parallel, a second Langley bill was in the offing in the early months of 1922, which was expected to pass and release $17 million in new construction funds for veterans hospitals. Those funds were not earmarked for control by the Veterans Bureau. Forbes was determined that the bureau would be granted this appropriation. A military leader needs control of his materiel, and so, in his view, did he.

Behind the politics were fundamental differences about the need for a large increase in hospital beds. What hospital services did World War I veterans need? What kind of facilities should government provide? Who should be in charge? Colonel Forbes's answers were different from those of General Sawyer. The war risk insurance program had been based on principles similar to those of workmen's compensation in industry, that is, as compensation for working in an extra-hazardous occupation during wartime. The public image of a war veteran was that of a plucky man without an arm, eye or leg, who would take full advantage of excellent facilities for physical reconstruction and occupational retraining before leaving military service, emerge cheerfully and get back to work. President Harding singled out such a man for special praise: Carl Bronner, a navy veteran, blind in both eyes, his hands blown off by a grenade but nevertheless a "happy, self-reliant young fellow with abundant confidence in himself." The Veterans Bureau had provided him with a special typewriter and he planned to study law. Many who needed physical therapies, however, chose demobilization instead, putting unexpected demands on hospital services for veterans. What of other ex-servicemen whom war had disabled or made sick? Was the veteran with mental illness to end up living on the streets, or was the man with a retching cough from tuberculosis doomed to wander aimlessly in the Colorado highlands? And what about the more than 70,000 draftees who had passed cursory medical screening tests at hastily assembled local draft boards and entered the military but then were rejected for medical reasons after they arrived at their respective base camps? Did they get free health care, too, assuming they qualified as disabled? (Yes.)[2]

Forbes sought advice from leading medical specialists and made his position clear: Tuberculosis and neuropsychiatric cases were products of war; therefore, most of the government's ongoing responsibility would be for long-term care, and proper hospital facilities must be provided. "Proper" meant specially designed hospitals with medical specialists and trained nurses for tuberculosis and mental illness, respectively, as well as for general medical and surgical cases, each backed up by relevant lab and x-ray diagnostic technologies, plus treatments such as massage, electrotherapy, hydrotherapy, thermotherapy, actinic ray, and exercise, all under physiotherapists, plus occupational therapy and other special treatments. Occupational therapy services included among other possibilities work with textile, reed and cane, woodworking, leather and bookbinding, cement and plastic; academic, commercial, agriculture, and metal work; music and photography.[3]

He also supported free choice of health services by the World War I veteran: "I believe this: That no man knows how a man feels better than himself. If a man goes West, goes East or South, and if he is a tubercular patient, and feels agreeable and contented there, that is 75 per cent of his treatment." He wanted to build hospital and dispensary services for tuberculosis, mental illness, and general medicine and surgery to serve veterans through both the acute and chronic phases of their illnesses; in short, offer them a comprehensive health care system. If his plan were implemented in full, he would provide better services for disabled war veterans than were available to other disabled members of the population. The word *hospital*, as applied to well-equipped mental and tuberculosis hospitals at the time, meant building self-contained hospital campuses on substantial acreage, complete with housing for staff, garages, and road systems among other amenities. Each was a major project. Questions of policy, as well as authority, were thus involved, as they are to this day: How much and what kind of health services do war veterans deserve, and for how long?[4]

General Sawyer argued on grounds of principle against an expensive, long-term, specialized, permanent hospital system for war veterans, many of whom had had noncombat assignments. He was against building specialty hospitals for neuropsychiatry and tuberculosis: "It is absolutely senseless to build separate institutions for the various classes of patients." Surely it was possible to make do by using decommissioned military hospital beds and barracks, even if they were not fireproof, rather than spend millions more? Federal budget estimates for the end of January 1922 showed an approved net increase of more than $20 million over budget for the Veterans Bureau (though this was mostly because of expansionary changes made by Congress), and now Forbes was seeking more. For Sawyer, less pampering would produce better, more manly citizens: "Let us give them punch and determination rather than dependence and lack of character." Everything to do with hospital location, construction, and policy, he argued, should be in the hands of someone who subscribed to these tenets—and that, in his view, was his role as chief coordinator of the Federal Board of Hospitalization. Sawyer had no independent authority, however, via an assigned budget or means of enforcing his views unless approved by a majority of the board. And members of the Federal Board—the surgeons general of the army, navy, and Public Health Service plus other federal officials with hospital responsibilities—at this point stood with Forbes.[5]

Congress had given the Public Health Service $9.05 million in 1919 to construct new hospital beds for ex-servicemen, a measly sum to attempt to meet an estimated need for 30,000 beds. No funds came forth in 1920. The Public Health Service had to cope as best it could, garnering considerable criticism for failing to meet the need. After the first Langley Act provided $18.6 million to the Treasury Department in 1921, Secretary Mellon's group of consultants, the White Committee, launched twenty-one construction projects across the country. Besides the nine new hospitals, the committee funded additions to existing Public Health Service hospitals, to military facilities where beds were being leased for veterans, and to government-operated soldiers' homes, which were primarily residential centers for veterans of earlier wars. Two noteworthy large ventures were the purchase of an impressive Roman Catholic orphanage in the Bronx, New York City, to be turned into a hospital for mentally ill World War veterans; and a new hospital for "Negro ex-servicemen" at Tuskegee, Alabama, built on the committee's assumption that African American veterans would get better treatment in an all-black facility than in racially segregated veterans hospitals. The cost of construction per hospital bed fluctuated widely, depending on where they were built: from $722 per bed to add to the facilities at Fort McKenzie, Wyoming, to $4,342 for additions at Jefferson Barracks.[6]

The second Langley bill, introduced in December 1921, recognized that the first did not go far enough. The major sponsor of both bills, Republican Congressman John Wesley Langley, chair of the House Committee on Public Buildings and Grounds, was in his early fifties, a little portly, with neatly parted, slicked-back hair, a cleft chin, chubby cheeks, a broad smile, and a friendly and accessible demeanor. Langley was pushing legislation to appropriate new funds, no matter which government agency would be responsible for spending them.[7]

Forbes made a good case for additional funds, which would be placed under his control. At the end of 1921, a third of hospitalized veterans were being treated in private and nonfederal public hospitals on a lease or contract basis (collectively known as contract hospitals). The facilities varied in quality from excellent to terrible. There were admittedly 8,000 unoccupied beds in government institutions, but these were generally reserved for acute medical and surgical conditions, while the chief need was beds for patients with tuberculosis and mental illness. Roughly 40 percent of the 30,000 veterans hospitalized had tuberculosis as their primary diagnosis, and another 30 percent suffered from neuropsychiatric disorders as a primary condition, leaving 30 percent in all other medical and surgical categories. The White Committee was creating more than 6,000 new hospital beds, but these were balanced out, Forbes said, by the need to drop an equivalent number of beds in unsatisfactory contract facilities as their leases expired. The Veterans Bureau controlled the leases. In short, the first Langley Act would provide no net addition in beds, but the second Langley bill would provide $17 million to construct 9,000 new ones in better facilities overall. The critical question from Forbes's perspective was which of three interested entities would allocate and control these funds: the Treasury Department, advised by the

White Committee; the Veterans Bureau, which had its own advisers for tuberculosis and mental illness; or the Federal Board of Hospitalization (part of the oversight apparatus of the Bureau of the Budget) chaired by General Charles E. Sawyer.

In January 1922, the Federal Board agreed that it would go along with the Veterans Bureau recommendations for further hospitals and declared that such hospitals would be known as US Veterans Hospitals. Forbes let it be known that if given the responsibility for hospital construction he would act with the advice of the Federal Board. Sawyer graciously agreed on behalf of the Federal Board to accept recommendations from the Veterans Bureau, "since no one could know better the needs of hospitalization." Left open were what, in practice, "advice" and "recommendations" meant. For an administration devoted to efficiency, there were too many cooks in the kitchen. The White Committee remained active, working on its independent agenda, but was to be terminated once that task was done. Forbes was willing to work with the committee, assuming they worked together. Sawyer said flatly that the White Committee had served its purpose, which was to allocate funds appropriated under the first Langley Act, and that was that; it was no longer needed. Competing claims for the second Langley funds were ahead.[8]

Medical experts added their views to the debates. There was no definite cure for tuberculosis in the 1920s, though some patients were fortunate enough to recover. Treatment for acute pulmonary tuberculosis required boring months of bed rest, special diets rich in milk and cream, rigidly programmed schedules and exposure to the outdoors for rest and sleeping. The modern tuberculosis hospital had rows of sleeping porches or verandahs to which beds could be moved out for a while and then pushed back into patients' rooms. Over and above its ongoing program, the White Committee recommended two or three more sanitariums, each costing between $3,000 and $3,500 a bed.

Some of the facilities in use were appalling. In February 1922, Forbes and his team of tuberculosis specialists struggled to shut down a damp, leaking Public Health Service facility on Staten Island, New York, known as Fox Hills—an old wartime debarkation facility consisting of "shack buildings of beaverboard and lumber, badly situated, unsanitary and drafty," with some

of the wards known as "Death Valley." The White Committee was not building new facilities for tuberculosis in New York. Closing Fox Hills meant
moving most of the 800 patients with tuberculosis out of state. Forbes wrote
President Harding to convince him of the huge amount of adverse criticism
of Fox Hills over the previous two years: "Roofs are leaking and occasional-
ly with a storm, a roof will be blown completely off. The heating plant is in
poor condition and would have to be completely remodeled if the hospital
were to be continued. Without extensive improvements it would be entirely
impracticable to continue Fox Hills as a hospital through another winter."[9]
This was not a popular stance to take. The Fox Hills patients were moved by
mid-April at the cost of considerable criticism of Forbes and his team. Doctors, attendants, and other employees organized to keep the hospital open,
flaws and all. Local merchants objected. The American Legion denounced
the closure and New York congressional leaders jumped into the fray. A
hospital guard shot and wounded a soldier, who threatened to sue. It was
pointed out quite frequently that New York State had furnished more than
half a million soldiers for World War I but had not seen its "fair share" of veterans' benefits. Forbes suggested setting up tent hospitals for tuberculosis in
New York State, but the National Tuberculosis Association objected. Wom-
en's charitable and civic groups caused him particular irritation: "There are
forty different female organizations in and about New York City, every one
having different views and ideas," he remarked at a meeting with legislators
to discuss the New York situation in April. "Some are fire-eaters and raise
hell and you can't hold them down and they insist they know more about
the TB situation than anyone else and peddle bunk that is damned rot."
Colonel Patterson, the bureau's medical director, backed him up: "If there
is anyone more harassed by women on this subject, it is the Director. They
mean well, but they are pernicious and dangerous." Members of such groups
went into the hospital and incited patients, making a bad situation worse.
Forbes spent some of his personal time looking for a site for a new tuberculosis hospital. He mentioned a possible site near Liberty, New York: "I got
half way up there Sunday night," he reported, but "my car broke down and
we spent the day fixing it and then came on back."[10]

Mental and neurological disorders—lumped together under the term
"neuropsychiatry"—raised problems of definition. Lester Rogers, a future
chief medical adviser to the Veterans Bureau, admitted to confusion about

the diagnosis of anxiety neurosis: "It is a term used by neuropsychiatrists, and I am frank to say that if I met it face to face I might not know what it is." Psychiatrist Thomas W. Salmon, former director of psychiatry for the American Expeditionary Force and a postwar adviser to Forbes and to the White Committee, told bemused members of a congressional committee that 90 percent of mentally ill veterans suffered from war-induced or aggravated psychosis (possibly related to concussion, shrapnel, or other injury to the brain and sometimes from triggering or the exacerbation of a hereditary condition, or both). "I think in the main you can tell pretty well whether a man has a nervous disease or is insane," Salmon instructed them: "You can tell the difference between a man who has a mental disease and is suffering from a nervous disorder. You can tell the difference between a man who has a mental disease and a man who has a leg or arm shot off, and a part of a nerve shot away." Many mentally ill veterans were in contract facilities, hidden away in small public or private "homes" or huge state mental asylums that acted as holding pens or were inappropriately placed in general hospitals. "I have visited those hospitals in nearly every part of the country in the last three years," Salmon declared, "and I have never before had an occasion to be ashamed of the fact that I am an American," but he was when he saw young men newly admitted to some of these hospitals looking around with apprehension and seeing "demented faces, many of them temperamentally insane."[11]

Hearings on the second Langley bill began in January 1922. Forbes, ably backed by his staff, expressed his considerable frustration: "You charge the director of the bureau with the responsibility for treatment and care of these men; you charge him with the responsibility for treatment and proper hospitalization; you provide in the act that he is responsible for their proper housing; you charge him with everything having to do with the rehabilitation of these men, and yet you do not give him the tools with which to do the work." A senior staff member who took over from Forbes when his voice gave out, offered a down-to-earth version of these views: "When the building operations are proceeding very slowly [under the White Committee], who gets the telegrams and kicks and inquiries? We do. You gentlemen [congressmen] write down and say, 'What about the hospital at so-and-so?' The Senators write us, the American Legion writes us, they come down, and we are obliged to say, 'Gentlemen, we have nothing to do with it. It is true that Congress has made the bureau responsible for hospitalization of these men, but we have nothing to do with saying where the hospital is to be or anything of that kind.'" All the bureau's leadership wanted to do was to eliminate this buck passing. Control must go with level of responsibility and that meant construction of hospitals through the bureau.[12]

February 1922 was a difficult time personally for Forbes. After testifying ably to the Langley committee and leaving with a hoarse voice, he started on a business trip to New England but returned home on doctor's orders. He missed a meeting of the Federal Board of Hospitalization at which Sawyer claimed that the Veterans Bureau should be regarded as part of the board but was present at another, when he was able to get his agenda moving forward. He had spoken with Treasury Secretary Mellon, he said, and Mellon had no objection to the new Langley funds going to the Veterans Bureau. The board approved this policy and that the hospitals should be fireproof, which eliminated the use and renovation of wooden buildings in the old cantonments. Though some differences in views were expressed in discussion, the vote was unanimous. Bit by bit, sick or well, Forbes made his case.[13]

His wife, Kate Marcia Forbes, was suffering from a periodic, undiagnosed malaise that had plagued her from her time in Hawaii and had come to aggravate her spouse. Kate Forbes, elegant in appearance, lacked the reassurance of a "mission" or of full-time work. She had come to Washington, DC, as the author of a published book and a number of articles and with entrée to the White House and had reason to expect her life to be exciting in the capital. Florence Harding had given her the opportunity to shadow her and write about life as the First Lady. Kate Forbes published a syndicated newspaper series of five articles (six were planned initially), with the first two appearing together on Christmas Day 1921, the others in January. These were well-written, complimentary descriptions that humanized the White House and its occupants, but press editors wanted more personal information, ideally some "dirt." The series gave Kate Forbes valuable name recognition. She was listed in 1922 as one of five promotional directors of the National League of American Pen Women. However, she was not asked to write more for the press—a bitter blow. The sardonic, hard-boiled style adopted by many postwar writers was not her métier, and tuned-in women were already in the field. Mrs. Harding entertained thirty-six women reporters for tea in July 1921 and forty-five in March 1922. While Colonel Forbes was focused on establishing a modern hospital system for veterans, Mrs. Forbes was without a place for herself.[14]

Nor was she much interested in politics, large or small. The hierarchical social world of officialdom came with a lofty aristocracy, with Alice Roosevelt Longworth, daughter of the late President Theodore R. Roosevelt, at the top, and beneath this, a constant in-and-out flux of legislators, officials, lobbyists, and others who required sorting out, some to be recognized, others not. The system included prescribed visits and calling cards (with a certain corner to be turned down in a specific way for different purposes) and complicated arrangements for seating at dinner. Intelligent women agonized over whether to seat the chief justice or the Speaker on the right side of the hostess at dinner. (The answer was not to invite both at once.) Kate's official name, Mrs. Charles R. Forbes, was noticeably absent from the social pages.[15]

Husband and wife were quickly reaching an impasse. His ideal of womanhood was his mother, who kept her family safe and optimistic through years of hardship, demanded nothing from him, and was always there for him when needed. His older sister, Marie, was a professional nurse who cared, sequentially, for her younger siblings, ailing husbands, and then her widowed mother. In 1922, Marie Forbes Judkins was living in the Boston area with her fourth husband and holding the important position of chief nurse for District 2 of the Veterans Bureau. Outside of the home, Forbes treated individual women on more or less equal terms. Unlike many men of the time, he talked with women, was interested in their work, and joked with them, making him popular among the "telephone girls" he worked with in France, clerks in the Veterans Bureau, and indeed with Florence Harding—the two of them conducted a jocular flirtation. Marriage, however, was a different issue. When Kate Forbes was away, it seemed, she felt much better. She seems to have protected herself by taking their daughter on visits to her widowed mother or to see friends. At home, she felt trapped. Her health fluctuated; she lost and gained weight and was often listless or in pain. In mid-February 1922, she was on the upswing and seemed more cheerful and then down she went again. She was hospitalized at Johns Hopkins Hospital while the second Langley bill was in process. Here was a clear sign to her husband that she was indeed sick. The stay clinched the argument about her next step; she must get away to restore her health.[16]

Harding's younger sister, Carolyn Harding Votaw, the official liaison between Public Health Service and the Veterans Bureau, wrote Forbes from out of town to give him a boost when he was feeling down. She was a striking, gregarious woman with prematurely white hair, girlish enthusiasm, and a strong social conscience, who gave little attention to the political nuances involved in being sister to the president. A Dr. G. R. Cole sued her for libel for writing a letter to the judge in his divorce suit in support of his wife: "terribly wronged by Dr. Cole," Mrs. Votaw wrote. She refused to sever her connections with African American organizations at the time Harding and his siblings were rumored to have "Negro blood." And she continued her friendship with Harding's secret lover Nan Britton, whom she had known for years. On one occasion, when Miss Britton's sister and brother-in-law visited Carolyn "Carrie" Votaw at the Veterans Bureau with two-year-old Elizabeth Ann (whom they adopted), Mrs. Votaw introduced them to Colonel Forbes, who reportedly "took quite a fancy" to the child.[17]

Votaw was serious about her work. She had spent nine or ten years in Burma with her husband, a Seventh-day Adventist missionary, where she worked with sick dispensary patients. On their return to the United States, she ran a police program for unwed mothers in Washington. In 1920, she joined the Public Health Service to work in its new Division of Venereal Diseases, lectured on sexually transmitted diseases and disease prevention to women's organizations, and worked with war veterans, and was then seconded to the Veterans Bureau, where her forte was connecting people and spreading news across the constituent organizations.

Her letter to Forbes was to mark his birthday, celebrated on February 14, Valentine's Day. Carolyn Votaw was characteristically chirpy and cheering: "Well how does it feel to be forty five and director of everything in view? A big job is yours Col. C.R.F. but I have not doubts about your ability to handle it. You ask me if I had faith in you – I surely have!!! some valintine [*sic*]. I wish you many happy returns of the day and all the joy and success that is due you a lot I say!! God knows how much." She invited him to come out of town with her husband, the superintendent of prisons, to pay a visit and recuperate: "Hope you get Heber and have him join you to come right up here." Adding in some government news, she ended, "God bless you and help you is my prayer. Most sincerely, Carolyn H. Votaw." This letter later appeared in print as an insinuation that Forbes and Mrs. Votaw were romantically involved (impossible to prove, and doubtful in any case). Its writer was a kind woman and a known eccentric, and Forbes was a family friend as well as a fellow combatant in bureaucratic trenches. Moreover, a friend of his wife, she knew that similar support was not forthcoming from Kate, who was struggling with her own low spirits. It was not easy to come from outside Washington into a culture that relied excessively on social place; nor was it easy to know how to act as a woman in one's forties in the youth-oriented culture of the postwar years.[18]

The Langley bill raced to conclusion. In short order, Harding directly endorsed the bill and the Federal Board of Hospitalization unanimously agreed to urge Congress to pass it. Forbes testified before a subcommittee of the House Committee on Appropriations to explain the costs of the Veterans Bureau, including vocational training and hospitalization. At the bureau's recent conference with leading psychiatrists, "seven of the biggest men in the United States," he said, it was concluded that 12,200 beds were needed for neuropsychiatry alone, compared with fewer than 9,000 that were then occupied (and many of these were well below standard). Legislators expressed surprise about how the bureau worked: "You mean that the Government has leased hospitals?" (Well, yes, for years.) He was also asked about rumors circulating about unhappy bureau employees, who were complaining to congressmen in their efforts to hold onto their jobs or get a new one, as jobs at headquarters were cut. Forbes agreed that there was indeed "very general unrest." Because of the decentralization to district offices, he was "declaring people surplus" at headquarters—a statement the legislators no doubt appreciated—and transferring many out to the districts. He had a standing committee on personnel changes and had made a net reduction of 2,000 employees at central office. No wonder there was unrest at the base, while Forbes pushed on with his hospital agenda.[19]

Showdown time before the Langley committee was in March, when Forbes gave an irritable and combative performance as he battled head-to-head with the Treasury over whether veterans hospital construction would be managed by the Treasury's supervising architect and his staff (who were geared up to do the new work), or by the Veterans Bureau. He criticized the White Committee for moving too slowly, bragged he could build hospitals much more quickly, and stressed the economic advantage under his management of letting out work under fixed-price contracts rather than on a cost-plus basis, which he did, imposing penalties for builders who did not meet contractual deadlines. New York Representative Hamilton Fish, noting that the White Committee had not provided one bed for tuberculosis in New York, where there was a "tubercular emergency," declared: "I believe if this money had been placed in the hands of Col. Forbes and he had selected the sites and turned the building operations over to large contractors . . . that they could have built these modern hospitals in eight months and have them ready for occupation last December." These were big claims to make—and unlikely to achieve—in a government system. Nonetheless, Forbes won this battle. Both location and construction decisions were given to the Veterans Bureau in the bill.[20]

President Harding returned from his Florida headquarters at St. Augustine to face a congressional campaign for the soldiers' bonus, which passed the House for the third time, 333 to 70. American Legion Commander Hanford MacNider toured the country pressing for the bill. These renewed calls made it urgent to get the Langley bill passed and signed quickly as a major political gesture toward veterans. Langley informed Harding that "the hospital situation has grown steadily worse," and urged passage of the hospital bill "as a matter of justice as well as of party policy." On March 31, 1922, the second Langley bill passed the House with a record vote. The Senate followed unanimously, and the bill became law on April 20, 1922.[21]

While his wife was making plans to leave the country with their daughter, Forbes worked furiously to get the new construction program up and running. His initial moves did not suggest someone who was thinking about personal financial gain. Quite the reverse. There was to be no money involved in the acquisition of hospital sites. From the beginning, as a matter of principle as well as cost savings, Forbes refused to buy land for the new hospitals, relying instead on donations from government agencies and private sources. General Sawyer brought an early request to the Federal Board of Hospitalization: "The Vice President, Mr. Coolidge, has asked whether it would be possible to get one of these hospitals at Northampton [Massachu-

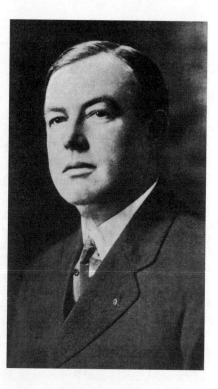

1. Charles R. Forbes as an official in Hawaii, ca. 1916.

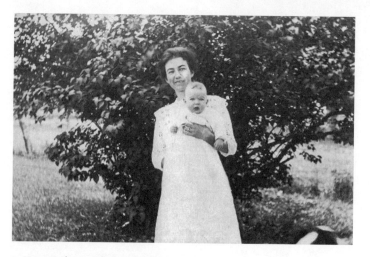

2. Kate Forbes with daughter, Marcia, in Hawaii, ca. 1913.
Courtesy Joan Barry Marsh.

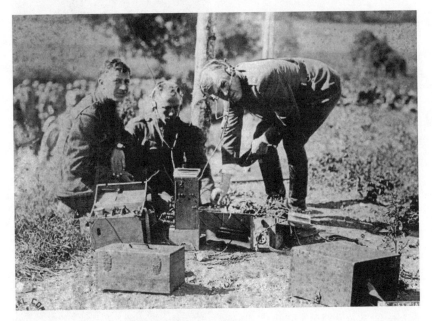

3. Major Forbes, Thirty-Third Division signal officer, testing field radio with men of the 108th Field Signal Battalion, September 1918. Courtesy Barry D. Marsh and Joan Barry Marsh.

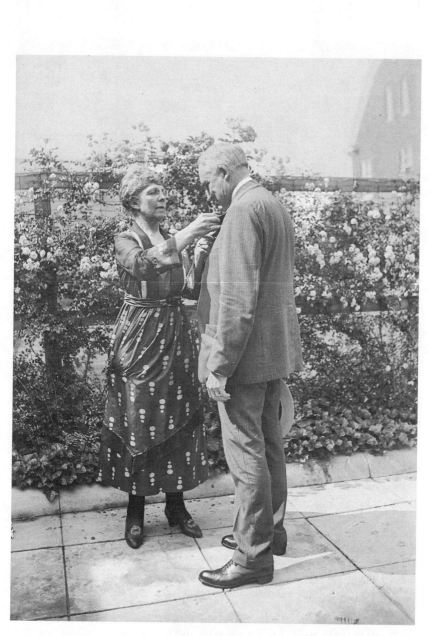

4. Senator Warren G. and Mrs. Florence Harding, June, 1920, presidential
election year. Library of Congress, http//www.loc.gov/pictures/item/hec2013000646/.

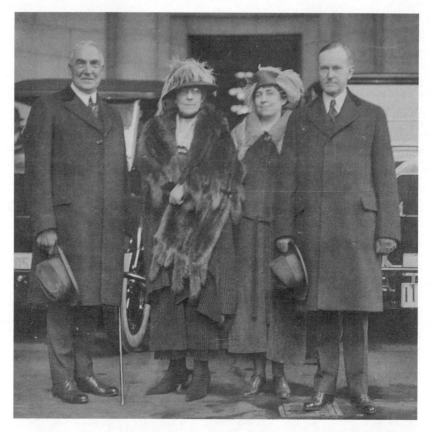

5. President Harding and Mrs. Florence Harding, and Vice President Calvin Coolidge and Mrs. Grace Coolidge meet at Union Station on arrival for Inauguration Day, March 1921. Library of Congress, http://www.loc.gov/pictures/item/94511979/.

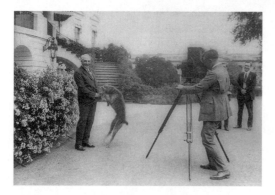

6. Harding and the exuberant Laddie Boy, June 1922. Library of Congress, http://www.loc.gov/item/96522830/.

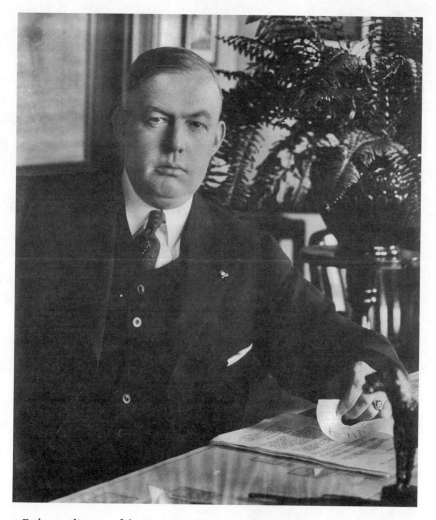

7. Forbes as director of the US Veterans Bureau, 1921.
Courtesy Barry D. Marsh and Joan Barry Marsh.

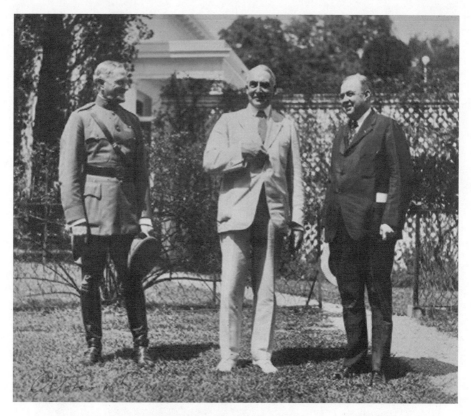

8. *Left to right,* John J. Pershing, Commander of the American Expeditionary Force in Europe in World War I, President Harding, and Colonel Forbes, Director of the US Veterans Bureau, October 1921. Courtesy of Richard F. Barry.

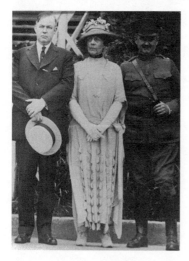

9. Florence Harding, Forbes, and an unidentified military office at a reception for veterans. National First Ladies' Library.

setts]." Northampton was Coolidge's hometown. Forbes: "We are investigating that now and think very favorably of it." The Northampton land (240 acres for a neuropsychiatric hospital campus with multiple buildings) was put together by the local Chamber of Commerce. Donations of land were achieved for all the proposed new facilities except for the anomaly of Livermore, California, purchased by the Treasury: the case where the bureau's chief lawyer, Charles Cramer, had negotiated a deal with the approval of the White House.[22]

The first list of proposed new hospitals was quickly completed. Forbes called a meeting of the Federal Board of Hospitalization early in May, while Sawyer was out of town. "Gentlemen, the President requested me to call this meeting," Forbes announced, presiding in his role as vice chair. He presented a detailed list of hospitals and locations to be approved and put up a map to show the location of the White Committee hospitals, in progress and planned, together with the Veterans Bureau proposals. He and Colonel Patterson went through the list systematically, district by district. The two colonels ran the meeting with the efficiency of a military briefing. Forbes came in well prepared, moved the agenda, and got what he wanted. Decisions to recommend the bureau's proposals to the president were unanimous. He proposed that the army and navy do most of the architectural work on the new hospitals (which they did). Also, "I would like to see some real competition between commercial concerns and the Government." The bureau had standard plans for tuberculosis and neuropsychiatric hospitals, which Forbes said would be modified as necessary to fit specific locations. The meeting ended with Forbes's initial hospital proposals in place.[23]

The next day was eventful: Congress approved the second Langley appropriation, making it possible to get contracts under way. Forbes dispatched his report to President Harding listing the Federal Board's recommendations, and Sawyer returned to Washington to find he had been outmaneuvered. Harding, the ultimate decider, was faced with recommendations for eleven new federal hospitals and one purchase (a fully operational, well-regarded general hospital in Memphis)—a program, if completed, that would provide more than 4,000 beds, three-fourths of them for mental illness (in eight locations), with most of the others for tuberculosis. And this was only a partial list. Decisions for several districts were still to be made. Sawyer wrote immediately to Harding. The Federal Board had been called in his absence, he complained, and only three regular members of the board were present (they sent substitutes, but there was not a quorum of active members). He had been trying to talk about the issues with Forbes "almost daily . . . whenever Colonel Forbes was in town," but had not been able to meet with him. He had tried again without success before going out of town the previous Saturday. Sawyer was particularly worried that Forbes's use of the Federal Board had placed blame for the bureau's hospital location decisions on the board and thus on his shoulders as chief coordinator for hospitals in the Harding administration. Sawyer made this point quite clear; he was not "disturbed in any way by the course hereto followed by Colonel Forbes, providing I am not expected to be responsible for things ultimately resulting." He was quite upset.[24]

Faced with congressional pressure for the Bonus Bill, Harding quickly approved the Veterans Bureau plan for seven new hospitals out of the eleven recommended, including the hospitals at Northampton and Livermore, and approved purchase of the Methodist Hospital in Memphis. Locations for the other hospitals recommended by Forbes and the Federal Board were on hold. Two days later Sawyer sent Harding competing recommendations: "Looking from the position of Hospital Coordinator for the Budget Commissioner, it seems inconsistent to throw away these valuable properties and locations [military cantonments] and build in new localities." Sawyer called the president's attention to the fine Soldiers Home in Marion, Indiana, whose managers told him all they needed were a few more beds to take care of patients in the district—they had "splendid laboratories, etc. . . ." Other soldiers' homes could also be better used, he thought, including the ones at Sawtelle, California (despite its coastal fog, which experts discounted as a problem for the disease, but prospective tuberculosis patients viewed as the kiss of death), and Leavenworth, Kansas. Leavenworth would be "much more economical" than a new institution at Kansas City, Fort Dodge, Sawyer wrote.[25]

There was no room for compromise. Forbes was unwilling to use soldiers' homes because, he said, the homes needed their beds for domiciliary use; because insane men were truly sick and needed special quarters; and because the homes were largely filled with Civil War veterans who were decades older than most veterans of World War I: "You can't put these old men in there with these young fellows." According to Forbes, Sawyer "kept talking about 9,000 vacant beds, but these were mostly in these rotten fire traps."

Sawyer was still pushing for the public welfare bill, in which the Veterans Bureau would theoretically be placed, and "was for the cantonment type of hospital," to which other members of the board were opposed. Sawyer later reported: "I should say that Colonel Forbes ordinarily regarded our board as a sort of interference, if you please, with his conduct of affairs, and I don't mean to say that disrespectfully of Colonel Forbes at all. I think that was his opinion. He was given by the law the authority to operate these hospitals and do this business and he felt, therefore, that it should not be necessary for him to have any restrictions or handicaps in carrying out his own ideas."[26]

As a concession, Forbes offered Sawyer an office in the Veterans Bureau for the Federal Board to use, but Sawyer moved in with a vengeance, parlaying his invitation into a hospital headquarters for himself, expanding his space to multiple rooms, and setting up a secretary. To Forbes's chagrin, he also commanded the services of Veterans Bureau employees. Sawyer had no qualms saying of something he did not want that "he did not believe the President would approve it." Forbes claimed later that Sawyer interfered with every department, sending for staff, "quizzing them," ordering information, sending out messengers, "wanting his own way." Forbes was quick to say that he wanted his own way too—"because I was charged with the responsibility, and I so told him." Battle lines were drawn.[27]

On May 20, 1922, Kate Marcia Forbes, aged forty-two, five feet three tall, with blue eyes and black-gray hair, applied for a passport for herself and her daughter, Marcia, giving her occupation as "housewife." (She had it sent to a friend's address in New York.) She planned to travel in the British Isles, France, Belgium, Holland, and Germany, sailing on the SS *Cambrai* on June 9. In leaving home for Europe to revive her troubled health (which did recover when she was away), and armed with letters of introduction to foreign dignitaries, for she was, after all, the wife of a senior US official, Kate Forbes took a leaf out of her husband's playbook: when things get rough in life, move on and out. Kate and Marcia Forbes were away for fifteen months—critical months for Charles R. Forbes as director of the US Veterans Bureau.

New problems for Charles R. Forbes were already evident. One major, apparently unperceived, problem for him was that Harding would not always back Forbes's recommendations, no matter how rational Forbes considered

them to be. In approving the proposed list of new hospitals, Harding largely followed Forbes, whose proposals encompassed those of the American
Legion, but in the absence of the American Legion and other political pressures, Harding's views were nearer those of Sawyer's, who shared his conservative, cost-conscious outlook and remained close to Harding, seeing
him every day in Washington to check on his health. A letter reporting on
the president's urine examination in June pops up oddly in correspondence
on national political issues. Sawyer prescribed a dose of soda water at least
three times a day, "and no matter what the condition of the bowels this
morning would have you tonight take the two pink pills which I left on
the dresser." When push came to shove, Harding would favor Sawyer over
Forbes.[28]

A second big problem accompanied the completion of the hospitals built
under the first Langley Act. Four of the White Committee hospitals had
been transferred to the Veterans Bureau at the time of Kate Forbes's departure, with others in the pipeline. In April, Forbes had joined other dignitaries at the dedication of the White Committee's expensively renovated,
majestic old orphanage situated on a rise on Kingsbridge Road in the Bronx,
reconceived as a neuropsychiatric hospital for World War I veterans—a
splendid institution in many ways, with a seventy-five-foot gym, two audi-
toriums, baseball diamond, basketball and tennis courts, plus quoit pits and
croquet lawns. The dedication included a live radio broadcast of a medical
consultation with staff on a naval vessel seventy-five miles out to sea. Unfortunately, according to the Veterans Bureau, essential "equipment" was
missing, including fencing to keep outsiders off the grounds of a psychiatric facility and to prevent mobile ex-soldiers from taking off to town at
will. Forbes estimated that another $825,000 was needed for this institution
alone. Colonel Patterson considered the situation "acute" in all of the four
hospitals, "and we will get all the blame if the equipment is not put in there."
Dr. William Charles White, chair of the White Committee, told the Federal
Board that his committee had initially been informed that "not a cent would
be necessary for equipment," but that was not what the bureau understood.
Forbes was becoming testy and stacking up a pile of influential foes. In his
view, the White Committee was intentionally forcing the Veterans Bureau
to fund completion of their institutions: "This fellow White repeatedly
states he is doing what the Veterans' Bureau asks him to do," Forbes said.

"The Veterans' Bureau has not a thing to do with his activities." White had made a "great fiasco about his whole proposition."[29]

Anxiety marked all aspects of the Harding administration by mid-1922, as eyes turned to the midterm congressional elections in November. Hospital issues remained red hot. In June, General Sawyer fought with a prominent figure in the America Legion, Colonel A. A. Sprague, the dedicated head of the legion's hospitalization efforts, after Harding decided to locate the hospital the Veterans Bureau had designed for Great Lakes, Illinois, in Battle Creek, Michigan, instead—allegedly on Sawyer's advice. Hostile telegrams flew between Sprague and Sawyer. Sawyer proclaimed that the decision to suspend the recommendation in favor of Great Lakes at a recent Federal Board meeting was at the president's suggestion: it was Harding who raised the "comparative merits of the claims of Michigan." Sprague stood behind the legion's experts who favored a hospital in or near Chicago, Illinois, declaring, "Chicago is absolutely center of the Eighth District." And so it went.[30]

The power plays between Sawyer and Forbes had turned into a larger set of struggles: Sawyer, backed by the president, versus Forbes and the American Legion; Forbes at loggerheads with the Treasury Department's White Committee; Congress pushing for the soldiers' bonus while the Treasury remained adamantly against it on grounds of cost; Harding struggling with Congress; Democrats looking for Republican weaknesses to exploit during the run-up to the elections. Summer was threatening, with the oppressive heat of Washington rising once more from its pavements.

Forbes was physically and mentally exhausted. He had underestimated Sawyer as a high-stakes opponent and fought with other participants in his field, including members of the White Committee, to the point of lasting enmity. He had been reinvented as a single man with a wife living it up in foreign parts who had removed his daughter from his care. In his hospital mission, he had been successful. All he needed now to complete a dismal cycle of his life was to fall in with a charming con man and his equally charming wife.

6 HYPE, HOOCH, AND THE ART OF THE CON

Given the political and budgetary importance of the US Veterans Bureau to the Harding administration, Colonel Forbes had little stature in Washington outside of his job. He was not a cabinet member attending regular multidepartmental meetings with the president. He did not enjoy participating in political and social gossip networks. He was focused on his work at the bureau. He had tricked General Sawyer by holding the key meeting to select the location of new veterans hospitals while Sawyer was away but was evidently impelled to do so by the urgency of his cause, not by a self-congratulatory Machiavellianism. Far from it. He had an overly optimistic, engineer's perspective on the world. He was an idealist rather than a cynic. Yet in America cynicism raged. There was an air of "looseness" everywhere in 1922: not only in the sense of moral order but also of a people let loose in an unforgiving marketplace; loose practices, loose money, loose lips.

Prohibition encouraged new forms of crime. Federal agents arrested 42,000 individuals for prohibition violations in 1922, but state controls were generally weak, laws flouted, federal enforcers could not keep up, and one of every twelve federal prohibition agents was reportedly dismissed for corruption. This was a nation of capitalists, corrupters, patsies, and marks, or so it seemed. Modern psychology suggested that human behavior was morally fluid. Literature followed up. Manners were more important than moral codes. *Character* could be learned from self-help experts. A postwar American could go a long way by projecting a trustworthy and endearing surface, whatever motives lurked beneath. The scenario was tailor-made for con men. Forbes was vulnerable and did not know it.[1]

Gaston Bullock Means and Elias Harvey Mortimer were products of the time. Means came to symbolize Harry Daugherty's laisser-faire attitude to dirty tricks at the Department of Justice. Mortimer destroyed Charles

Forbes's reputation and sent him to the penitentiary. Means was a large, merry-looking, fleshy, flamboyant man in his forties: a former salesman and teacher who had left North Carolina for bigger opportunities. The so-called Great Detective William J. Burns had hired him for his private detective agency in 1915, and through that source, Means became a spy for the Germans and a useful source for Burns, someone to be remembered when Burns took over the Bureau of Investigation (FBI) at the Department of Justice in 1921. (By that time, Means had gained control of the fortune of a Mrs. Maude King of Chicago, and had been prosecuted and acquitted of a charge of murdering her. She had died of a shot in the back of her head.) His biographer described Means as a man who needed constant excitement. Bribery, blackmail, and other forms of corruption fit the bill, as did searching offices without a warrant, stalking witnesses, and other illegal practices.

In the spring of 1922, Means worked in Washington for Daugherty's associate Jesse "Jess" Smith, investigating congressmen and senators who were attacking Daugherty, in order to dig out information that could be used against them for political reasons. Means, like Mortimer, worked with bootleggers, spreading the word that he could "fix" prosecutions for a hefty fee by tampering with official files. Later, Means was a prominent, damaging witness against Harry Daugherty in Senate hearings on the Department of Justice but then recanted. He was a colossal liar. It was "difficult for the lay mind to distinguish between trained dissimulation and lying . . ." was how he put it. Eventually, he was to overreach, beyond anyone's powers of credulity, but in 1922, he was in his element.[2]

Elias H. Mortimer was one of a crowd of lobbyists, publicists, and fixers who descended on Washington during the wartime boom in industrial production and stayed on during postwar readjustment. Means was more flamboyant, Mortimer more subtle. He projected appealing eagerness and an air of can-do sincerity and had helpful information at his fingertips, relevant contacts, the ability to convince, and (where necessary) a penitence so moving that he was usually forgiven. Before World War I provided opportunities to exercise his talents as a middleman hustling for war contracts, he lived at his parents' home and worked as a contracting agent and salesman for iron and steel companies in Minneapolis. He liked to party on a lavish scale, was "prominently identified with Minneapolis night life," and spent money freely. Shortly before he departed for the East Coast in 1917, he declared bankruptcy in US District Court. Among his creditors, besides various saloons, hotels, and clubs, his parents sued him for $215 for the cost of his room and board. His father made additional claims on two loan notes issued in 1914, which were still on file as unpaid in US District Court in 1924. Mortimer's lawyer and old schoolmate Augustus Dowdall sued Mortimer for an unpaid fee of $508. Yet on the surface he was as sweet and lovable as anyone could be. The president of a roofing company in St. Paul took his word that he was an engineer and hired him as a consultant: "I fired him." A general contractor: "He tried to swindle me out of $800 in a business deal, in 1916." The contracting manager for the American Bridge Company in St. Louis offered himself as a mentor in the belief that he was only "rather wild," not "anything vicious." All attempts failed. Mortimer had a slippery quality, constantly given new chances and almost invariably escaping punishment. Chicago investigative reporter Philip Kinsley summed up Mortimer's pre-Washington experiences, together with some similar ones later: "Mortimer held many jobs as salesman and estimator, traveled a good deal, and seems to have left a trail of disappointment and disillusion."[3]

A good government-industry contract fixer could make money as military-industrial production scaled up for war. Mortimer fit right in. He conveniently forgot to register for the draft. By 1919, he had perfected a slick one-two punch method: (1) corrupt officials and others by friendship and guile; (2) destroy the chief target's reputation if he refused to play. Where Means sought red-hot excitement, Mortimer was a puppet master. Affection and friendship were tools in a transactional relationship. He was a dangerous man to know.

Two recorded instances of his method show him as an established master of the con game well before he met Charles R. Forbes. The first centered on Captain Leo V. Lannen of the US Army Flying Corps and predated Forbes's encounter with Mortimer by about three years. The second revolved around Congressman John W. Langley, sponsor of the Langley Acts for veterans hospital construction, who met Mortimer a year or so before Forbes did. In both cases, Mortimer became a cherished friend. Lannen and Langley had their reputations destroyed and their lives upended, as did Forbes.

In March 1919, Captain Lannen became chief of the Building and Grounds Section of the air service (the fledgling US Air Force), responsible for government purchasing. Almost immediately, "not more than a day," according to Lannen, Mortimer appeared at his office and invited him to lunch. They became so friendly so quickly that the captain was best man for Mortimer at his wedding at the end of April. Mortimer subtly invited Lannen to join with him to rig bids for supplies by reporting a "rumor" that Lannen's fellow officers were "crooked" and that his predecessor had made off with a fortune—between $100,000 and $200,000 (a million or two in twenty-first-century terms). Lannen did not rise to the bait, but the friendship continued. Then, one day in 1920, Lannen learned that Mortimer had flat-out lied to him and ended their association. This triggered phase 2. Mortimer let it be known that Lannen was a crook who had a "very bad reputation" in his hometown of Buffalo and lodged an official charge that the two of them had worked together to rig bids on the government's purchase of 1.5 million nuts and bolts. Mortimer reported that he had persuaded a company that was not interested in the contract to put in a high bid so that the American Dump Company, which wanted the contract, could raise its own bid and still be the lowest bidder. Lannen protested his innocence. After military intelligence investigated, the War Department charged both men with conspiracy to defraud the US government. Mortimer made sure he could slip out of danger by using his contacts to get his file from the Department of Justice and make sure "they were unable to pin anything on me." Lannen was eventually exonerated, but his military career was destroyed. He spent years trying to bring Mortimer down, calling him a "fiend" and an "insane criminal." Mortimer continued as before.[4]

Congressman Langley had a twofold value for Mortimer. He came from Kentucky, a major whiskey-producing state (which was still producing whiskey under permit for medical purposes), and he chaired the House Committee on Public Buildings and Lands, where construction appropriations were negotiated. Langley had represented the Tenth Congressional District in the southeastern mountains of Kentucky since 1907. His wife, Katherine Gudger Langley, daughter of a former congressman, worked with him, staffed the committee, and ran his office. At the very least, Mortimer might use Langley to get introductions to prohibition officials in the hope of procuring illegal withdrawal permits for liquor from bonded warehouses. He could also get early news about where federal construction money would flow and which agency would control it. Langley was affable and, like Lannen, easy to reach. A story made the rounds that on one very hot August day in Washington

Langley bet a fellow Republican congressman that it was hot enough to fry eggs on the Capitol steps. Langley got two eggs from the House restaurant, cracked them on the steps, waited, flipped them over—they were cooked. He looked after his people back home in Pike County. Sometimes he was called Pork Barrel John. He played the banjo and enjoyed a drink but was officially "dry" (like many of his fellows in Congress); he had voted for the Volstead Act.

John Langley was sitting in his committee conference room with his wife one day in 1920, when in walked this charming man in his late thirties. They invited him to sit down and chat. Langley remembered Mortimer boasting of his acquaintance with the president and some members of the cabinet, "which was the main subject of our conversation." They observed when he departed that he drove a magnificent, costly automobile (a Packard Twin Six special car, nickel-plated), driven by a uniformed chauffeur. A few days later he returned with a friend, discussed politics in Langley's state of Kentucky, told Langley he was connected with Kuhn, Loeb and Co., a prominent investment bank in New York, and mentioned that he was in the coal business—a matter of interest to the congressman because Kentucky was a major coal-producing state. Although Mortimer did not know Harding or have access to the White House, and was extremely unlikely to have been connected with Kuhn, Loeb, it never occurred to Langley to check him out. Why would it? It became Mortimer's habit to drop by the office, supplemented by chance meetings in the House building. Langley wrote in his memoir that he was impressed with his "evident gallantry and refinement" and soon came to regard him as a good friend.

In 1921, when Langley told him he was in financial difficulties Mortimer made him a generous loan of $6,000 (more than $80,000 in twenty-first-century terms), giving the impression he had money idling in the bank. What Langley actually did or did not do for Mortimer in return for the loan is unclear, apart from introducing him to Kentucky's "dry" prohibition commissioner and others whom he knew. In May 1924, Mortimer was the unindicted coconspirator and star witness against Langley when he was tried and convicted of conspiracy to violate the National Prohibition Act. Langley eventually went to prison. (His wife succeeded him in Congress.) The story involved the use (and abuse) of official whiskey permits and the withdrawal of 1,400 cases of medicinal whiskey from the Belle of Anderson distillery in Kentucky. Langley's view of Mortimer had shifted from warm comradeship to icy loathing. The formerly "nice-looking, well groomed, smooth talking fellow" Langley had first met had become a man who was a "paragon of mendacity," comparable to a rat. Mortimer went free.[5]

The Langley case showed Mortimer's use of loans to reel someone in. Among Mortimer's known victims was Republican Congressman Frederick N. Zihlman of Maryland. Zihlman's encounter apparently began with a mere $8 from Mortimer to Mrs. Zihlman, which Mortimer recorded as "to pay maid never has been repaid." One day Zihlman telephoned him, Mortimer recalled: "He came over the same night telling me Margaret his wife had lost quite a sum of money and had pawned her diamond Rings [*sic*], etc and the money had been lost by her on card games." Zihlman's good friend Mortimer made out a $900 check to Margaret Zihlman (about $12,600 in twenty-first-century terms) and received a promissory note from her husband in exchange. Mortimer's stated reason for writing such a large check was that Zihlman "could help me in many ways"; notably because he was a "very personal friend and supporter" of a certain Mr. Budwitz, the newly appointed prohibition director for Maryland, who could grant "many favors." Among them were issuing blank whiskey withdrawal permits for legal withdrawal of alcohol from bonded warehouses. When Department of Justice investigators examined Mortimer's remaining bank accounts (some were mysteriously stolen or lost), they found the cancelled check paid to Margaret Zihlman for $900 dated August 9, 1921, plus another one for $500 dated August 30 (a total of almost $20,000 in twenty-first-century terms). Fred Zihlman finally broke with Mortimer after the latter's attempt to involve him in a scam. A Mr. Edward Robinson, who had a drugstore in Baltimore, found himself in trouble with prohibition officials and talked with Mortimer about it. Mortimer told him he would get Congressman Zihlman to "fix" his problem, but this would require a fee of $5,000 or more. After Zihlman dealt with the problem without money changing hands he leaned on Mortimer to return the money he had received. Mortimer's version was that Zihlman had taken money and that he, Mortimer, was trying to get Zihlman to return it. A congressional committee believed Zihlman and exonerated him in 1924, but the experience must have been unpleasant.[6]

Mortimer's surviving cashed checks included one for $25 to the president's sister, Carolyn Harding Votaw, who was a friend of Mortimer's wife. According to Mortimer, he offered Mrs. Votaw $5,000 (about $70,000 in twenty-first-century terms) if she could fix a pardon for a Charles Vincenti of Baltimore, who had been convicted for violating the prohibition law and sentenced to eighteen months in the Atlanta federal penitentiary. Vincenti and his associates D. L. Delancey of New York and Herman Geltzriler of New Jersey were (said Mortimer) offering him a princely sum for his release from the judgment. Mrs. Votaw took the problem to her brother at the White House—a good idea. Harding told her that "the papers would have to come through in the regular way," and that they must include the consent of government officials and the sentencing judge, Federal Judge John Carter Rose of Baltimore. Mortimer's friend Sidney Bieber duly approached the judge. Nothing doing. Judge Rose opined, "If he had to do it over again he would give Vincenti 18 years in place of 18 months." Every deal could not be won.[7]

Elias H. Mortimer had enhanced his social credibility by marrying Katherine Bulkeley Tullidge in April 1919 (with Captain Leo Lannen as best man). Her father, Dr. George Bowler Tullidge of Philadelphia, was a highly educated, well-connected, philanthropic physician with a well-regarded private medical practice in Philadelphia. He served on the staff of six of the city's hospitals. Her devout Roman Catholic mother was a prominent Philadelphia clubwoman. Attachment to the family offered Mortimer the protective clothing of upper-crust respectability. His contribution to the family was strictly negative. Before long, Katherine and other family members became enmeshed in the deviousness and lies of their new family member—a process that eventually led to Dr. Tullidge and his wife testifying against their son-in-law and in favor of Charles R. Forbes in federal court. Mortimer became particularly close to Katherine's aunt, Margaret (Mrs. James) Williams. He lent her money—a total of $760 via three checks in 1921 alone (more than $10,000 in twenty-first-century terms) and provided her with liquor. James and Margaret Williams became strong supporters of Mortimer, pitting them against other members of the family. Katherine Mortimer's sister Margaret, who lived with the Williamses, was apparently the only family member not to get caught in Mortimer's schemes.[8]

World War I had disrupted expectations across the United States. For George and Katherine O'Donnell Tullidge and their five children the war had brought catastrophe. Mortimer was the final straw. Forbes was to get to know all of them. The eldest Tullidge son, dashing, blue-eyed, dark-haired, enterprising, arrogant Dr. Edward Tullidge, homosexual in a homophobic society, gravitated toward the military. He traveled to Austria-Hungary and Italy late in 1914 to visit war zones and observe front-line military medicine for six months and report on it in the US medical literature. He suffered a nervous breakdown and was hospitalized and went to England, where he was briefly held as an enemy spy. Back home, in 1916 he served as a lieutenant in the National Guard on the Mexican border. Then, with American entry into World War I, he volunteered for the US Navy Medical Corps. As an assistant surgeon crossing the Atlantic aboard the troopship USS *Birmingham* his career imploded.

Edward Kilbourne Tullidge, MD, was arrested at sea on September 2, 1917, and convicted by a navy court-martial on board the USS *Sacramento* for inappropriate behavior during medical examinations, officially interpreted as disciplinary infractions. Summarily dismissed from the navy for what the records show to have been sexual transgressions, he was sentenced to five years imprisonment with hard labor, with his term to be served in the New Hampshire state prison. The verdict went up the line to President Wilson, who confirmed it. Between the court-martial and confirmation of sentence, Tullidge's article on motor-operating field theaters was published in the US Navy Medical Bulletin. Back on firm ground in the United States, Tullidge escaped his guards and fled to Mexico, where he lived for the next five years. He had pleaded not guilty on all counts. When Elias Mortimer joined the family, Edward Tullidge was an escaped convict in unknown mental and physical health, forced to live in exile to avoid hard labor.[9]

Katherine Bulkeley Tullidge, Mortimer's bride, began work as a laboratory technician in the US Army on September 1, 1918, when she was twenty-two years old. Fort Oglethorpe, a military post near Macon, Georgia, had suffered in the first recognized wave of the influenza pandemic that swept through congested military camps in March 1918. At Fort Oglethorpe, she worked in the biological laboratories of US Army General Hospital 14. Lab tests were crucial in identifying and controlling infectious diseases. Suddenly, tragedy struck back home. Mary Louisa, the oldest of the three Tullidge daughters, working as a Red Cross nurse, died of pneumonia brought on by influenza in the second virulent wave of the influenza epidemic, which hit Philadelphia in September and October 1918. Mary Louisa died at the Tullidge home, 843 North Sixty-Third Street, on September 25, twenty-four hours after reporting her first symptoms. The mother's faith in God had not been enough to keep Edward out of trouble; the father's medical skills did not save Mary Louisa. Katherine rushed home but arrived too late to say goodbye. Philadelphia newspapers, having pledged (with others) to keep public morale high during the war, emphasized upbeat news: the heroic role of American troops in St. Mihiel, France, the famous Bryn Mawr Horse Show, and the return of (well-heeled) Philadelphia families to the city after summering away. In this surreal context, Mary Louisa Tullidge was laid to rest. Her brother Edward, in Mexico, was reportedly "overseas on a Government ship."[10]

Katherine's decision to leave the army and marry Elias Mortimer seven months after her sister's death offered an upbeat change for the family. Bride and groom misread each other from the start. Mortimer had clearly wanted a young, pliable bride who would do his bidding and look like a wealthy society woman. She claimed to be twenty-one but was actually twenty-three, a determined young woman with a mind of her own. He had her dress conservatively in close-fitting hats and a long, expensive fur-trimmed coat. She was tall, dark-haired and elegant, with a square determined jaw, a Philadelphia lady through and through. When she was not smiling she could look remote, even intimidating, but when she laughed she sparkled. She was bound to be critical of her new husband when she heard him lie to others, let alone discovered his misdeeds. He was bound to be vindictive. The marriage took place at the Ritz Carlton Hotel in Philadelphia on April 30, 1919, when all seemed well. With her sister Margaret, a dietitian, as a bridesmaid dressed in pink chiffon, Katherine appeared in white satin and tulle trimmed with pearls, with a long train, her tulle veil held in place with orange blossoms. Teenaged George, the fifth and youngest sibling, serving as an usher, was about to graduate from the Staunton Military Institute in Virginia and embark on a course in engineering. (He, too, like the others, will reappear in Forbes's story.) The newspaper description of the wedding made no mention of Mortimer's parents.[11]

Mortimer's new wife and in-laws apparently accepted without question his claim to work in the coal business as vice president of the Campbell Corporation in Philadelphia, with an office in the Real Estate Trust Building, and also to represent various contractors. He also claimed a connection with the reputable Mulford pharmaceutical firm of Philadelphia. According to one report, Katherine Mortimer called on Colonel Campbell to ask about her husband's interest in the Campbell firm and was told he had none except for a commission on any sales he might make. (Wife passed this information on to husband, who was in New York at the time, and he, in turn, fired off a letter to Campbell "accusing him of trying to date up his wife and threatening to get him for it.") Katherine Mortimer was valuable as a legitimating prop for her husband, not unlike his luxurious automobile. He had no compunction in introducing her to B. G. Dahlberg, president of the Celotex Company, as President Warren Harding's niece, which she was not. By remaining silent, she became complicit in the "con." Dahlberg testified later that Mortimer "wanted to arrange to have us presented to 'Warren'" and have Warren "arrange a dinner for us at the White House." Later, having been taken in, Dahlberg commented on the fact that the apparently upright Katherine Mortimer did not contradict these statements. She was in an impossible situation. Objecting was no good. Mortimer's reaction was to hit her. She had been raised in the Roman Catholic faith in which marriage was an unbreakable bond. Elias and Katherine Mortimer separated after three months of marriage, then reconciled, and then separated again.[12]

Early in 1922, as prohibition enforcement became more effective, Mortimer saw new sources of potential income in the money expected to flow to the Veterans Bureau for hospital construction. Katherine and Elias Mortimer were only recently reunited when Mortimer met Charles R. Forbes. Mortimer was a predator, and Forbes his latest prey.

Colonel Forbes, looking warily over his shoulder at General Sawyer as his hospital plans took shape, was unprepared for a threat arising in his nonwork domain. For Forbes, the two spheres were unconnected: work was work, and play was play. He recalled his first meeting with Elias Mortimer in April 1922; Mortimer put the date back to February, when the hearings on the second Langley bill were being held. Both may be correct: a casual meeting in the House of Representatives in February and other possible conversations in March but Mortimer's serious campaign in April, when Forbes was poised to seize control of veterans hospital construction. All it would take, in the Mortimer scenario, was to find Forbes's weak spot so that he would willingly participate with him and others to scam the federal government through loans, bribes, and kickbacks. Carolyn Votaw had introduced Forbes to her friend Mrs. Mortimer. The scene was nicely set. There was Mortimer waiting for his wife with his magnificent car outside the Veterans Bureau at the end of the day and Forbes coming out in the company of Mrs. Mortimer and Mrs. Votaw, ready to be introduced. Kate Forbes was away or incapacitated in the weeks before she left for Europe in June 1922. Forbes recalled only one occasion when the two couples, Mr. and Mrs. Mortimer and Colonel and Mrs. Forbes, were together, sometime in April or May 1922, and another when Kate went driving with Mortimer and Forbes.[13]

Elias Mortimer figured in Forbes's social life from springtime to the fall of 1922. He offered Forbes, at a trouble-ridden time, the balm of an apparently uncomplicated friendship, as he had to Captain Lannen and US Representatives Langley and Zihlman. He radiated confidence and wealth, was intelligent and well informed—sometimes surprisingly so—and appeared fascinated with Forbes's ideas. He was a great listener, sympathetic and eager to help in whatever way he could—the perfect friend. Colonel Forbes, relying on his own assessment of others and typically brushing off divergent views, did not stop to ask whether Mortimer was too friendly, too helpful, too available or whether he himself was too uncritical or trusting. Mortimer maintained an illusion of respect in his form of address. He called Forbes "Colonel," rather than "Bob," "Charles," or "Charlie," while Forbes usually called him "Mort." For Forbes, the friendship was one of congenial off-duty companionship, friends to relax with over meals and on trips. He described Mr. and Mrs. Mortimer as "very sociable" and liked to "ride out with them" in their car in the evenings when he was free, play cards, and have dinner with them. Mortimer later characterized their relationship as business oriented from the start. Forbes consistently said it was "purely social." He liked both of his new companions and gave them a photo of himself, inscribed in his handwriting: "To Eli and Katherine Mortimer—Friendship should be lasting memories. Value them and remember me among those you love. Sincerely, Charles R. Forbes." Elias H. Mortimer, Katherine T. Mortimer, and Charles R. Forbes became a trio.[14]

By mid-April 1922, Mortimer had identified clients for whom he planned to act as middleman in his campaign to set up construction contracts for veterans hospitals. His chief targets were John W. Thompson and James W. Black. Thompson, a self-made millionaire about sixty years of age, was a contractor in the railroad and related construction business who was familiar with federal contracting. He had received a $3 million wartime contract to construct a camp for Canadian aviators near Fort Worth, Texas ($42 million in twenty-first-century terms). He lived in St. Louis and had an office in Chicago. Mortimer claimed that Thompson "was rated at an estimated wealth of $15,000,000 and could put up any bond that was necessary and give any references through any New York or Chicago bank that was necessary." Jim Black had major business interests in St. Louis, Chicago, New York, Portland, and other cities. Sometime in April, Thompson and Black made a formal agreement to work together for mutually rewarding business. Documents produced later showed that both of them stayed at the Shoreham Hotel in Washington, DC, on April 4–14 and April 19–20, 1922, and involved Mortimer in at least part of their discussions. On April 19, the day before the second Langley bill became law, Thompson contacted Owen Hughes in Dallas, president of one of his associated companies (Hughes-O'Rourke Construction Company), telling him to write Forbes with a copy to Mortimer that he had read press reports about a hospital to be constructed and that Hughes could handle the work.[15]

Thompson entertained Elias and Katherine Mortimer at the Ambassador Hotel in New York on April 22, when Black was also in New York, at the Belmont Hotel. It is reasonable to conclude that Thompson, Black, and Mortimer were developing plans for hospital contracts. Mortimer was to testify at Forbes's trial that the three men agreed in mid-April 1922 (sometime between April 12 and 14, Mortimer said with characteristic precision) to seek a commission of 34 percent of the profits on all contracts they might receive from the Veterans Bureau. He described this as a "fair and perfectly legitimate transaction." Neither Black nor Thompson corroborated this. (They were not asked, at least for the record.) But even if the discussions were as Mortimer reported, Forbes did not participate in them. Mortimer reported that he formally introduced Forbes to Thompson and Black sometime in April 1922. Forbes reported that he had met both of them before. Carolyn Votaw had introduced him to Thompson, and Forbes had known and liked Black for a number of years. "He was a very unusual man, and anybody would be interested in him," Forbes said. "He was a man, I should say, of around 60 years of age, unmarried, and he had an old mother that his whole life was wrapped up in, and he had a couple of little nieces that he was very fond of." Black's devotion to his mom would have appealed to Forbes. He had met Black and his nieces in Seattle.[16]

The master spider wove his web. With the addition of Thompson and Black, Mortimer had a full deck of potential coconspirators for Forbes to work with, with Mortimer as the pivot. Thompson, Black, Mortimer, Forbes, and, for never fully explained reasons, Charles F. Cramer, the Veterans Bureau lawyer, were the five conspirators named at indictments in 1924, though Mortimer might have had a different array in mind in the spring of 1922. As he did in other cases in which he served as a government informer/snitch, Mortimer deflected blame away from himself. On one occasion he declared, "The idea of bribing and corrupting Forbes originated with Black and Thompson—and I followed along in fine shape." Elsewhere Mortimer said that Forbes had corrupted *him*.[17]

Why James Black and John Thompson needed a middleman to get contracts is a mystery, as the proposals for hospital building contracts were advertised in the usual way. Either of them could have approached Forbes directly and asked him what he hoped to get out of any deal for himself, if anything, citing Mortimer as their informer. There is no evidence that they did. Thompson and Black, two successful midwesterners, apparently accepted Mortimer's word that kickbacks and corruption were normal practice at the Veterans Bureau. But here's the rub: why should they *not* believe Mortimer when Forbes was from all appearances Mortimer's friend? Forbes was entangling himself in the web. A government official who forms a close relationship with an individual who seeks or is likely to seek business advantages from that relationship is on a slippery ethical slope, even if no favoritism or corruption is intended by that official.

While Forbes in work mode was preparing plans for the US national veterans hospital system, reviewing the medley of hospitals inherited from the US Public Health Service, and casting a baleful eye on ongoing construction by the White Committee, Mortimer found Forbes's Achilles' heel: his love of civil engineering. Fortuitously, Mortimer had come across just the opportunity to entice Colonel Forbes. Black and Thompson were interested in railroad construction and other development prospects in Colombia, South America. (Mortimer had no role in the project.) Forbes was happy to bring his development experience in Hawaii to bear on this case. With the US debt to Colombia with respect to the Panama Canal finally paid and relations eased between the two nations, Colombia sought American capital to develop its coffee, oil, gold, and mining industries. Black and Thompson were members of an American business syndicate formed to pursue these goals and to develop necessary infrastructure, such as roads, bridges, and railways. The president-elect of Colombia, American-educated General Pedro Nel Ospina, visited the United States in April and May 1922. Forbes went with Thompson, Black, and businessman B. G. Dahlberg, the disbursing member of the syndicate, to call on Ospina in New York on April 28. They reportedly discussed matters of interest to the syndicate for about an hour. Members of the syndicate were impressed by Forbes. James Black raised the Colombia project with him on four or five occasions. No one disputed that there were subsequent discussions to offer him an appointment as consultant engineer. Forbes prevaricated: "I couldn't consider it. I couldn't stand the Tropics," but he would consider consulting if there were an opportunity to do this in the United States.[18]

Though there was no evidence that an offer of employment was contingent on awarding hospital contracts, a large sum of money was mentioned as the salary Forbes would get as a consultant. Mortimer's inflated figure was $100,000, corrected at the trial to the more realistic but still enticing sum of $25,000 a year (more than twice Forbes's government salary). Mortimer gave his version for involving Forbes in the Colombia project: To "keep him coming along in good shape for the hospital contract. We hung out some bait to Forbes and he bit it and took it, hook, line and sinker."[19]

Throughout all of the discussions, Forbes seemed unaware of the concept of conflict of interest and deaf to the need for a public figure to build and maintain a pristine reputation. He visited Ospina as a private person and development engineer, but he was also a senior US government official. His visit could be construed as lobbying for the interests of one syndicate on a matter of private commerce with a soon-to-be leader of a foreign government. He also discussed career opportunities with Thompson and Black, which might bias his decisions in their favor with respect to government hospital contracts. Dr. Joel Boone, Sawyer's White House medical colleague, commented on the effect of professional gaffes made by Forbes in 1922, including taking Mortimer with him on relatively short trips to see potential hospital sites: "He conducted himself in such a way as to make him a suspect of wrongdoing." Quite apart from anyone else's machinations, Forbes was digging a hole for himself.[20]

Part of Mortimer's version of their friendship, as told later, was that Forbes spent most of his free time with him and his wife and that the amount of time was substantial. How substantial is unknown. When Forbes was in town, he enjoyed Harding's poker parties at the White House, to which Mortimer had no chance of being invited. Cabinet member and classicist Herbert Hoover described these low-stake poker evenings, extending well into the night, as the president's "greatest relaxation," though Hoover disliked the game and refused to attend—"it irked me to see it in the White House." There were poker parties outside the White House as well plus other White House events and Washington gatherings of various kinds, and Forbes enjoyed going to the theater. Mortimer, too, must have had other business to pursue. Nevertheless, it is fair to say that Mortimer garnered as much of Forbes's attention as he could, and that Forbes made the process easy. At some point, presumably after Kate and Marcia Forbes left the country early in June 1922, he moved from their family apartment on Connecticut Avenue to quasi-bachelor status in room 111 at the 2,000-room Wardman Park Hotel, where the Mortimers lived. It was a good place for legislators, staff, and lobbyists to mix with one another when in town. Mortimer aptly described the Wardman Park as a "very nice hotel, with considerable ground around it" and, with a little puffery, as "the most fashionable and aristocratic of residential hotels in Washington." Interior Secretary Albert Fall lived there too, as did Attorney General Harry M. Daugherty and his associate Jess Smith, and the controversial head of the Bureau of Information, the "Great Detective" William J. Burns.[21]

Mortimer was to testify that he told Forbes as early as March 1922 that he was "very much interested" in hospital contracts: "We used to talk hospitals up there so much I thought I was in a hospital." Forbes said that he did discuss some Veterans Bureau matters with Mortimer as part of other discussion, but "I never discussed or gave him information that would lead him to believe that at any time he had any entrée to my bureau or any advance information of any of our work, and he knew that I would not entertain any such proposition." Mortimer let potential building contractors know that he was Forbes's close friend. His view of friendship was chilling. "I knew how I stood with Forbes at that time," he testified. "I knew how friendly he was, and everyone else in Washington knew how friendly I was with him and how friendly he was with me, and that is what half the game in Washington was during that time, was friendship." Was Mortimer selling friendship, he was asked, or "your ability to corrupt?" Mortimer: "Well, if it was necessary I would have sold both."[22]

Colonel Edward C. Stockdale, who had known Mortimer in the war years, tried to warn Forbes about him in mid-April after seeing them together one Sunday evening at a party. Charles and Kate Forbes had been invited, but she was not present, and Forbes brought Elias and Katherine Mortimer instead. Stockdale remembered greeting Mrs. Mortimer mistakenly as Mrs. Forbes. Stockdale, who was also interested in federal contracts, was suspicious of Mortimer's presence with the head of the Veterans Bureau and warned Forbes that the association might lead to trouble. Forbes gave an astonishingly naive response. He told Stockdale that he had no business relationship with Mortimer, *and* knew he was an unfit person to do business with. Obviously, these views had not been transmitted and received by his friend Mort. A more cautious Washington official would have dropped Mortimer like a red-hot poker at this point. Forbes acted like a babe in the woods. In his view, there was no danger, no crossover between the spheres of work and play. He waved away Stockdale's concerns. Sometime after the party, Stockdale became disgusted with Forbes after Mortimer told him that he was handling construction proposals for Forbes (which was untrue), and Stockdale learned that Forbes and the Mortimers were still partying together. Forbes had clocked up one more hostile critic.[23]

By the end of April 1922, the state of play among the key figures interested in veterans hospital construction was that each was bent on fooling at least one of the others. Mortimer was playing Colonel Forbes as a potential victim/cash cow, while ingratiating himself and his wife as his intimate friends. Forbes was playing Mortimer by welcoming him as a friend but not taking him seriously as a colleague or partner in business. What Mortimer had not observed was that Forbes, too, had a shell; he was a past master of withholding part of himself from others. General Sawyer was open about his policy differences with Forbes but expected to outwit him on hospital planning and control of supplies through exerting authority in his role as chief coordinator of the Federal Board of Hospitalization. Forbes, determined to get his program approved and implemented, played Sawyer by excluding him from the Veterans Bureau hospital planning process, neglecting to inform him when the list of proposed hospitals would be ready for the Federal Board and speaking independently to President Harding. Harding played an equivocal role by listening to both Sawyer and Forbes without directing their relationship. He was a practical politician who kept his options open.

In the last week of May 1922, Forbes conferred with President Harding, Republican Congressmen Martin B. Madden of Illinois, and Daniel R. Anthony of Kansas (fiscal conservatives) on whether it would be better policy to enlarge existing hospitals rather than to build new ones (no, in Forbes's view); kept the president on track on the hospital construction program; reminded the Federal Board of Hospitalization that they had already allocated $12 million to $13 million of the second Langley funds, including new buildings at Northampton and Livermore; and hosted a national conference on rehabilitation. Before going to New York and saying goodbye to his wife and child, who left for Europe in early June, Forbes wanted to get away for a restful weekend. He asked Mortimer to suggest a good place to go. Mortimer named the Traymore Hotel in Atlantic City, New Jersey, fashionably located at Illinois Avenue and the Boardwalk and overlooking the Atlantic Ocean and invited himself and his wife to come too. Forbes and the two Mortimers traveled to the coast together by train. Abandoning hope of a complete rest, Forbes sent a telegram to headquarters summoning his secretary Merle L. Sweet, who took business papers to Forbes at the hotel on June 1 and stayed on to work with his boss.[24]

Mortimer also arranged for the actors Francine Larrimore and her sister Stella, members of a prominent New York theater family, to be there at the same time. Enter the "actresses," as they were called in later attempts to suggest Forbes was sexually involved with Francine. (Whether he was or not is undetermined.) Forbes said she had asked him to help her get a US passport (she was born in France), but he declined. Francine Larrimore, with her ingénue blue eyes and cloudy mop of reddish hair, played the lead as racy flapper Theodora "Teddy" Gloucester in the comedy *Nice People* at the National Theater in Washington in the first week of May after a successful run in New York. The Mortimers and Forbes had been at various gatherings with the sisters, including a party hosted by Francine Larrimore and attended by President and Mrs. Harding, followed by a reception Miss Larrimore gave for Forbes, the Mortimers, Stockdale, and others at her suite at the Shoreham Hotel. Charles Forbes, Elias and Katherine Mortimer, and the Larrimore sisters had dinner together one night at the Traymore Hotel. Again, Forbes walked into a situation that was later construed as dubious on several fronts. There was of course the implied sexual frisson of intimacy with actresses, particularly with one who played a sexy role onstage, but beyond that, Forbes was both on vacation and working, mixing up his work / play roles, and he let his apparently rich friend Mortimer pay his hotel bill at the Traymore, raising questions of accepting favors or a bribe. The hotel record for the rooms showed that the two rooms used by the Mortimers and Forbes, numbers 614 and 615 (for check-in May 31, departure June 4), were paid for as one amount. Forbes argued that, if Mortimer did pay his bill at the Traymore, he could not remember; it was in exchange for something else, such as paying for dinners, but as an explanation that is weak. It was definitely not true, as some accounts later alleged, that Forbes took over a whole floor of an Atlantic City hotel for partying.[25]

As on other occasions, Katherine Tullidge Mortimer was on the Atlantic City trip as a silent supportive wife, merely the "and Mrs. Mortimer," an addendum to her husband's name. She was not actually silent, of course; rather, her actions and words were not recorded. Sometime in the spring or summer of 1922 her father, Dr. George B. Tullidge, went to Mexico and stayed there for about a year, ostensibly for his health (he had a heart condition) but also to check on his exiled son Edward, leaving his wife in an empty house in Philadelphia and his daughter Katherine, in her mid-twenties, without male protection from her abusive husband. Not surprisingly, she would turn to her friend Charles R. Forbes, a comfortable man in his mid-forties, for help when she needed it. The Mortimers stuck to Forbes so intensely that it was only a matter of time before he would see some evidence of Mortimer's physical abuse of his wife.

It happened soon. One day early in June, Katherine Mortimer telephoned Forbes on the house phone at his first-floor apartment at the Wardman Park Hotel and asked him to come up to hers on the fifth. "I found her crying and pretty well hammered up," he said. "Her dress was torn, and up here, this part of her eye [indicating] was swollen pretty badly." Mort had gone down to get some cigars or sundries, and returned shortly. Forbes duly "took him to task." Mortimer said he felt bad about it, was sorry, and it wouldn't happen again. Forbes accepted this statement and invited Mort and Katherine down to dinner in the Wardman Park dining room. He had done his duty and spoken "just as a man would call one down for beating a woman up," he said, and then they had a meal together.[26]

Colonel Forbes had planned an overdue four-week working trip to Veterans Bureau districts in Chicago and on the West Coast from mid-June to mid-July 1922. Travel would allow him to get away from the craziness of Washington's intrigues, critiques, and rumor mills. Gossip was becoming unpleasantly pointed, including general attacks on the Harding administration. In January, New England textile workers had gone on a six-month strike. In April, a major coal strike had begun. In June, twenty strikebreakers were killed by armed miners at Herrin, Illinois. In July, railroad shop workers struck. Harding's speech before Congress in August against the miners' and shopmens' strike was called the "most scathing indictment ever laid upon any body of workers in America." At the same time the president was criticized for doing nothing, for seeking to impose government control on business, and for wasting time on unnecessary investigations.[27]

A cynical response to congress and the presidency was by no means unreasonable. This was a fruitful time to "debunk" (expose the underbelly of) government and its minions and to engage in character assassination. H. L. Mencken described politics in the United States as "incomparably the greatest show on earth," with its "ribald combats of demagogues, the exquisitely ingenious operation of master rogues, the pursuit of witches and heretics [and] the desperate struggles of inferior men to claw their way into Heaven."[28]

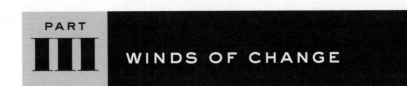

PART

III

WINDS OF CHANGE

TAKING A FRIEND ON A
BUSINESS TRIP WEST

Elias Mortimer was like a limpet. Once attached, he was difficult to dislodge. As a result, Forbes's four-week working visit to western Veterans Bureau districts in the summer of 1922 was filled with unanticipated drama: plotting behind the scenes, slights and misperceptions, conflicting accounts of off-duty activities, and the shedding of tears. This trip involved much more than the director's usual heavy round of inspections, exhortations, conflict resolutions, speeches, and meetings, though it was all of this as well. The drama followed a last-minute error of judgment and was almost entirely of Forbes's making. Mortimer pleaded to come with the traveling party, bringing his wife with him. He had never been to the West Coast, he said. Forbes said yes. "We left so hurriedly," Katherine Mortimer remembered, that she was not able to pack all she needed and had to go shopping when they reached Chicago, where she got "one or two gowns and a wrapper, dinner gown." Mortimer, meanwhile, got a last-ditch opportunity to snare a hospital contract for his rich clients.[1]

John B. Milliken, a senior member of Forbes's office staff, was assigned as his personal assistant for the first part of the trip instead of Merle Sweet, whose father had died. Sweet joined the party later, in Denver. Milliken liked Forbes: "He treated me fairly and squarely, and I endeavored to render him the best service I could." Part of that service was to caution him about the impropriety of bringing friends on business trips. Milliken said he told Forbes he did not like the "aspect of things . . . that he as a Director of a Bureau of the United States Government should be more circumspect, that his indiscreetness should not be misunderstood by parties who might put an improper construction upon it and in turn reflect upon him as well as the Bureau and likewise those associated with him." Milliken and Veterans Bureau tuberculosis expert Dr. Stanley Rinehart, a member of the party, discussed such concerns, together with rumors that were circulating in Washington about Forbes and his travel companions.[2]

As a group, the individuals on the overnight train to Chicago could have served as the cast of a mystery story. Here was the able, erratic, charismatic boss whose wife had left for an independent life overseas; the worried civil servant, distinguished by a sense of proper behavior; the disappointed doctor (with a famous wife offstage) who was trying against major odds to improve the quality and availability of services to veterans who were patients and constantly being thwarted; and the slick bootlegger-fixer and his attractive wife whose marriage was marred with violence and deceit. In the train's well-lit cocoon, streaking across a nation scarred by strife, black attendants served the white passengers with courteous efficiency. The travelers were engrossed by the multiple problems of the Veterans Bureau and the tenure of its chief. Milliken reportedly heard Forbes say he expected to go into the cabinet (as interior secretary, Mortimer said later), though Forbes denied making any such claim. Forbes knew he was demonstrably not in good health. Nevertheless, he kept up a full work schedule. Milliken suggested to Forbes's old boss Charles B. Hurley of Seattle who met the group in San Francisco that Forbes should resign: "I told him that I thought his health was being impaired, simply because he was not temperamentally fitted to the position." Then Hurley told Forbes what Milliken had said, but Forbes dismissed the idea and ignored Milliken, which did no one any good.[3]

Washington gossip had him on his way out. Late in the trip, Dr. Hugh Scott, one of Forbes's senior aides, sent him a telegram from Veterans Bureau headquarters to the Davenport Hotel, Spokane: "Persistent rumor around Washington that you are to resign soon. This is disconcerting to your loyal friends." Forbes shot off a telegram to President Harding the same day: the rumors were without foundation. He listed his efforts on the trip: "Since leaving Washington have inspected hospitals in Illinois, Washington, Oregon, California, Colorado and Idaho including District and Subdistrict offices. Have also inspected all hospital sites offered the Government in the Western Section on [sic] the country. Have submitted reports to the office for consideration by Federal Board on [sic] Hospitalization. Will inspect the sites in Minneapolis thence return to Washington arriving about twentieth. Tuberculosis expert accompanies me." In Chicago, he talked about a potential job for himself with a Chicago company, which reportedly offered him $20,000 a year (twice his government salary) plus expenses, but did not accept.[4]

Newspapers east and west reported that President Harding had reached the point of showdown with Congress. The midterm congressional elections were looming in early November. Democrats were programmatically split but united by their common enemy: Republicans. Republicans were split and worried about losing seats. Harding was assailed for being too weak or too strong. The *Oakland Tribune*: If Harding remained a "hands-off" president, distant and aloof, the unsympathetic attitude of the public toward Congress would grow into "such a storm of protest as to threaten republican supremacy in the House of Representatives and discredit the entire administration." The *New York Times*: "President Harding is not the same easy-going Executive that he was.... Today the President is the leader of his party and he intends to exert his influence as other presidents have done, when it appears necessary to get legislation through." Harding was having difficulties in getting his ship-subsidy bill through Congress, designed to alleviate the problem of the surplus ships built for the war. The Republican chair of the Senate Finance Committee, longtime Senator James McCumber, announced he was going to delay Harding's tariff bill in favor of passing the Soldiers' Bonus Bill, which Harding had threatened to veto if it did not come with a revenue stream to fund it. Porter James McCumber of North Dakota needed to deliver votes for Republicans in his state in November by passing a popular bill.[5]

Harding had shown he could be tough. In March, following an inquiry made by the Treasury Department, he issued an executive order directing the firing of James L. Wilmeth, director of the Bureau of Engraving and Printing, plus thirty-one other high officials in the bureau, including all agency chiefs. There was a message here for other government executives, and particularly those regarded as weaker members of his administration, including his old political associate Attorney General Daugherty, his brother-in-law Superintendent of Federal Prisons Heber Votaw (husband of Carolyn Votaw), and his Ohio doctor Charles E. Sawyer. And then there was his old comrade in the senate, Albert B. Fall, and his younger friend, Charles R.

Forbes. Senator Truman Newberry of Michigan, who had been investigated for overspending in the Michigan primary election against Henry Ford,
was finally seated in the Senate, only to become an anti-Harding target.
Newberry was tarnished by comments about "purchasing" a Senate seat
"obtained by corruption." In the spring and summer of 1922, there was a
not-so-subtle suggestion that Harding was in the grip of big money interests.
Harding was under considerable stress. Opinions varied about how he was
handling it. Seasoned Washington journalist Mark Sullivan noted in his diary in July that Harding "made the impression of a cool capacity." A young
southern journalist, Thomas Stokes, described him during the almost daily
conferences at the White House over the summer crises as a man whose
nerves were wearing raw.[6]

Representative Langley's reputation was safe for the time being, as was
that of Charles R. Forbes. Interior Secretary Albert B. Fall and Attorney
General Harry Daugherty were on shakier ground. Having been Harding's
friend and source of information about Mexico when both were in the Senate, Secretary Fall expected to play a central role in national policy making
on Mexico and other issues. Not so. The president had "grown away from
Fall," the *New York Times* reported as early as March, and was leaning more
toward Secretary Hughes (State) on foreign problems and Secretary Hoover
(Commerce) on domestic policies. Fall also assumed, unrealistically, that the
"business" of the Interior Department, with himself as CEO, was to control
the development of all of America's natural resources, not only oil and other
extractive processes but also forests and watersheds. Having maneuvered
successfully to transfer oil leases from the navy to his department, he announced that he was planning to lease contracts to drill on government
lands in California and was leasing the so-called Teapot Dome reserve in
Wyoming to oilman Harry Sinclair. Harding supported Fall on the oil leases. In mid-April, Democratic Senator John Kendrick of Wyoming called for
an explanation of the leases and Attorney General Daugherty's failure to
question the legitimacy of the executive order that allowed the leases to
proceed. Later in the month Senator La Follette (Progressive Party) introduced a resolution to investigate the leases. Thus began the case called Teapot Dome, though nothing of import was to happen for months.

Fall's campaign to acquire the Forestry Service, part of the Agriculture
Department, failed dismally. Forestry was backed by influential conserva-

tionists and fought back, casting Secretary Fall as a tool of capitalism who would ruthlessly exploit the forest reserves in Alaska for business gain. Fall made an arrogant riposte: "I know that my ideas do not meet with the approval of certain narrow-minded and biased bureaucratic Government officials and their followers." In a parallel blow for Albert Fall, Harding assigned Herbert Hoover (an engineer) rather than Fall (a rancher) to head a new commission to explore and plan for irrigation projects in the region served by the Colorado River. Secretary Fall, firmly (and accurately) labeled anti-conservationist, was a potential suspect for investigation well before the oil leases became a major focus of the Harding scandals.[7]

Attorney General Harry M. Daugherty was besieged by a backlog of cases of alleged fraud in wartime purchasing contracts, each to be investigated and moved to legal action as justified. There was suspicion that the Republican administration was deliberately downplaying these cases to do favors for big business. In May 1922, Daugherty appeared before the House to urge approval of half a million dollars to cover the costs of war frauds investigation, and in June, he gave it as his belief that corporations doing business with the government during the war years were honest, and there were some "honest mistakes in bookkeeping." This judgment may have been reasonable. The cases were complicated, with contracts rushed to completion for wartime needs, each case handled separately. It made sense to let them go. Simultaneously, Daugherty had the challenge of investigating and prosecuting prohibition cases under the Volstead Act, responding to continuing antiradical sentiments for which draconian remedies were prescribed, and finding effective ways of dealing with major coal and railroad strikes. Daugherty had informed the press that there were large stocks of coal on hand and a short strike could be tolerated, but the government had the authority to act if necessary to maintain the production of coal. Later in the year, he was to use the same logic to stop the strike of railroad employees.[8]

A weak spot for Daugherty was the presence of his acolyte from Ohio, younger businessman Jesse "Jess" W. Smith. There were no suggestions, at least in public, that this was a homoerotic relationship—more like a benevolent father and appreciative son. Lucy Walker Daugherty, Harry's wife, was crippled by the combination of rheumatism and failed attempts at curing it and stayed in Ohio. Their two grown children were troubled and addicted. During the Harding years, Jess Smith traveled and went on vacation with

Daugherty, joined him at social events, had a desk at the Department of Justice though he was not on the payroll, dispensed favors as Daugherty's assumed representative, and acted as his general factotum. The combined presence in the department of Smith, with an unclear portfolio, and Burns, with a cast of dubious agents, gave it a disheveled, unpleasantly rakish air. Smith was to be remembered in history as Daugherty's bagman and Burns as the employer of the slickest of slick agents, Gaston B. Means: liar, burglar, swindler.

By selecting assistant attorneys general on political rather than qualitative grounds, Daugherty missed the opportunity to raise standards at the Department of Justice. There were two notable exceptions, as biographer James N. Giglio has pointed out. Both of them became accusers in the Harding scandals. The first, Mabel Walker Willebrandt, was an astute, politically attuned lawyer from Los Angeles who took responsibility in the Department of Justice for prohibition and taxation cases, a massive undertaking. Willebrandt played her female role brilliantly, was popular in Washington, and strongly supported by leading California politicians. Newspapers tended to stress her looks. Willebrandt was "pretty" and "young," with "well-molded features, wavy chestnut hair, a fresh complexion, expressive gray eyes and a slender, graceful figure." She was married but separated, had a young daughter, and was committed to her work: ambitious, tough, and ruthless. The second promising appointment, John W. H. Crim, was a private practice lawyer with a strong courtroom presence and a wide span of expertise. Within four years, both would play essential roles in the fate of Charles R. Forbes.[9]

In Chicago, the Forbes party stayed at the new, magnificent Drake Hotel, occupying a suite of rooms. The group expanded with the temporary addition of building contractors John W. Thompson and James W. Black, for whom Elias Mortimer had as yet produced no sign of a hospital contract. Mortimer and Thompson were cool to each other in Chicago. As a result, Katherine Mortimer shed the western trip's tears. Mort had told her not to speak with Thompson, she said: "They had a very unfortunate affair. I could not see anybody." Thompson found her crying in the Drake Hotel on June 19. "Mr. Thompson just spoke [to me]," Katherine explained later: "I was placed in an embarrassing position." She knew nothing about any business transacted between them. Mortimer's abuse of his wife continued. One day at the

Drake Hotel, Forbes testified, before he went out on his round of official visits, he heard a woman scream and headed toward a hotel room that was not far from his own, diagonally across the hall, "and as I went out the door was a bit ajar, and I saw who was in there." Mortimer was "beating up on his wife." On another known incident of abuse, this time in San Francisco, a temporary member of the extended party (Albert L. Lindley) intervened. Forbes was still taking a hands-off stance: "I did not want to get mixed up in the family rows." There was also little he could do without fanning Mortimer's rage, which was often alcohol related. Mortimer got drunk and unpleasant several times on the trip, Forbes reported, and after he "admonished" him, Mort "seemed to delight in taking it out on his wife." Yet he was always so apologetic afterward.[10]

Despite all their reported conversations, Mortimer had little knowledge about the process of hospital contracting Forbes was following. The sites for the new hospitals were already selected on government-owned or donated land, meaning that there was no room for a third party to make a profit from the purchase. Before he left Washington, Forbes arranged for the bureau's hospital construction program to be handled by the military. The heads of the navy's Bureau of Yards and Docks (the "most efficient engineering department in the Government," Forbes said) and the Army Quartermaster General's Office had agreed to take responsibility for drawing up the plans and specifications for the new hospitals, advertise for bids, award them, and supervise construction. Forbes urged them to act with speed. He did not expect to see the plans or specifications until they were finished: "I put the job entirely in their hands." However, as a legal matter, the Veterans Bureau director had to sign the contracts, and even on the western trip, he could not let go of his intense commitment to the hospital program. While he was away from Washington (from mid-June to mid-July 1922), the specifications, advertisements, and bids for the first new hospital were in motion: a multi-million-dollar complex for neuropsychiatric patients at Northampton, Massachusetts, to be built on a large undeveloped site. James W. Black and John W. Thompson were potential bidders, together with Elias H. Mortimer, their purported agent. When the formal bids came in, all else being equal, Forbes might prefer one contractor over another. However, the budgets promised to be tight—too tight for the profit margins Mortimer expected.[11]

Instead of reporting profitable results when he met up with Thompson and Black in Chicago, Mortimer asked them for more money, specifically, $15,000 (more than $200,000 in twenty-first-century terms)—in cash. Thompson's coolness toward Mortimer probably had something to do with this. Nevertheless, Thompson and Black approved the loan as a formal business arrangement: a time-limited, interest-bearing loan at 6 percent interest, guaranteed on Mortimer's signature. Thus, they justified their investment, or so they thought. Mortimer later claimed that the money was to cover expenses for the trip and to bribe Forbes. With sleight of hand, Mortimer made most of the $15,000 vanish without a trace. He claimed, first, that he had made a secret handover of $5,000 in cash as a bribe to Forbes in Chicago, with no receipt or witnesses and, second, that he had spent almost as much in lavish expenses he shouldered on this government-paid business trip, again without producing receipts. Mortimer's ability to be believed was his single most important asset. The $5,000 he allegedly handed to Forbes would be central to bringing Forbes down (see chapter 13). Mortimer never repaid the $15,000 he borrowed from Thompson, from whose bank account it came, nor was he punished for reneging on the debt. There was no evidence of lavish entertainments, outside of events held by other parties to greet the visitors in different locations.[12]

Though the details of Forbes's work for the bureau continued to be barred to Mortimer, Mortimer watched Forbes's off-duty actions closely. Forbes assumed he was free to do unpaid and/or paid outside consulting while on the government payroll. He was still thinking about the Colombia project, dealing directly with James Black on this, not (Forbes testified) at any time through Mortimer. Forbes and his aide John Milliken went over a draft of a proposed Colombia contract as a favor to Black during the trip and wrote comments on the draft. Milliken said he made his notes on it "around Spokane." In a further mixing of private and public interests, Forbes agreed to help John Thompson find a lawyer to deal with the Navy Department about a ship the government had commandeered from him during the war without, Thompson said, giving due compensation. (The German tanker Gut-Heil had sunk and been abandoned in the Mississippi River near Baton Rouge, Louisiana, in about 1913, but in 1917, with wartime ships in short supply, it became a viable project for resurrection. Thompson raised, refloated, and refitted the ship on the basis, he said, of agreed government assurances and had received an offer from the French government for $1.5 million, which he was not allowed to accept.) Thompson planned to sue the US government for the $800,000 he believed he was owed (more than $11 million in twenty-first-century terms). Mortimer claimed there would be a substantial commission to be shared out if the case were successful.[13]

Work on the trip was heavily scheduled. In Chicago, Colonel Forbes had Veterans Bureau District 8 assign him an experienced stenographer to work in the suite at the Drake Hotel so that he could dictate letters, write memos, and draft speeches. (She was to become an important defense witness later.) His local rounds in Chicago illustrate his work at each stop: two days spent inspecting the district office with its executive officer Fred Hamilton, visiting veterans hospitals and vocational schools in the city, and talking with staff and residents as well as other visits and meetings. He was generally pleased by what he saw in Chicago, he wrote in a detailed report to President Harding on his return: the district office was working better than before, vocational rehabilitation was moving in the right direction, and he had directed the office's move to a less expensive location—expected to save $101,410 in fiscal year 1922–1923. The Edward J. Hines Jr. Hospital, US Veterans Hospital 76, with more than 700 patients, provided abundant and well-prepared food. He heard no complaints from patients there, and the Treasury Department's White Committee was constructing a deep well, which he would ask them to expedite. Drexel Boulevard Hospital, Veterans Hospital 30, with 425 mostly medical and surgical patients, was well equipped, and had a "splendid medical staff" and "fine morale." And so on. One meeting or visit followed another, duly reported to the president in an upbeat tone. On June 21, while he was in Chicago, the proposals for bids for the Northampton Hospital were advertised in the press. The same day, a Clinical Tuberculosis Section was officially created in the Veterans Bureau (Dr. Rinehart, who was on the trip, was one of its two leaders), and on June 22, a Section on Clinical Neuropsychiatry. Forbes's voice was heard on the radio in Washington at 10 p.m., on June 21, via NOF, the Naval Air Station, Anacostia, speaking on "The Employment of Rehabilitated Veterans." Contrary to the impression Mortimer gave later, this trip was far from a vacation.[14]

Similar visits were next made in Denver, where Colonel Forbes met with citizen representatives and with the Chamber of Commerce and then on to San Francisco, arriving on Sunday, June 25, a week to the day since they embarked on the trip. The San Francisco office (District 12), was trying unsuccessfully to cope with the serious problem of veterans with tuberculosis migrating to California, Nevada, and Arizona. Visits to bureau facilities seemed to go well in San Francisco. However, a disturbing note came during Forbes's appearance (and speech) at the annual convention of a major veterans' group, Disabled American Veterans (DAV), when the organization's commander, Judge Robert H. Marx, strongly criticized him—"attacked" was the word used in the press—followed by hostile speakers from the floor. One demand was that the national vocational training camp he had set up with such hope at Chillicothe, Ohio, be closed because it was overly "militaristic" and unnecessary. Veterans resented military discipline; they had had enough of it at war. According to one California newspaper, Forbes had his "back against the wall"; in another, criticism of the Veterans Bureau was "just opening." Forbes did not report the tone of this meeting in his report to Harding.[15]

A more pointed critique occurred during discussions with interested parties about the Livermore site near San Francisco, designated for a hospital for tuberculosis patients. Important local luminaries Judge A. E. Graupner and John R. Quinn shared their doubts about the Livermore purchase with Forbes at the Fairmount Hotel, San Francisco. (That was the botched negotiation initiated by Veterans Bureau lawyer Charles Cramer.) Graupner represented California on the hospitalization committee of the American Legion, and Quinn was commander of the legion's Department of California. Their views were worth taking seriously. The purpose of the meeting was to inform Forbes that Livermore "had been made the subject of graft" and to demand that he put matters right. Forbes's response was remarkably offhand when he recalled the meeting later: "Oh, I believe there was some mention made by Graupner that they thought there was something wrong with Livermore, but I don't recall what it was." He did not remember them using the word *corrupt*. Graupner became yet another of Forbes's enemies. Later, in a detailed statement for the Senate Committee on Investigation of the Veterans Bureau (1923), he was to recount a mix of facts and rumors that implicated Forbes. According to Graupner, Lucien B. Johnson, the owner of the former vineyard, had offered the property to the county of Alameda and the city and county of San Francisco at a much lower price than the government paid. Johnson, architect Matthew O'Brien, associate Thomas O'Day, and Veterans Bureau lawyer Cramer seemed to have a "very close connection." Johnson had allegedly stated that he had to make a kickback of $25,000 from the revised purchase price of $105,000, allegedly to split between Cramer and Forbes. It was claimed that in addition Johnson had sent one hundred cases of wine to Washington to be split three ways: between Cramer, Forbes, and an unknown third person.[16]

A second iteration of these rumors came from Major Grant, the director of the bureau's district office in San Francisco, who took Forbes aside to tell him what they were. His telling included the hundred cases of wine, this time with the third share going to President Harding. This seemed an unlikely tale all around. In characteristic form, Forbes thought the report "so ridiculous" and "so strictly absurd" that he paid no attention to it. A third warning came, in witchlike progression, at lunch with leading doctors at the Bohemian Club, where two members told him that there were "dirty rumors" about Livermore, though they could not come up with specifics. Forbes asked Major Grant to investigate. When Grant concluded that the transaction was "all right," Forbes regarded his task as done and dismissed these and other rumors he heard in Washington as "so much hearsay," without facts or attribution. (Likewise, he dismissed rumors he heard over the summer that Mortimer was a bootlegger.)[17]

Rather than worrying about a possible scam at Livermore, Forbes seems to have been shockingly disengaged, not fully "there." Judge Graupner reported that, while the charges of corruption were being made, Forbes "exhibited neither concern, anger, nor particular interest," nor did he offer any denials. He merely asked whether the property was suitable for a tuberculosis hospital. Graupner replied in the affirmative. Forbes then asked why it mattered to Graupner "what price was paid for it as long as it was a good site?" Graupner heard Forbes say that extravagance with taxpayers' money was immaterial, while Forbes's overriding goal was to get a hospital built and running, no matter what it cost, so that tuberculosis patients could be treated—a few thousand dollars here or there was immaterial. The meeting was a colossal failure of communication. After Forbes left, Graupner's criticisms of him escalated. According to one source (no supporting details given), Graupner reported that Forbes had been an "unspeakable beast" in making sexual advances to nurses, as well as making a huge profit on the Livermore site, and hosted an "orgy" in Stockton.[18]

Cramer's role, never properly elucidated in the Livermore dealings, was suspect for other reasons in California. There was report of a scandal in California in 1922, in which the Veterans Bureau reportedly paid $35,000 to the Mack Copper Company to prevent it from defaulting on a mortgage for land on which the Camp Kearney convalescent home was built. (Forbes described this as "a fire trap outside of San Diego," which had been run by the US Public Health Service as a stopgap measure for tuberculosis patients.) Cramer worked out the lease with Mack. The first annual rent payment for the home was allegedly more than the property was worth. According to one account, the American Legion decided not to publicize the murky details of the case because the Bonus Bill was coming up for approval and its leaders did not want to muddy the waters. However, the president of the copper company argued that he had a valid contract, that no one in his organization had engaged improperly, and that the government had been giving him a run-around since the land was originally leased by the Army—all probably true. Among the few who commented on Cramer later was Forbes's associate on the western trip, John B. Milliken, the upright, modern civil servant, who disliked Cramer and had no confidence in him. Milliken testified that, though he knew of "no crookedness, or graft," he left the Veterans Bureau in disgust for a lower-paying job in September 1922. Forbes had doubts about Cramer, too, though always reluctant to confront or accuse him. When he was asked at the Senate hearings whether he suspected Cramer of "taking graft," Forbes refused to say yes, no, or even maybe; he had "heard very many things," but that was it. By that time, as Forbes said, the man was dead.[19]

On June 28, 1922, Forbes's group left San Francisco for Rough and Ready Island along the San Joaquin River to inspect a vocational school with one hundred of the bureau's agricultural trainees and went on to Stockton, Livermore, and Santa Barbara, the latter reached on Sunday, July 2. A hotel looked at in Santa Barbara for possible use was too small. On July 3, the visitors were in Los Angeles, where Forbes inspected the suboffice of District 12 and made other visits in the area and then on to San Diego, where Forbes met, as usual, with local officials and made more visits. By July 9, they were in Seattle and Tacoma. Forbes enthused about the "ideal site" for a neuropsychiatric hospital at Camp Lewis on land bordering American Lake, in his old stomping ground, the State of Washington. More visits and meetings followed in Seattle, Portland, and Spokane, before moving back east via Minneapolis and St. Cloud (both in Minnesota) and Fargo (North Dakota). Forbes informed Harding, in concluding his report, that "better service can and should be rendered" to patients; called for "trained teamwork" and the application of scientific standards "supported by sufficient evidence and corroborated by practice" and urged that federal hospitals fall in line with the movement for hospital accreditation ("standardization") run by the American College of Surgeons. With Harding's approval, he wanted to go ahead and develop hospital standards for Veterans Bureau hospitals. These were sensible, modern recommendations, but Forbes could not do every new thing himself. He tended to bounce from one enthusiasm to the next, leaving disappointed allies, supplicants, and employees in his wake.[20]

The four-week business trip included some enjoyable nonbusiness experiences, notably the chance to see friends and acquaintances on the West Coast and travel by sea. The visit to San Diego culminated in a dinner at a General Terry's house, where Mortimer got drunk and insulted the host and his wife, followed by a trip on the ship *President* to San Francisco. There, courtesy of Forbes's friend Bert Alexander, they transferred to better quarters on the *H. F. Alexander* up to Seattle. Alexander hosted a luncheon on board at which Forbes, in what he later called an "impulsive act," formally presented him with a medallion (later referred to inaccurately as a medal) from the president. Forbes explained later that Harding gave him six inauguration medallions as mementos to distribute, "with my compliments," to "such friends as have been friends of mine." Forbes took four of them with him on the western trip. Alexander was no doubt pleased. In Tacoma, Joe Carman, "one of the biggest men in the west," said Forbes, gave a supper party at which Mortimer was drunk again.[21]

At Hayden Lake, a resort in Northern Idaho, Forbes had dinner with friends and afterward sat on the wharf and fished for what he called "little, wee fish." He had a reputation in the west for being a fisherman, and some of his "cronies out there from the club" teased him by leaving in his room a huge rod with the sign "Forbes's fishing pole" on it, together with a pair of overalls and a fishing hat. The pole was an enormous pole for catching shark. "They were putting up a little joke on me." He wore the overalls at the wharf. Someone suggested a swim. Forbes jumped into the lake into water about three feet deep with a friend who was a local resident (name and gender not disclosed). Assuming this happened as described here, we get a glimpse of a rambunctious, boyish Forbes having fun with friends. Elias Mortimer was not present on this occasion (he had left for Spokane), but Katherine Mortimer was there and once again her version was not recorded for posterity. This incident and the presentation of the medallion to Alexander were blown up at the Senate hearings via the testimony of Elias Mortimer, as conduct unbefitting the director of the Veterans Bureau; namely, unauthorized use of the president's name in presenting a medal and engaging in risqué parties, including fully dressed plunges into a lake.[22]

Mr. and Mrs. Mortimer left the party at Minneapolis to visit his family. He presumably still had some of the $15,000 he had borrowed from John W. Thompson and could show them he was rich, but there is no account of the impressions of those concerned. In Forbes's reported memory of events, nothing extraordinary happened from April through July 1922 (and beyond), or at least nothing sufficiently critical to force his resignation. There was little news about the Veterans Bureau in the national newspapers. He had dealt with numerous administrative problems, but that was par for the job, as were hostile rumors. The hospital construction program was finally under way. President Harding acknowledged receipt of his report on the western trip in a reassuring note on his return: "I have no doubt [the trip] was highly advantageous to you. . . . I fully realize the tremendous problems which are confronting you. I like to say to you that I have confidence that you will handle them to the very best advantage for the service and for the war veterans in whose cause the government is deeply interested."[23]

Bids for the construction of the first new hospital, at Northampton, were opened at the Veterans Bureau while Forbes was away. He had asked the Army Quartermaster General's Office, which was handling the Northampton contract, to divide the project into two parts for reasons of speed: one contract for the foundations and a separate contract for the aboveground structures. As an experienced builder, he wanted to get the foundations in before the ground froze in the Massachusetts winter, with the rest of the construction ready to go up as these were completed. Otherwise, the whole project might be stalled until spring thaw. Colonel Edward S. Walton and Captain Frank C. Starr of the army initially demurred, but then agreed. The same plan was put into effect, for the same reasons, for the construction of a 500-bed tuberculosis hospital at Tupper Lake, New York, with work done by the navy. The lowest bid for the Northampton foundations, which involved a number of buildings, was from Northeastern Construction Company: $133,000 with completion in 120 days. This was a longer time than Forbes wanted, but Northeastern refused to budge on the time needed. Opinion was divided in Washington whether to accept Northeastern, the winning bid, and put up with a serious delay in getting the hospital finished and in operation, or negotiate on the basis of time with the second lowest bidder, the Pontiac Construction Company, a company organized and controlled by James Black, which bid $160,000. The time was negotiated down to sixty days with Pontiac. Charles Cramer sent a telegram to Forbes in Tacoma on July 10 recommending Pontiac: "Speed is what you want and these people will give it to us and that is worth more than a few thousand dollars difference."[24]

Forbes delayed a final decision until he was back on July 19 and then came up with an ingenious arithmetical reckoning that imposed a high per diem penalty charge on Pontiac—$450 a day for every day the project was not completed over the contracted sixty days. If these daily penalties were calculated for Pontiac, and assuming, for argument's sake, that the firm hit the far less desirable completion goal of 120 days (Northeastern's time estimate), the two contracts evened up in monetary terms. Pontiac also agreed to eliminate extra fees for moving rocks and boulders. As a result, though Forbes may well have favored Pontiac as a contractor all along, he gave the firm a fearsomely difficult task. Pontiac had every incentive to put on extra shifts and do whatever else was necessary to avoid penalties and finish quickly. The Army Quartermaster's Office, handling construction, agreed to these terms. The result was that the foundations were finished in seventy-six days, but Pontiac lost money on the contract. Work was also completed for the much larger contract for the superstructures (the aboveground buildings, which could not be started until the foundations were in). The George A. Fuller Company, which received that contract, without any connection to Mortimer, started building before winter set in. Forbes's goal for building as quickly as possible had been met.[25]

This was a good outcome for Forbes and the disabled veterans he served. Forbes reckoned the government saved forty or fifty days. However, in no way could the outcome be seen as a sweet deal for James W. Black, whose company lost money. Mortimer claimed, rather weakly, that Black got the contract because of graft but then Forbes changed the rules on him, and thus Forbes was a "double crosser." Implausible. The contract terms were hard, but Pontiac accepted them.[26]

The manner in which the bids were considered for the foundations at Northampton, and what happened to them, were to become critical in evidence for the Senate investigative hearings and subsequently the joint trial of Forbes and Thompson, which took place after Black had died. Jim Black left no notes for posterity on what had occurred or who said what.

By the time Forbes returned from the western trip, Harding had heard complaints about him from three influential members of the American Legion: Assistant Secretary of the Navy Theodore Roosevelt, Jr., Bill Deegan, and Lee Garnet Day. Over breakfast at the Willard Hotel these three New Yorkers "conferred on the hospital situation in New York, which is bad," Roosevelt wrote in his diary. Though Forbes had plans for a new hospital under way at Tupper Lake, New York, this could not be raised up overnight. Tuberculosis cases were not being adequately served in the state. There were problems in the district office in New York City, and criticisms were coming from all sides, from furious, frustrated veterans to angry, demoralized employees. Later in the day Roosevelt accompanied Deegan, Day, and John J. Wicker, another legionnaire, to the White House. "The President listened to their troubles, in his pleasant affable way, and said he would try to rectify them," Roosevelt observed. "Personally I feel that no rectification will come except of a temporary nature. The real problem lies with Forbes. He is a 'blow-hard.'" Day later reported his frustration. "Frankly, I could not tell at times whether [Forbes] was acting on his own instructions or was receiving word from higher up." Day said he told Harding the Veterans Bureau situation "was rotten from the core out" and that Forbes acted in haste, as though hospitals "could spring up overnight." Roosevelt waged a continuing campaign to oust Forbes as untrustworthy and inept, aided by Deegan, who was running for the position of national commander of the American Legion. On the first Saturday in July, Roosevelt went to Gettysburg to watch military maneuvers with the president, and afterwards dined with him: "We lallygagged on every conceivable subject. I lived up to my reputation as harbinger of woe by telling the President I felt he should get rid of Forbes." A week or so later Roosevelt reviewed the New York situation with Deegan: "Forbes, I am afraid, is no good. There is no question but what we want is action, unchanging action." Later in August Roosevelt met Deegan at the Harvard Club in New York and the two went off to lunch at the Biltmore. Roosevelt was backing Deegan, "an awfully good fellow," as the next commander of the American Legion. Both men believed that the legion had been putting too much emphasis on the soldiers' bonus rather than the sick and wounded.[27]

Criticisms of Forbes's character and management style fanned the flames of dissatisfaction about veterans' services, and vice versa. The establishment of the Veterans Bureau was supposed to create an efficient organization to solve problems that were evident in 1919, but many of the problems were still there in 1922, in many, if not most, parts of the system: slow responses to applicants, red tape, lack of jobs, inadequate hospital services. Forbes's promises had stirred enthusiasm in the early phases of reorganization, but those not (yet) delivered became false claims. It was not Forbes's fault that New York lacked hospital beds for tuberculosis, but who else was there to blame?

Those in the spotlight are vulnerable to dissection of their moral character, manners, and private life, and speculative gossip can be entertaining. Was Forbes a bad man? Did he have a disreputable past? Rumors flourished. Federal Judge Horace Worth Vaughan of Honolulu sent a vitriolic letter to US Senator Morris Sheppard of Texas (both Democrats), which circulated among a number of his congressional friends in Washington in mid-1922. The letter reported Forbes's desertion from the army in 1900 among other criticisms and ended with a flourish: "You better keep track of what this fellow is doing. He was regarded here [in Honolulu] as slick and shrewd, crafty and resourceful, unscrupulous and unprincipled." Good stuff for Democratic gossip networks. In July, Vaughan's letter was passed on to the American Legion, accompanying a letter from the legion's post commander in Honolulu to National Commander Hanford MacNider, which described Forbes as a "four-flusher . . . ungrateful and unreliable . . . absolutely unscrupulous and lacking in honesty." He was alleged to be a man who caved in when cornered, yet also someone with sufficient cunning to destroy his War Department files to protect himself if necessary, and someone who might end up either rich or in the penitentiary. The more such stories circulated, the more fantastic they became.[28]

Because of the rushed processes by which Charles R. Forbes had been appointed as director of the Bureau of War Risk Insurance and then confirmed as director of the Veterans Bureau, there had been few public reports on his origins, education, and experience. Forbes continued to offer up false tidbits about his life with the gusto of an old-style raconteur. Had he really sailed before the mast to Australia on a square-rigger as a young boy and been beaten by a sadistic captain? (No. Yet this story was attached to an official photo.) Why, when gazing out of thirteenth floor windows over the Connecticut Valley during a satisfying inspection of the Bureau's well-run subdistrict office at Hartford, did he say he was born in the Berkshires? Over the Massachusetts state line, he said; one can imagine him waving in that direction as he spoke. He was a second lieutenant in the cavalry when he was last in Hartford, in 1896, he added. Neither claim was true. The drama of the moment was more important to Forbes than the cloudiness of years past. Even Forbes's secretary, Merle Sweet, had scant information about his boss's past: "I have heard it said that Col. Forbes was married before and had some children, but I have never sent a check to any of them." In fact, his first wife, Sarah "Sadie" Forbes, who had not remarried, was working as an operative and foreman ("forelady") in a shoe factory in Brooklyn, and their two grown children, alive and well, read about him in the newspapers. Forbes was by no means alone in camouflaging his past. (F. Scott Fitzgerald made this a pivotal theme of *The Great Gatsby* in 1924.) However, members of the burgeoning business and professional classes were sticklers for exactitude. An ungraspable past and drifting memories were bound to damage the reputation of a senior government official when serious criticisms of his character were raised. And now they were.[29]

Three days after he returned from the western trip, Forbes traded in his 1921 Cole automobile for a new machine, a Stutz six-passenger convertible, serial number 12080, from the Stutz sales offices at 1507 Fourteenth Street in Washington, DC. Within months, federal agents were scrambling to connect this purchase with the money Mortimer allegedly gave him in Chicago as a bribe. They were unsuccessful, but the timing of these incidents seemed convincing in itself. Forbes traveled on district office work in Eastern Districts 1, 2, 3 and 4, between July 31 and August 6, mostly by car, billing the government for his expenses on gas and oil. On the open road, the stifling summer air swirled back over the open car as welcome breeze.

The augurs for Forbes still did not look too bad. He had sidetracked General Sawyer on most of the hospital construction program. While Forbes was on the western trip in June and July 1922 American Legion officials turned on Sawyer because of Harding's decision, which Sawyer strongly endorsed, to build a veterans hospital for neuropsychiatric patients at Battle Creek, Michigan, instead of Illinois, thus favoring the former state. Hostile telegrams flew between Sawyer and A. A. Sprague, the legion's expert on hospital affairs. In July, Sawyer sat down and wrote Sprague a condescending, five-page, single-spaced letter, in which he deplored the influence on government of "outside organizations." Sprague fired back: Sawyer was a noncombatant who could not really know how men "lose their nerve, their health and their minds in their devotion to duty." Sprague told him to "stand aside." President Harding intervened, declaring that he was as capable of making hospital location decisions as Colonel Sprague, and that General Sawyer was "answerable to me." These salvos between the American Legion and the White House gave Forbes some temporary breathing space.[30]

Forbes gave the impression that his relationship with the president was fine and told one audience early in August that on a recent evening, "despite the worries of the rail and coal strike and other pressing problems, President Harding talked with me concerning our hospital plans for caring for disabled service men, from 10 o'clock in the evening until 2 the next morning." Later in August, Forbes wrote his wife, Kate, in Great Britain that while Harding was "head over heels" with the labor controversies, he (Bob Forbes) had a "very nice visit" with Mrs. Harding. Kate Forbes sent intermittent letters but kept her travel plans largely to herself. Armed with letters of introduction from the US State Department and the US Veterans Bureau arranged for by her husband, and living on American dollars in war-torn Europe, she was living the life to which she had aspired. This included attending a garden party at Buckingham Palace and later, in full court dress, attending a royal reception in Holland. She was considering wintering in Italy. Back home, Colonel Forbes needed a recuperative break; it was difficult to sleep; he was taking a battery of medications for his heart and for pain (neuritis) and had trouble with one arm. Merle Sweet saw half a dozen bottles of prescription pills and medicines on his office desk and in a drawer. In August, too, Harding turned down Forbes's request to make a trip to Honolulu and the Philippines on Veterans Bureau business. Forbes had hoped to travel by ship from New York via the Panama Canal to get a rest along the way. He wrote Kate early in October that Harding preferred him to visit Europe rather than the Philippines, and felt "very kindly" to the prospect because there was a "great deal at stake in Europe." But his plea for any foreign business trip was nixed.[31]

In the absence of his wife and daughter, Mr. and Mrs. Mortimer acted as substitute family members. Katherine Mortimer returned to Washington seriously ill, was hospitalized, and operated on (for reasons undisclosed) but recovered. "She looks much better and feels a great deal improved," Forbes wrote in early August to a friend they had met on the western trip. Later in the month, the Mortimers met up with Forbes at the famous Greenbrier Hotel in White Sulphur Springs, West Virginia, where Forbes planned to take a week of rest. The three were outwardly all on good terms. Forbes drove down with Sweet so they could check out two possible sites suggested by Howard Sutherland of West Virginia, the Republican chair of the (weak) Senate committee on veterans. (Sweet's report on one of the sites, recommended for mental patients: a "dump of an old hotel above a bluff 200 feet above a railroad [the C&O], a very dangerous place." The second was also rejected, as a training center.) The colonel had spent the week "loafing in the mountains of Virginia," Sweet wrote Mrs. Forbes, and taken a "real rest," compared with the rigors of the western trip, where he had only a three-day rest in Seattle with "old cronies and friends."[32]

Forbes's break with Mortimer came in September. Sometime after Labor Day, a special agent from the Department of Justice came to Forbes's office to ask him about Mortimer and a man called McChesney, seeking the pair of them on a liquor deal. A flurry of activity followed. Forbes sent a Veterans Bureau agent over to the Department of Justice for more information; Forbes and Sweet met with William J. Burns, the director of the Bureau of Investigation, to discuss Mortimer, and Agent McInerney of the Veterans Bureau investigated Mortimer independently and made a statement to both Forbes and Burns. The Department of Justice brought Forbes what he ac-

cepted as the "real information": Mortimer was the "social and professional bootlegger of Washington." Like Captain Lannen, Mortimer's best man,
before him, Forbes experienced a sudden transformation. . . . Suddenly his
eyes were opened. All seemed clear. He learned that Mortimer was seeking
information, mostly but not always about liquor, from "every department of
the Government." The man was smooth, radiating probity and spewing out
lies.[33]

One day in October Mortimer appeared at the office shared by the two military liaison officers at the Veterans Bureau, Lieutenant Commander Charles
R. O'Leary of the navy and Major John P. MacDonnell of the army. Mortimer
wanted to know whether the Sutherland construction company, which he
professed to represent, was going to get the contract for additional work
on the tuberculosis hospital at Tupper Lake, New York. MacDonnell and
O'Leary reported to Colonel Forbes, who sent for Elias Mortimer and William M. Sutherland of the Sutherland Company. A Sutherland vice president, George W. Williams, was also present. Forbes asked whether Mortimer
was representing the company, and Sutherland said no. Mortimer claimed
he was representing the company on other contracts. This too was firmly
disavowed. Forbes still could not rage at Mortimer to his face. Only after
Mortimer had left did Forbes say he had been hearing things about Mortimer and advised the contractors to have nothing to do with him.
    In the evening, Sutherland and Williams dined at the Occidental Restau-
rant, where they ran into Mortimer. Williams later described Mortimer's extraordinary projection of affability and trust. He and Mortimer left Forbes's
office together in a "friendly" way, Williams said: "It took me from that time
until I met him in the evening to get into a mood where I wanted to call
him a liar." According to another witness at the restaurant, Williams, after
calling Mortimer the biggest liar and four-flusher he had ever known, proclaimed, "I am through with you." Whereupon Mortimer smiled and said,
"Well, I have got to be going," and left. He did not play by normal rules.[34]

The colonel and Mortimer were no longer friends. But what about his other
friend in the trio, perhaps more than a friend, the marriage-trapped, abused
Katherine Tullidge Mortimer, whose family could not be counted on to
protect her? Her father and older brother were settled in Mexico for the

duration, where Edward was prospering as a doctor, living on a ranch, and meddling in Mexican politics. Her mother was emotionally unpredictable. Forbes and a certain Sidney Bieber, a Republican national committeeman in the District of Columbia, joined forces. Oddly, Forbes had first met Bieber in Washington when he (Forbes) was a teenage apprentice musician at the Marine Band School, but then, after a long gap, they met again. Bieber had known Mortimer and members of the Tullidge family for years and worked with Mortimer before turning against him. Both men attended the wedding of Katherine's sister Margaret Tullidge to Dr. Robert Porch Sturr in Philadelphia in September. While they were there, Katherine's aunt Margaret Williams (sponsor of the ceremony) and Katherine's friend Carolyn Harding Votaw (matron of honor), asked Forbes and Bieber to look after Katherine because of Mortimer's brutality. Forbes and Bieber became her protectors.[35]

Soon after the wedding Forbes accompanied Katherine Mortimer, her aunt Margaret Williams, and family friend Mrs. Thomas Hogshead to Staunton, Virginia, to consult a shrewd lawyer, Stephen Timberlake, who gave them advice and the name of a divorce lawyer in Philadelphia, where the petition should be made. Back at the Wardman Park Hotel in Washington, Forbes helped Mrs. Mortimer look for papers that might incriminate her husband, finding, among others, two blank whiskey withdrawal permits. She went back to Philadelphia, joining her mother in the Tullidge family home and filed for divorce, claiming "cruel and barbarous treatment" and "indignities to the person."[36]

While Forbes's struggle for authority with Charles E. Sawyer over the Veterans Bureau and veterans hospitals continued, Mortimer became a dark presence in his life—a man imbued with sociopathic charm and guile, and the ability to upend a former friend's life. The first phase of his method, co-opt an individual in the hope of mutual profit, was over with respect to Forbes. The second kicked in: annihilate his reputation and career. Forbes's willingness to help Katherine Mortimer added fuel to Mortimer's cold fire. The western trip had given Mortimer a rich source of material to be manipulated, when the time was ripe, for the role of a lifetime as a courtroom star.

8 HARDING RESURGENT

White House versus Forbes

On September 19, 1922, President Harding vetoed the Soldiers' Bonus Bill and sent a strong message to Congress along with his veto: Congress was providing "a very dangerous precedent of creating a Treasury covenant to pay which puts a burden variously estimated between four and five billions upon the American people . . . to bestow a bonus which the soldiers themselves while serving in the World War did not expect." Services to disabled veterans were another matter. The government provided funds "gladly and generously" to meet the binding obligations to ex-servicemen, he said. The House of Representatives voted to override the veto, but the Senate did not. Harding won. A more forceful Harding was in evidence. The same month, at Attorney General Daugherty's request, James H. Wilkerson of Chicago, a newly appointed federal judge, issued an injunction to stop the strike of railroad shopworkers. The strike was stopped. Harding accepted responsibility for the controversial use of an injunction and survived the wrath of organized labor and criticism in the press.

With the soldiers' bonus shelved, Harding turned his attention to the US Veterans Bureau, which, by virtue of the failure to achieve a department of public welfare and a merchant marine, was the most visible achievement of his administration. Major veterans' groups were objecting to White House adviser General Sawyer's "interference" with Forbes's hospital location decisions, and Forbes was acting as though he were running an independent corporation with stronger ties to veterans' groups than to the White House. Harding had made his view plain in dealing with the politics of the bonus, namely, that money for the Veterans Bureau to care for disabled veterans was a better policy (and much less costly) than giving everyone who served in World War I a sum of money. Without the countering pressure for the bonus, a significant question arose. Were all the costly new veterans hospitals being developed really needed?

American Legion delegates were spoiling for a fight in the fall of 1922. Sawyer's slanging match with American Legion hospital leader Colonel A. A. Sprague in the summer had begun as a disagreement over Harding's decision to locate a veterans hospital for neuropsychiatry in Battle Creek, Michigan (supported by Sawyer), rather than in Illinois (as Forbes wanted, supported by his medical experts), but had escalated to a battle in which lines were drawn. Sawyer, on behalf of the White House, saw the American Legion as a private group that should play no part in policy making. He was supported by General Charles G. Dawes, the former budget director, as well as by Harding. Dawes backed Sawyer as a voice for federal economy and told him there was no need to jump when the legion said jump. The American Legion, which considered itself the founder, technical adviser, and watchdog of the Veterans Bureau, supported an expansive hospital agenda, and worked closely with Colonel Forbes. The National Commander of Disabled American Veterans put the view of the veterans' lobby simply: "We want conditions to be such that Colonel Forbes will be responsible for anything and everything pertaining to the disabled men." Forbes was out on a limb, while Sawyer was recognized as part of an increasingly activist White House.[1]

Harding called in Colonel Sprague to meet with him and General Sawyer shortly before the American Legion's national convention in mid-October, and got them to declare a public truce. Legion delegates drawn to New Orleans from across the country cheered at reports of a gradual improvement in the operation of the Veterans Bureau, despite Sprague's 250-page report to the convention that described problems in every Veterans Bureau district. Fury rang through the hall when they heard about the truce. A resolution to demand Sawyer's removal as chief coordinator of the Federal Board of Hospitalization passed by 601 votes to 375. Harding's name, in addition, was followed by a "roar that was more of a 'razberry' than a tribute." Harding held firm. Sawyer continued in his position.[2]

Forbes went to the legion's convention with several aides, expecting to give a speech. The White House called them back to Washington by telephone. Forbes explained in a letter to his wife that William F. "Bill" Deegan of New York, a candidate for the position of national commander (and by then one of Forbes's major critics), had described the presence of Forbes and his staff as a deliberate attempt to inject Republican politics into the legion to get a commander acceptable to the president. Maybe so. Forbes was lying low after he returned to Washington, "out of reach of the telephones and pernicious visitors." His star was on the wane.[3]

The weight of the legion's wrath fell on Sawyer. A scathing resolution accused him of hampering Forbes as director of the Veterans Bureau; as unable to understand the need for immediate action to build hospital beds and completely ignorant of existing conditions; of being more interested in the economy than in saving the lives of disabled veterans; of publishing inaccurate statistics, and being "temperamentally unfitted" for his position. Sawyer was at the White House with his colleague Dr. Boone when the resolution was adopted. Boone reported that he "felt the sting very deeply," and left for Marion, Ohio, to recover. Forbes felt battered too. His once-trusted friend Elias Mortimer had tricked and wounded him. A lasting friend, Wallace Farrington, then governor of Hawaii, wrote to ask when the Forbes family was coming to visit. Forbes answered despondently: "My small family is presently in Holland, so if, as you observe, we were but in the same place, we might have a jolly time together. As it is, my official duties keep me pretty well tied down, and too weary to enjoy the little social relaxation for which I find time." In an unguarded moment, Forbes told Sawyer that the Veterans Bureau was "the biggest lemon ever given to an hombre to run." Still, neither of them would cooperate with the other.[4]

The 1922 midterm elections on November 7, 1922, left the Republican Party with only nominal congressional majorities for the Sixty-Eighth Congress, which began in March 1923. American voters showed little comfort in President Harding's efforts to take bold decisions and seize leadership of the Republican Party—if, indeed, they were even aware that he had tried. Harding's inspirational book, *Our Common Country: Mutual Good Will in America*, had foreseen an end to jealous rivalries and a move beyond congressional stalemate. Published less than eighteen months earlier, it seemed to have been written for a different nation. The *Washington Post* explained the election results as a general dissatisfaction with business, social conditions, and life in general and as part of the psychological aftermath of the war, but such analysis carried little weight. Warren Harding and his administration had suffered a blow. Turnover of seats in Congress meant an unusually large break in continuity, a throng of new members seeking to make their mark, and a scuffling for new alliances. Historian Frederic Paxson wrote: "It would be misleading to assert that the Republican Party was in control of either house." Nearly one-third of the US legislators in the Sixty-Eighth were "new, noisy and ambitious," while "Democratic hopes fattened on Republican troubles."[5]

Democracy worked: the country, too, was noisy and unstable, tinged with paranoia. Attorney General Daugherty's anticommunist, antiradical point of view echoed that of the 1919 Red Scare, namely, that Moscow-driven enemies of law and order were "sowing the poisons of lawlessness . . . scattering and propagating their vicious theories of government" and instigating strikes and fomenting revolution in order to overthrow the US government by force. Why not accept that it was not only Bolsheviks, radicals, and immigrants who aimed to destroy the US government but also heartless government officials? From recognizing corruption in the procurement and supply of liquor, why not assume the likelihood of widespread corruption elsewhere? There were promising opportunities for legislators, old and new, to launch investigations into suspicious and wasteful activities in government.[6]

For weeks, Sawyer had been warning Harding that Forbes was going too far. Sawyer prepared a list of complaints: Forbes's inappropriate conduct of hospital affairs (bypassing Sawyer where possible); his allegedly ill-chosen medical advisers; the serious consequence of differences between the Veterans Bureau and the Federal Board of Hospitalization; neglecting to consult with Sawyer on the disposal of surplus supplies at the bureau's depot at Perryville, Maryland; and Forbes's objections to using independently run soldiers' homes as a base for new hospital construction. Sawyer noted that the veterans hospital service was already of such magnitude (ninety-nine hospitals) that it deserved a special board of directors (a good suggestion). Behind all of these were fundamental questions of value and costs, which Sawyer set out succinctly for the president: "If the policy of making these great, ornate, elaborate and high-powered hospitals is pursued, we shall finally find that we have wasted a large part of the money."[7]

Harding called a special meeting in his office at the White House one evening in the week following the November elections, to deal with contentions over veterans hospitals. Forbes and Sawyer were there, as were Treasury Secretary Andrew W. Mellon and members of the White Committee (the Treasury Department committee that was building hospital beds under the first Langley Act) and members of the Federal Board of Hospitalization (specifically, the surgeons general of the army, navy, and Public Health Service and the commissioner of Indian Affairs). Forbes's immediate problem was that the White Committee was turning over inadequately equipped hospitals to the Veterans Bureau, which did not have the funds to complete them. Sawyer sought greater control over decisions in the bureau. Harding was reviewing the policy dimension.[8]

Asked by the president to make an opening statement, Forbes gave the disastrous performance of a man who has nursed a grievance for too long. For more than an hour, he laid out what he called the "deficit of the White Committee," an estimated $3.8 million (more than $50 million in twenty-first-century terms). By the time he finished, it was after 9 p.m. Harding turned to the smooth and subtle Dr. William C. White of Pittsburgh, chair of Mellon's "consultants on hospitalization," the White Committee. As if flicking a small insect from his sleeve, White demolished Forbes's various statements as misinformed, inaccurate, or based on reasonable differences of opinion. Indian Affairs Commissioner Charles H. Burke pointed out that if Forbes were correct and more money were needed, the president would have to go to Congress for an additional appropriation, an unrealistic political move. Furthermore, Burke questioned the justification for the planned extensive hospital construction. In his view, building all the facilities under the existing Langley appropriations—for the White Committee plus the Forbes program—"would probably exceed the needs of the Government." As the evening grew late, there was no collective resolution.[9]

Harding invited a select few for an executive meeting the following evening to get the problem solved: Secretary Mellon, General Sawyer, Colonel Forbes, Dr. White, and a second member of the White Committee, Dr. John G. Bowman, an expert on hospital standards. The solution was simple. The White Committee agreed to turn over to the Veterans Bureau a site they had purchased and argued over at Chelsea, New York, with the understanding that Colonel Forbes "might build on it any type of 'hospital, shack, or bunk' which Colonel Forbes and the Federal Board of Hospitalization may desire." Forbes in turn would not purchase an alternate New York site, Arcadia Farms. The White Committee would use the appropriation for Chelsea and any other unexpended funds to equip hospitals already built under the first Langley Act, in consultation with Colonel Forbes.

Forbes had won the battle but not the war. He now had the funds to equip hospitals to his specifications, but the political and personal costs to him were huge. Secretary Mellon, who had reportedly liked him, told a reporter that after this experience his "confidence in Mr. Forbes dwindled." The White Committee went out of its way to dissociate its $18.6 million program of hospital construction under the first Langley Act from the $17 million second Langley program run by Forbes and his medical advisers. Secretary Mellon recalled that one of the difficulties had been "the zeal of the various heads to forward their own particular organization." The White Committee's final report, which circulated in draft a few weeks later, took the view that too many hospital beds were being built. Sawyer was on the bandwagon, declaring at a meeting of the Federal Board of Hospitalization in January, in Forbes's absence: "Really, men, we have no actual need for building this $17,000,000 worth of hospitals." Army Surgeon General Merritte Ireland clarified the point by stressing the political importance of veterans hospitals: "Do you think the Administration could have lived without building these hospitals?" The expected answer was "no." Sawyer told the Federal Board that the bureau was "one of the greatest menaces to the character and results of the administration." In this casual way, Sawyer and other like-minded critics dismissed—as at best political window-dressing—much of the work Forbes and his hard-working medical staff had achieved on the veterans hospital system. Forbes was no longer taken seriously.[10]

Absent other pressures, President Harding was as frugal as Sawyer. At the second November meeting at the White House, Harding criticized plans for lavish living quarters for hospital officers "with considerable emphasis," according to the minutes: "I lived in a frame house for thirty years; it was good enough for me, and it's good enough for any of the officers." Sawyer reported to the Federal Board that the president "lost his patience entirely." Forbes, in contrast, was proud of thinking big. His new hospital campuses included "storehouses, garages, [staff] quarters, vocational training, recreational buildings, fire protection, roads, landscapes, side-walks, water-works, railroad spurs" and were "completely mechanically equipped in every degree." He hired Katherine Mortimer's younger brother George Tullidge, who had studied mechanical engineering at Lehigh University, to travel to each district and survey equipment according to Forbes's specifications. "We have had a good deal of trouble with mechanical installation," Forbes explained. He also brought in a nationally recognized civil engineer as an adviser, Francis Betts Smith, familiarly known as "Dry Dock" Smith, for completing the second-try dry dock at Pearl Harbor after seawater pressure blew out the first.[11]

To critics, Forbes needed to be restrained. General Sawyer lost no time in extending his authority. On November 20, 1922, he called the first meeting of the Federal Board of Hospitalization to be held in the space he had appropriated at Veterans Bureau headquarters. There would always be some member of "our force" at the bureau, Sawyer said. "It looks now as if we would be very nicely domiciled here." Forbes was absent. Dr. Hugh Scott, the bureau's executive officer (on detail from the US Public Health Service), stood in for him at this meeting and endorsed Sawyer's agenda for economy. Scott reported that he had just had a "set-to" with Colonel Robert U. Patterson, the medical director, on the matter of employing a "high-end landscape gardener." Scott shared Sawyer's concerns about lazy, exploitative veterans who were not well served by being coddled. These were "gold brickers and fakers," the crowd that stirred up dissatisfaction outside.[12]

Forbes's inner circle at the bureau was falling apart. American Legion journalist Marquis James claimed that a triumvirate of Dr. Scott, executive officer; Colonel Patterson, medical division head; and Charles Cramer, Esq., chief counsel, were the "powers behind the throne" at the Veterans Bureau, but then they fell out. In James's telling, Scott thought Cramer and Patterson were leading Forbes astray and went to complain to Forbes, without result. Scott then went directly to the president, an act Forbes considered grossly disloyal. Scott's support of Sawyer suggested that he was trying to build a necessary rapport between bureau officials and Sawyer, but he was also maneuvering to become the next director of the bureau. (Sawyer wrote a letter of recommendation for him to the president.) While James did not apparently talk to Forbes, Cramer, or Patterson to get their perspectives, his conclusion that Forbes banished Scott to Muskogee, Oklahoma, is credible, though Scott recorded no complaints about his leaving when questioned later. (Scott had a soft landing. Oklahoma was his home state, and he was welcomed ecstatically to run a brand-new local government hospital for veterans.) At the very least, the story shows how confused the scene was at Veterans Bureau headquarters. Scott testified later that there was a lack of "esprit de corps" at the bureau, but he was unable to deduce why that was.[13]

Some staff members groused about poor conditions in the bureau and spread negative rumors, attributing them all to Forbes's ineptness. (In contrast, there were no reported charges from staff at headquarters that he was corrupt and lining his own pockets.) Most of the staff apparently accepted him as a complicated, out-of-kilter man, blamed the impossible conditions imposed on him (and them), or put up with him out of respect, affection, or concern. He could be unpleasantly authoritarian at times, as when he accused his hard-working, by-the-book chief clerk, William C. Black, of disloyalty in front of Black's own staff and members of the legal division. Black, who knew Forbes well, let this outburst roll over him. He continued to give Forbes helpful advice and made no criticism of him at the Senate hearings, when he was a witness and free to do so.[14]

Nuances and shifts in the political environment whisked by Colonel Forbes like flurries of dust while he stuck to a by-then outdated understanding of his mission: namely, to act as the director of an independent federal organization, free to cut through red tape and make executive decisions without entangling consultations. Kate Forbes sent him intermittent letters from Europe. She instructed him to send various items to her, including a Corona typewriter, books, and a corset, for which she included the measurements. (He mislaid this letter and had Merle Sweet, his assistant, write back for details.) In November, she wrote that in a picture she had seen of him he looked about sixty years old (he was forty-five), and he wrote back that he felt about ninety, "but that is the price of public office."[15]

The first, exhortative phase in the establishment of the Veterans Bureau was over. A period of assessment and readjustment had set in. There was a wistful quality to the speech Forbes gave his staff at the second annual conference of district managers and officers for medical and vocational services, in which he cited the obstacles, problems, and constant criticism they all faced: "It may be that all I hoped to do has not been possible. . . . These conditions, however, are a part of the job. . . . Your reward will be that comfort which comes from a job well done." He ended with a preacher-like exhortation: "do not ease up on your endeavors to bring back the great opportunity to those whose wounds and ills resulted from the service given that our nation might live on forever."[16]

In December 1922, he broadcast a radio message to the 24,000 veterans then in government hospitals, promising them that the bureau would work night and day to settle outstanding claims by Christmas and wrote an appreciative end-of-year letter to the bureau's staff, scattered in their thousands across the nation, which cited decentralization, vocational rehabilitation, and the hospital construction program as major achievements of the year, as indeed they were. "I am perhaps thinking not so much of what we have done as about how full of fallacies is life—and how during the history of this great Bureau we have made our mistakes! But another thought follows quickly—it is a proud realization that the errors progressively have grown fewer as the months rolled by." He emphasized this point: Making mistakes and learning from them was "at once the secret, and the explanation of our progress." And added: "This, my friends, is YOUR work and I recognize that in its performance you have given of yourselves not only without stint but in many instances with real sacrifice." The same month Forbes published his one and only annual report for the US Veterans Bureau (for fiscal year ended June 30, 1922), measured in tone but carrying a sense of urgency for expediting the hospital program: nine of the hospitals used for veterans, with 3,700 beds, were in seriously deteriorated condition.

For Forbes, the Veterans Bureau was first and foremost a consumer-oriented, full-service program. He put himself on the line for the adequacy of services given (or not given) to World War veterans; and they, as was their right, generated a constant buzz of complaints. As Forbes pointed out, every unhappy veteran having problems with his claim was a "walking propagandist against the Government." In the views of some, he had been overly optimistic, a "blow-hard," but at the same time much was expected of him. When the calendar shifted to 1923, he had been responsible for a national system of veterans hospitals, some woefully inadequate, for a mere eight months.[17]

Joseph "Joe" Sparks, the new head of the American Legion's National Hospitalization Committee, told the Federal Board of Hospitalization in December, "So far as the Veterans' Bureau is concerned, the operation of it throughout America was never better." Sparks wanted to push the hospital agenda urgently—"step on the gas and go down the line just as fast as we can"—because there was a "storm brewing." That is, a storm of political opposition.[18]

Forbes seemed to be on the edge of sanity in early January, 1923, when he visited the office of District 1 in Boston, which had been in general disarray for months. There he suspended the district director, Dr. Arthur E. Brides, former football player and coach at Yale—a heavy drinker who had expressed disloyalty to President Harding while inebriated (one of Forbes's charges against him). Forbes also accused the chief medical officer Dr. David Flanagan of disloyalty. Flanagan brought fiery lawyer Brigadier General John H. Sherbourne to the hearing, Sherbourne asked Forbes to retract the charges. Forbes refused. Things went downhill from there. Sherbourne shouted: "I am shocked and horrified" and later compared the investigation to a "star chamber." Forbes, furiously: "I am running this bureau and I don't propose to have anyone show me how to run it." Sherbourne: "I am not trying to show you how to run it, but how it is being run." A *Boston Globe* reporter described the argument as of "such intensity that spectators feared the two men would come to blows." Eventually, Sherbourne stalked out from the room, "his fists clenched, and his color high." Forbes "unclenched his fists, lit his pipe and opened the hearing." He was confined to bed sick the same night. In the end, after a hearing filled with accusations and counteraccusations, Forbes accepted Brides's resignation, ordered Flanagan and another staff member to Veterans Bureau headquarters for reassignment, made other staff changes, and told the office to move to less expensive quarters. As quoted in the press, he had found "intrigue and false ambitions" throughout the office. Forbes's sister Marie (Mrs. Harry) Judkins, the chief nurse of the district, was noticeably absent in press accounts of the hearings. Stella Marks, an assistant in Forbes's office, informed Laura Harlan, assistant to the First Lady, Florence Harding, that Forbes was "a very sick man" and needed immediate hospitalization. In all likelihood, she was correct. Harding did not act. At a meeting of division heads on January 22, Forbes told his senior staff that there had been "politics," "gumshoeing," and "intrigue" in the bureau, and he had taken measures to stop it. He also told them he was there to stay.[19]

In parallel, during the fall of 1922 and into 1923, Brigadier General Charles E. Sawyer fought Forbes for control of hospital supplies. Sawyer had his eye on the major depot at Perryville, Maryland, which held masses of military surplus goods (inherited from the Public Health Service in May 1922). Forbes and his military officers at the bureau saw piles of junk comparable to other piles the military had offloaded in France and the United States. Sawyer, chief coordinator of federal hospital supplies for the Bureau of the Budget, saw pearls among the deteriorated dross, including medicines and canned food that could still be used. Forbes considered turning over known narcotics at Perryville to federal prohibition agents for destruction, he said, buying new when necessary. Sawyer wanted to save them as an economy measure: "Now Colonel, if you have morphine, that would be just as good at the end of twenty-five years and codeine would be just as good at the end of the century." Forbes told the Federal Board of Hospitalization that it made no sense to keep the Perryville depot open. The cost of operating the depot was $643,000 a year (the equivalent of more than $8 million), and there were other such depots elsewhere. At a short meeting in September, members of the Veterans Bureau planning committee (which did not include Sawyer) voted unanimously to get rid of the goods and shut Perryville down. Scott wanted to destroy much of the goods. "Damned if we will destroy them," Forbes said; they would sell. But first, there needed to be some kind of inventory.

As Chief Clerk Black put it later, "You couldn't very well expect any of us to know what was contained in a conglomeration of eight or ten million dollars' worth of property." Partial attempts followed—for years—to assess the value of the goods sold in this enormous mess of stuff—"everything from square-rigged ships to twine," Forbes quipped. He moved toward a negotiated sale without a reliable inventory and without consulting Sawyer, ignoring or oblivious to the political ramifications. Maryland politicians had an interest in keeping the depot open and its staff on the job for economic reasons; Charles Cramer, chief lawyer at the Veterans Bureau, wanted the support of these same politicians as he sought the position of assistant secretary of war; and Sawyer was riding a potent theme, "waste of taxpayers' money," which could readily slide into charges of fraud.[20]

In November 1922, Forbes instructed Naval Commander Charles R. O'Leary, newly deputed to supervise the Perryville depot, to take steps immediately to dispose of surplus stocks at Perryville and cut the number of staff there as quickly as possible. O'Leary made a rudimentary inventory of the property, kept sufficient stock in hand to last the Veterans Bureau for a year, deducted 20 percent of usable goods for the Public Health Service as previously agreed (though it was not made clear on exactly what supplies the 20 percent was based), with the rest to be sold. O'Leary submitted Forbes's official request for clearance to the coordinator of the Bureau of the Budget in charge of surplus property (Major Sidney G. Brown), who checked with other government departments about whether they needed the property (the answer was no) and then submitted it to the chief coordinator, who cleared the list for sale. Forbes testified later that there were three potential bidders on the Perryville supplies, although this was not a regularly advertised sale. He had the name of the most promising candidate—an experienced Boston firm, Thompson and Kelly—checked out with the army and navy, and asked the chief of the Veterans Bureau Finance Department to check out the firm with banks. Although there was no reliable inventory, the Veterans Bureau quickly closed with Thompson and Kelly at a price of 20¼ cents on the dollar of assessed invoiced costs, with specific prices for some items, such as bed shirts, soap, and safety pins.[21]

For a civilian government operation, the process moved so rapidly it seemed suspiciously slick. Approximately fifteen loaded railroad cars went out from Perryville to Boston on November 15, before the agreed 80:20 physical division of usable goods had been finalized between the Veterans Bureau and the Public Health Service. When this news reached the Public Health Service, Surgeon General Hugh Cumming, accompanied by Dr. Frederick C. Smith, head of the Public Health Service Hospital Division, marched over to Sawyer's office at the War Department to report that goods were being shipped out that might have been used by the marine hospitals and relief stations under his command. Moral indignation was not enough; for Sawyer this was an emergency. The three men rushed over to the Veterans Bureau and had, in Sawyer's words, a "quite heated conference" with Forbes. Sawyer then went to the president, who approved military transport for Sawyer, Cumming, and Smith to proceed to Perryville forthwith. There Sawyer, exercising the president's authority, demanded the shipping stopped. Forbes's recollection was that the meeting in his office had been harmonious and that he had agreed to give the Public Health Service whatever they wanted. Hearing from Sawyer about the stop order, Forbes sent a telegram to Perryville to stop shipping, which was done.[22]

At a Federal Board meeting early in December, Forbes was furious at Sawyer's proprietary stance over supplies that were under Veterans Bureau jurisdiction. "I don't propose to pass the buck to anyone," he said: "It is up to me to make decisions." Sawyer countered: "I will not have this property that has been stored away at the cost of thousands of dollars disposed of until I know what our needs are." The uses of "I," "me," and "our" were instructive. The argument was fundamentally about control. Forbes said the bureau went through regular channels at the Bureau of the Budget and that he had talked with the president and told him he wanted to be relieved of this responsibility for both narcotics and liquor and put them under medical custody.[23]

In mid-December, Forbes and O'Leary, his chief of supplies, met with President Harding and Major Carmody, chair of the board of revision of the Bureau of Sales at the War Department, to discuss the amount the Veterans Bureau was getting for the surplus property. (The conclusion, after months of arduous work by federal accountants and investigators, was that the price was not unreasonable.) According to O'Leary, Harding was eager to know the details and was cordial when he and Forbes left the meeting. Forbes ordered shipping to resume. By then, Sawyer was darkly suspicious. His colleague at the White House, Dr. Boone, noted in his diary that Sawyer "wanted to know about Comdr O'Leary of Supply Corps. The General fearful that there is some crookedness in the Veterans' Bureau. Forbes & O'Leary do not look like a good combination." Sawyer had heard that O'Leary had a bad reputation in the navy.[24]

The relations between Harding, Sawyer, and Forbes had some of the characteristics of a family dispute between two hostile brothers, each wanting to please their father. According to Forbes, the president asked him to explain the troubles at the Perryville depot, and Forbes replied that there was no trouble: "It seems to be General Sawyer's hobby to object to anything moving out of Perryville." Harding told him to make an appraisal and bring it to him, Forbes said, and Harding added, "'We will settle this thing'—in a happy frame of mind and speaking in a kindly way." O'Leary had done an initial appraisal, which was turned over to the president with some samples of the goods, as requested. Forbes remembered that Harding objected to disposing of some of the towels. However, much of the stuff had deteriorated, including rotten catgut the Public Health Service had taken and hoped to use. Forbes said he had "a couple more" interviews with the president after this, at which Harding showed none of the indignation later reported by Sawyer, though he was concerned about selling surplus property that could be used.[25]

In December, Sawyer, writing as chief coordinator, Federal Board of Hospitalization, went to Commander O'Leary with a request for about $460,000 worth of items at Perryville (more than $6 million in twenty-first-century terms) for the use of the constituent homes run by the independent federal National Home. When Sawyer put in the required requisitions, these included the following: 20 barrels of whiskey and another 20 barrels of ethyl alcohol, 100,000 yards of gauze, 50,000 bath towels, 50,000 blankets, 100,000 gauze bandages, 40,000 pounds of absorbent cotton, 100,000 sheets, and 50,000 other towels. Forbes refused Sawyer's requests. He made matters worse for himself on December 28 by instructing his assistant director in charge of the supplies to release the loaded railroad cars that were sitting at Perryville, if "agreeable to the representative of the Public Health Service at Perryville."[26]

In January (1923) there was a second order to stop shipping. General Sawyer said he had been informed by Dr. Smith (of the Public Health Service) that mattresses were being loaded, which the Public Health Service needed. Sawyer called O'Leary, who denied mattresses were being shipped, but Smith confirmed that they were. Sawyer complained to the president that the Public Health Service was being "disregarded entirely." (Smith later testified that he had some "minor difficulties" over the mattresses but these were adjusted. He also said that in making the selections for the 20 percent for the PHS, the Veterans Bureau was "exceedingly courteous, and my belief is that they did give us the pick [i.e., first choice of the goods] in a great many instances.") The Perryville situation was ripe for probing by a Senate investigation. The president of a veterans' organization in Massachusetts asked Harding to order a special committee to investigate the Veterans Bureau "thoroughly, without fear or favor," charging that it was a "cesspool of corruption," but apparently supplying no supportive evidence.[27]

Sawyer's younger medical colleague at the White House, Dr. Joel Boone, supported Sawyer's views of Forbes and the Veterans Bureau. He wrote in his diary in late January: "Things look rotten at Veterans Bureau." "Talked to Mrs. H[arding] about Forbes, Director of Veterans Bureau—am pleased that she seems to have had eyes opened to him. . . . Detective Burns [of the Bureau of Investigation] called told Gen'l Sawyer that steal at Veterans' Bureau one of greatest in government history." "Forbes apparently on descent. . . . He is and always has been a 'nut' in my estimation. Believe his record will reflect adversely on Administration." In his unpublished memoirs Boone remembered that he and Sawyer had various conversations with Harding at this time, sometimes at meals, and Boone also discussed Forbes with the president privately. Boone sometimes wondered "whether the man was mentally sound; yet I felt that he was probably just plain crooked." Sawyer and Boone both tried to get the president to "get rid of Forbes." Harding listened patiently. According to Boone, "The President with his kindly, generous, patient disposition was always loath to believe anything ill of his fellow man. He wanted to get all the facts and unbiased facts and accurate facts, as far as he could, before he was willing to take drastic action." By the time Forbes asked [again] for permission to go abroad, Harding was becoming "very suspicious" of him and would only let him go after he left his written resignation. Forbes wrote Harding an undated letter of resignation for him to hold in reserve, with a sixty-day delay period, arguing simply, "After nearly two years of strenuous service, I find my own health so endangered, that retrenchment is necessary to safeguard it, and I realize that only a partial service is impossible."[28]

Harding, too, was suffering from a debilitating bout of illness, diagnosed as influenza. Nevertheless, in January 1923, it was not too early to begin maneuvering for the 1924 presidential elections. Problems in the Veterans Bureau had become overly visible and Forbes a political liability. Theodore Roosevelt, Jr., wrote in his diary in early February: "I don't think [President Harding] is at all awake to the seriousness of the general situation. He discussed with me in general the Veterans Bureau and told me of his troubles with Forbes. . . . Matters have gone so far that he is not even sure that he has not been financially crooked." Roosevelt added: "The President is fooling himself. He thinks that the last autumn election was not a repudiation of the national administration. It was."[29]

In January 1923, there was noticeable backlash against so-called military influences in the Veterans Bureau. The fighting had been over for more than four years. Army and navy officers were quietly withdrawn, Colonels Patterson and Rees to the army, Commander O'Leary to the navy. In parallel, veterans' organizations criticized the bureau's chief legal officer Charles F. Cramer for not being a veteran and as "un-American" because his division did not employ more veterans. The executive committee of the American Legion passed a resolution in mid-January demanding Cramer's resignation.[30]

Forbes continued to assure Harding that all was well. On January 12, he wrote Harding to request his absence for six weeks to go on an official trip overseas to investigate the advisability of training men in Europe, where thousands of Americans were still stationed. The award of hospital contracts was practically completed, he reported, the more pressing problems of the bureau had been settled, and "in view of the highly developed and effective service which the bureau is giving," he felt able to take time away. He would take merely his secretary, Mr. Sweet. Harding, discouraged and unwell, refused the request. Forbes decided to go instead on a short personal trip to Europe, where he could at least see his wife, Kate, and his daughter, Marcia. In his passport application, he gave his address as the home he shared with Kate on Vashon Island.[31]

Charles Cramer resigned on January 26, amid rumors about irregularities in the purchase of the hospital site at Livermore, complaints about his effectiveness as chief lawyer at the Veterans Bureau, and general criticism about Veterans Bureau contracts, which went through his office. Cramer submitted his resignation after Forbes had a conference with President Harding in which Harding clearly gave the order to remove him. Cramer took the blow hard. He had hoped to move on to become an assistant secretary for war. Now he would be jobless.[32]

A final blow for Forbes's deteriorating reputation was that rumors about his character and messy life history were filtering into official documents from different sources. One extraordinary meeting took place just before he left for Europe; extraordinary because of those involved: Katherine Mortimer's emotional mother (Katherine O'Donnell Tullidge), the disaffected wife of Charles Cramer whom Forbes had fired (Lila Cramer), and the deputy director of the Bureau of Investigation (J. Edgar Hoover). Mrs. Tullidge had heard a rumor that her twenty-seven-year-old, still married daughter was going off to Europe with Charles R. Forbes, a married man. She contacted General Sawyer, who telephoned J. Edgar Hoover and asked him to meet with her, which he did, making notes that were duly filed. "Mrs. Tullidge was in a highly nervous state," Hoover wrote, "and several times during the course of the interview burst forth in tears." She had heard "in a round-about way," from unnamed individuals who thought she knew this already, that her daughter was planning to go to Europe with Forbes. The two had been intimate for some time, she revealed; she thought her daughter was under the influence of "dope" and thus not responsible for her behavior. Mrs. Tullidge wanted federal agents to find Forbes posthaste. Hoover said he would tell Director Burns, assured her there would be no publicity, and got in touch with Special Agent Edward Brennan in charge of the office in New York at 15 Park Row. A special agent found that Forbes had cancelled his reservation at the Army and Navy Club, located and interviewed Katherine Mortimer at the Pennsylvania Hotel, and concluded that no further action was necessary. The FBI's standard incident forms, duly filled in and signed, were sent to headquarters. Case closed. In the process, Hoover's efficient filing system held information that Forbes was an adulterer who had a relationship with a married woman. Lila Cramer, who disliked Forbes, could spread the same news if she wished.[33]

An interesting coda to this incident is worth recounting here as an illustration of how stories mutate. Almost two years later, J. Edgar Hoover's memo appeared in the hands of the chief federal prosecutor at Forbes's trial, John W. H. Crim. He, in turn, jumped to the conclusion that Mrs. Tullidge had charged Colonel Forbes and Mrs. Mortimer with violating the White Slave Act (the Mann Act), with its sexual image of a man transporting a woman across state lines for immoral purposes. Hoover told Crim that Mrs. Tullidge made no such charge, though he could not vouch for what she may have said to General Sawyer. Nevertheless, the idea of Forbes as a seducer of women was firmly planted in Crim's head, so much so that he pressed FBI agents to find Forbes listed anywhere as a co-respondent in a divorce case, with no result. In fact Katherine Mortimer had made no plans to leave for Europe, for which she would require a passport (which she did not have). Forbes and Merle Sweet, his executive assistant, had their passports in hand.[34]

Charles R. Forbes, still officially director of the Veterans Bureau, left the United States for Europe on January 30, 1923, accompanied by the loyal Merle Sweet. Friends reported that the trip was "entirely for the ocean voyage," that he had been under continuous strain, had needed a vacation for months, had no thought of resigning, and expected to be back at his desk on February 20. Ill on the trip, he gave Sweet his money belt for safekeeping. The two men left at two in the afternoon on the Cunard Line's *Berengaria* for Southampton. The Bureau of Investigation, nothing if not thorough, ascertained that they checked no baggage, carried hand luggage only, shared state room D 113, paid $245 plus tax each for their tickets, and arrived in Southampton on February 5.[35]

TRANSITIONS IN 1923

Forbes's Resignation to Harding's Death

For six days, beginning January 30, 1923, Charles R. "Bob" Forbes sailed east across the North Atlantic. The voices of his many critics dimmed with the receding land: veterans and their organizations, opponents of the Harding administration, Washington insiders seeking to oust him, frustrated and ambitious legislators demanding change, and on a more personal basis, Charles E. Sawyer, Elias H. Mortimer, and their supporters. In a statement published while he was at sea, Forbes described the progress made in veterans hospitalization under his directorship and reaffirmed his vow to give veterans the best possible care. Yet complaints about veterans' services were widespread. What was wrong with the Veterans Bureau? The *New York Times* identified two major problems, neither of which focused on its director: (1) the bureau's unwieldy organizational structure and (2) political interference: "The politicians with their meddling are always a demoralizing influence, but they are harder to shake off than barnacles from a ship's bottom."[1]

The Harding administration and the Republican Party needed to project confidence and show success as eyes turned to the 1924 elections, and the Veterans Bureau needed a new image and a visible overhaul to counter negative reports. Harding's struggles as president in the months January to August 1923 form an essential narrative in the history of Forbes, the bureau, and the scandals that were to come. But history is never simple. Three other relevant stories played out in parallel, each coming from a different perspective: Forbes and the Tullidge family, as he planned a new career; Elias Mortimer as he inserted himself into influential networks and crafted a vengeful agenda; and Congress in setting up a Senate investigation of the Veterans Bureau. This chapter describes these stories, disjointed though they are in this period; for in the end, after Harding's unexpected death in August, all of them merged together.

Forbes's departure provided a wonderful opportunity for speculation, inside and outside of the press. An official in charge of a major branch of government—in this case with the vital job of caring for ex-soldiers for the nation—must expect criticism in normal times. When he leaves the country for an unknown period to go on an unexplained foreign trip, tongues wag and rumors flow. Had Colonel Forbes fled the United States for good? If he was running, what, if anything, was he guilty of? Had he taken a woman with him? Rumors suggested that Forbes had "some connection" with charges against the Veterans Bureau and that he might not be on a ship at all, but hiding in New York. William J. Burns, director of the Bureau of Investigation, added to the speculation when he "would not comment" on whether he was checking on Forbes's activities. Forbes was traveling for his health, it was said, but his movements would have been more believable if he had checked into the Johns Hopkins Hospital, where he could be described as a man exhausted from overwork (true), and everyone would know where he was. Perhaps if he died he would be dubbed a hero. The comments were still gossip, nothing more. The national press did not suggest that Forbes had taken a bag of ill-gotten federal money with him. At the same time, this gossip belittled Forbes and made it possible, in a very short time, for legislators and others to consider more damaging stories about him and his role at the Veterans Bureau.[2]

Forbes arrived in Europe apparently oblivious to gossip about him. He met his wife and daughter, Marcia, in Paris. Mrs. and Miss Forbes were then living at the Hotel Witterbrug at The Hague: a "lovely hotel," Kate Forbes wrote her mother, "that seems to us almost like home." Years later Marcia told her son Robert that they traveled with Bob to the sites of the battles of the Somme: "My mother said her father wept. It was the first time she had ever seen him cry." Forbes cabled President Harding his resignation from Paris, but then, according to one account, "friends of Forbes cabled him, advising withdrawal of his resignation, as he was under fire." Forbes cabled to withdraw his resignation but was unsuccessful. By leaving the United States, he had put himself in limbo. He rushed to return—rushed to the port of Cherbourg, that is, for he was still more than a week's voyage away from New York City.

Harding made Forbes's resignation public on the day he received it, February 15, releasing the resignation letter to the press for publication. Kate

Forbes did not follow her husband to the United States but returned to The Hague, and then went to Italy. In May, she won three gold medals for her tiny miniature pinscher (weighing less than three pounds) at an international dog show in Rome. Marcia's life was upended by being both companion and appendage to her mother during the European trip, but she attended school in Rome and developed a close friendship with a young Italian girl to whom she wrote throughout her life. Kate and Marcia Forbes arrived back in the United States at the beginning of September 1923, fifteen months after they had left.[3]

Accompanied by Merle Sweet, Forbes disembarked from the SS *President Harding* at the port of New York on February 25, healthier but soon to be unemployed. (His last day was February 28.) He tried to explain his expedition. The Veterans Bureau "had operated efficiently during the two years of his administration," and he had gone away in an "unsuccessful effort to get rid of a cold which had bothered him for a long time." Too late. The day of his return, the *New York Times* published a devastating article on the bureau with headlines that tell all: "$2,000,000,000 Spent for Aid. But War Veterans Suffer—Critics Allege Waste—All Relief Agencies Overwhelmed in the Early Days—Many Men Lack Care—Inquiry by Congress Impends on Charges of Bungling and Political Influence." There were charges that senior officials in the bureau had engaged in a "whirlpool of excess." Joe Sparks of the American Legion reported serious unrest among legion constituents: "I can say a ton of brick is going to fall on this Bureau within the next year." Others took a larger view, namely that reform of the Veterans Bureau was a "test of President Harding." It was.[4]

The Harding administration received a serious blow when the lame-duck Sixty-Seventh Congress, fueled by opposition from the farm bloc, killed the ship-subsidy bill, which the president had strongly pushed for. It would be too much if the US Veterans Bureau were seen to fail. The danger was that somehow or other a scandal would emerge that would be damaging to the Republican Party, fueled by zealous politicians and imaginative journalists. "It doesn't seem you want facts," Sawyer said to a reporter, "you seem to be sent out to get proof for a position you take." Meanwhile, Sawyer was looking for proof of his own. On behalf of his role as chief coordinator for hospitalization for the Budget Bureau as well as White House counselor, Sawyer was determined to find evidence to support his suspicions of waste, dark deeds, and possible graft at the bureau's supply depot at Perryville. When Harding showed no interest in pursuing this topic, telling his old doctor, "You know as much about that as I do," Sawyer continued to investigate.[5]

Harding accepted the resignation of Interior Secretary Albert B. Fall in January 1923, to take effect in March. Fall's reasons for retiring seemed quite reasonable: obstruction of his plans for Alaskan development and the need up build up his finances and attend to personal affairs. Teapot Dome and other oil leases were not (yet) a major issue. During the summer of 1923, sixty-one-year-old Fall, freed from a government position and sporting his trademark mustache, accompanied oil baron Harry F. Sinclair on business to Russia and other countries, far away from the Washington crowd. Fall listed fifteen possible destinations in his passport application, ranging from countries in western Europe through Estonia, Latvia, and Lithuania. There were rumors Harry Daugherty would resign, but Harding vigorously refuted them. Foreign and international matters engaged cabinet members in the spring. Harding's reputation was largely in the clear. In March, there was some questioning whether a Republican candidate other than Warren G. Harding should be nominated for president in 1924, but he survived, and by June his status seemed assured.[6]

Harding was still recovering from his serious bout of illness (he did not fully regain his strength until March) when he talked with Forbes at the White House soon after Forbes's return, sparking speculations in Washington's gossip network. One story circulating with the power of myth presented a surprisingly strong Harding grabbing Forbes by the throat, thrusting him up against the wall, shaking him "as a terrier shakes a rat," and shouting, "You yellow-belly! You've double-crossed me again!" The image was so compelling—and tailor-made as a pro-Harding political anecdote for Republicans—that it had a wide and continuing circulation. Some accounts used "yellow dog" or "yellow rat" as more vivid terms than "yellow-belly," and at least one embellished the incident's color by placing it in the Red Room. Popular writer Samuel Hopkins Adams soon had Forbes "huddled against the wall," and then staggering away, "his face discolored and distorted." Decades later, historian Robert H. Ferrell found a document from Adams's friend Will Irwin, dating to about 1936, which stated that a confidential but unnamed reporter for newsman Adolph Ochs stumbled accidently into a room at the White House and saw Harding shaking Forbes, and at some point, Ochs told the story to Irwin. But by then Ochs was dead, and the incident could not be confirmed. Most probably it was fiction. Nevertheless, the image, once visualized, is difficult to erase. That is what good stories do.[7]

A couple of days after seeing Forbes, Harding wrote Senator Atlee Pomerene, Democrat of Ohio: "The affairs of the [Veterans] Bureau are not in such a discouraging state as a good many people incline to believe. There is not a state of chaos by any means, but there is an extremely difficult job there, and the Director who performs it with distinguished success is entitled to the plaudits of the country." The job called for "eminent ability, unfailing patience and endless tact." Harding reported that he had asked General John J. Pershing to take on the bureau, but Pershing declined after thinking about it for twenty-four hours, and then Harding turned to General Frank T. Hines, "who has an exceptional record as an organizer and administrator, and I believe you will find the Bureau has been placed in good hands." Hines began March 1. Forbes was no longer a player in the Harding administration.[8]

General Hines ran the Baltic Steamship Corporation in New York and was strongly backed by Republican Senator William M. Calder of New York and other members of the New York congressional delegation. During the war, he had done a superb job mobilizing US troops and organizing their transportation. He understood large-scale operations, was an effective, no-nonsense leader, and had a calm and tactful personality. The Veterans Bureau's initial phase of reorganization was disruptive and stressful. Its second phase of reorganization involved acceptance and routine. Both phases epitomized the management style of its director. In 1923, Forbes's style was usefully and negatively contrasted with Hines's style. Forbes was the past, Hines the future. Where Forbes issued challenges and berated staff, Hines smoothed. He was remembered for taking a bus to work, in contrast to Forbes and his splendid Stutz. Journalist Silas Bent described Hines as "one of the gentlest and most urbane persons ever you saw, slender and brown-eyed and candid, with the smile of a small boy." Hines talked with General Sawyer at Perryville early in March and suggested careful planning and consideration before any action was taken there. He resolved the political problem of Livermore by recommending that, instead of one large hospital in Northern California, there should be two smaller hospitals, one in the north, one in the south, as American Legion officials were recommending. The Federal Board promptly agreed. Hines provided a needed lift to employee morale. He said he found the bureau well organized, and with efficient information services: "Not once have I asked for information that has not been promptly forthcoming." He had no incentive, however, to praise his predecessor in any way. Quite the reverse. Hines's image was as a much-needed savior.[9]

Forbes issued a statement to the press wishing success to General Hines, made some recommendations for Hines to consider, claimed that the injection of politics was the bureau's biggest problem, and paid tribute to the "splendid support" of President Harding and to Mrs. Harding's welfare work for veterans. He was ignored. His assigned role was to be blamed for problems in the Veterans Bureau. Part of the charm of the "yellow-belly" story was that Harding was portrayed as a forceful president and Forbes as a good-for-nothing bounder.[10]

Forbes's two most damaging critics continued to campaign against him. General Sawyer continued to probe for fraud and waste at the Perryville depot, purportedly on behalf of the White House. Elias Mortimer developed a more devious set of strategies. He had a two-pronged agenda with respect to Forbes: first, get his wife back, and second, punish Forbes. His mother-in-law, the credulous Mrs. Tullidge, was one possible avenue to achieve his first aim, but by this time she was wary of him. This was nicely illustrated in the Philadelphia press soon after Forbes left for Europe, when a misnamed Mrs. "Catherine O. Pillage," aged sixty-eight, reportedly accused her son-in-law, Elias Mortimer, of assaulting her at his apartment at the Wardman Park Hotel. Someone she took to be a federal agent (and probably was) reportedly told her that, if she accompanied them to the apartment, they would "fix up some legal matters" concerning Katherine Mortimer. Mrs. Tullidge went with them. During their discussions, Mortimer reportedly attacked her. Sergeants McQuade and Davis of the Philadelphia police "created a stir" in the elegant lobby at the Wardman Park on February 11 looking for Mortimer and bearing a warrant for his arrest. According to the press, he was released on bail with a hearing in police court scheduled two days later. The charges appear to have been dropped, but the story was too good not to circulate. One version had Mortimer hitting his mother-in-law over the head with a shovel. As usual, Mort escaped scot-free.[11]

Mortimer was more successful in other areas of inquiry. The bootlegging business was less promising than it had been, because of an increase in prosecutions and the forming of conglomerates and gangs, but he found a role that suited him perfectly: building ties with federal prohibition agents as a government informer or "snitch," while continuing to work (and profit) as a bootlegger to give him plausibility and necessary evidence. A cagily written memo by J. Edgar Hoover in February 1923 showed that charges Forbes had made against Mortimer were meanwhile dropped. Specifically, FBI Director Burns had dropped an investigation of Mortimer that was based on Forbes's accusation that Mortimer was attempting to blackmail him. (He probably was.) Burns directed the case, Hoover wrote, detailing Special Agent Walter G. Walker for this purpose: "I do not believe any reports were made upon this investigation as it was of a confidential character and personally supervised by Mr. Burns." Hoover "seemed to remember" that Walker was "suddenly called off the investigation, for what reason I, of course, do not know." Effectively, Hoover claimed that the charges against Mortimer were dropped because Mortimer was useful to FBI Director Burns.[12]

Mortimer did not confine himself to government work. In May 1923, he was charged as "John Mortimer" for conspiracy for violation of the prohibition laws in a federal case filed in New York against Colonel John W. Clifton, a lawyer from Tennessee, and others in a sting operation with federal prohibition agents involved. One of the agents, Sol Grill, said he met Mortimer along with one of the defendants, Joseph Cadina (or Codina), at a New York hotel in February or March. Cadina and Mortimer had led him to believe that Clifton was related to Mrs. Harding, "and had assured him that all Clifton had to do was call up the White House and that everything would be all right and that Clifton was the right man to get the permit through the department in Washington, DC." When charged, Clifton claimed he was a victim, and took his case directly to Justice Department officials to exert pressure. Mortimer's lawyer was Thomas B. Felder, known for getting pardons and negotiating deals on behalf of Attorney General Daugherty. Supported by DOJ, Mortimer's indictment was quashed. "I gave a bond and it was released by Mrs. Willebrandt," he reported. Assistant Attorney General Mabel Walker Willebrandt, determined to crack down on the illegal liquor business, had gained a hold over Mortimer that she could use. If he did not play as her informant, she would toss him back into the court system. He complied, developing evidence for indictments against prohibition violators in different states. According to Willebrandt, he had a "great mass of documentary evidence." Through his association with the department, he attained a strange kind of respectability.[13]

While Mortimer was easing his way into government by the back door, at least one anonymous letter reached the White House revealing parts of Forbes's past. A letter that has survived, addressed to the president, was received two days before Forbes returned from Europe. It was not strictly anonymous but signed by an unknown "James Duryea" from New York, without further identification or address. "Dear Sir," it began, "Just a line or two to enlighten you a little concerning the affairs of the head of the Veterans Bureau—namely Mr. Chas. R. Forbes. . . . Before you appointed him to the office why didn't you look into his past a little. He was an army deserter, also a wife deserter." (True.) The writer claimed that the first Mr. and Mrs. Forbes were never divorced. He "dropped out of sight just as mysteriously as though the earth swallowed him up" and "came back the same way bubbling up in public life just like a weed." The first Mrs. Forbes, the writer noted, was still living in Brooklyn with her family. There is no way to know whether Harding saw this letter or whether it was taken seriously. Harding's executive files and private office files for "Charles R. Forbes" disappeared, most likely destroyed. A copy of this letter was filed in a folder dealing with veterans hospitals, and there it remained. What we can say, however, is that someone who was well informed was interested in getting potentially damaging information about Forbes into authoritative hands.[14]

Two similar letters, received later in 1923, have survived in other places, and there were probably more. The writer of all three known letters was most likely Forbes's son, Russell Forbes, an able, ambitious, thwarted twenty-one-year-old with mathematical skills who had to leave school at thirteen or fourteen to work in the mailroom of an engineering company, who read about his long-gone father's reappearance as a prominent government official, and harbored understandable (and lifelong) resentment against him. Family feelings can cross the generations. According to one source, Sarah Forbes, "a small, well-preserved woman of 50 or so," had walked unannounced into Forbes's office in the Veterans Bureau one day, and Charles Cramer, the legal chief, was called into consultation. A delayed divorce might have been the topic for discussion, or money to pay for Russell's education, or something else. Whatever the outcome, the theme of bigamy was included in the files of the chief investigator for the Senate investigating committee. A rapidly prepared, typed-up analysis of the law of bigamy (where there is a presumption of death) in the New England states has survived, with the names "Forbes" and "file under Forbes" written on the file. The investigation did not use this information overtly, but again suspicions were raised. Four points can be made here: (1) stories travel, (2) stories about Forbes were coming together from different sources in 1923, (3) there is no such thing as privacy in official records, and (4) Mortimer had fertile ground to seed stories of his own.[15]

Campaigning to get his wife back, Elias Mortimer felt free to change his stories at will, and typically got away with it. In November 1922, he had threatened to name Sidney Bieber and Charles R. Forbes (her two self-appointed protectors) as co-respondents in her divorce case, but then reversed direction in a letter exonerating Forbes, Bieber, and Katherine Mortimer of charges of improper conduct that clearly stemmed from him. He was writing "in good faith and with the idea of putting an end to all this foolish talk," he said, as if he had nothing to do with it. Such shifts in view were unnerving to those involved.[16]

When Katherine Mortimer's mother, Mrs. Tullidge, weighed her religious belief that husband and wife should stick together against the reality of marital abuse, and came out against her son-in-law, Mortimer concentrated his charm on Mrs. Tullidge's gullible sister, Margaret O'Donnell Williams, whose husband, James, ran a creamery business in Philadelphia. Mortimer's capture of Mr. and Mrs. Williams was a tour de force. Margaret Williams had supported her niece in her search for a divorce, but her husband was angry because he had not been told about the divorce action. Wife then joined husband and became committed to Mortimer and against Forbes—an allegiance that continued through their testimony at Forbes's trial. Schooled by Mortimer, the Williamses accused Forbes and Bieber of turning Katherine Mortimer against them and even of abducting her. James Williams said he had gotten the "facts" from Mortimer, whom they were fond of, whose word they believed implicitly, who was their cherished bootlegger, and from whom Mrs. Williams had borrowed a considerable amount of money. They accepted what Mortimer said as gospel truth and adjusted their memories to match his.

After Katherine Mortimer started divorce proceedings (late in 1922), Mr. and Mrs. Williams sat at the dining room table with Katherine Mortimer and Staunton lawyer Stephen Timberlake and launched into a conversation that Timberlake described as "wild, excited, and at times incoherent." Mrs. Williams told Timberlake that Forbes was to give a $3 million contract to Mortimer and Mortimer was working on the contracts; that Mortimer handed Forbes $5,000 in Chicago; that Forbes gave "millions" to another party; that Forbes lost money in a stock deal and had to leave the Wardman Park Hotel because he could not pay and was now broke; that Forbes had a rich uncle who would help him; that Forbes "was making a bluff on what he could steal"; and that Forbes wanted Mortimer to go in on a deal selling narcotics and liquor from Perryville, but Mortimer told him he could not do it and that it was a "dangerous proposition." Mortimer reportedly told the Williamses that Bieber and Forbes were working on this narcotics/liquor deal, and they wanted to get rid of him (Mort) and that Katherine knew all about this. Mortimer had briefed the Williamses well, whipping up their emotions. Mr. and Mrs. Williams remained unshaken when Timberlake told them he had a report from the Justice Department that Mortimer was a bootlegger and potential blackmailer. James Williams examined the two blank liquor permits (for the withdrawal of alcohol using illegally obtained permits) from among papers belonging to Elias Mortimer that Katherine Mortimer had taken. Mr. and Mrs. Williams did not change their views. They were sufficiently wound up that at one point they thought Forbes and Bieber were going to kill Katherine. Mortimer was developing ammunition in his anti-Forbes campaign. When convenient, however, he claimed that he did not believe the "lying statements" made by Mr. Williams. It was not a difficult job for Mortimer to suggest ways in which Charles R. Forbes had allegedly fooled and cheated the US government.[17]

In Congress, Democratic Representative W. W. Larsen of Georgia introduced a resolution in the House of Representatives for a congressional investigation of the US Veterans Bureau in mid-February 1923 while Forbes was in Europe. Larsen wrote Mortimer at the Bellevue Stratford Hotel in Philadelphia, asking him for a copy of an affidavit he had heard that Mortimer had written to President Harding, in which Mortimer accused Charles R. Forbes of proposing to a contractor, "J.N. Thompson of St. Louis," that Thompson should raise his construction bid for an unnamed hospital from $32,000 to $52,000, and the two men would split the extra $20,000 as a kickback, fifty-fifty. There was no such affidavit. Mortimer claimed he never met Larsen. However J. W. [not N.] Thompson existed, and the allegation was specific enough to be taken seriously. Mortimer did not reply to Larsen. He did not need to. The story launched his initial strategy to bring Forbes down. Sitting at his desk at the Bellevue Hotel the same month (February), he proceeded to write a four-page document in pencil that listed charges he could make against Forbes. In it, he accused Forbes of steering the hospital construction contract at Northampton, Massachusetts, to Pontiac Construction instead of the low bidder, Northeastern; of doing a "very irregular deal" in a contract let to W. M. Sutherland Company at Tupper Lake, New York; and of proposing a $5 million liquor deal at Perryville, where, he said, reportedly quoting Forbes, "we could clean up enough on this one job to retire for life." According to Mortimer, Forbes told him that he was going to do all the buying of drugs, equipment, and supplies personally and reiterated that "we could clean up a nice pile of money." Again, according to Mortimer, he had refused to do business with Forbes, a "bad egg," since the day after Labor Day 1922; also Forbes had been working with Sidney Bieber on illegal transactions. Mortimer's handwritten memo (which appeared in testimony for the Senate investigation) includes one accusation based on fact, the admittedly unusual contract for the Northampton hospital foundations, one that has no credence (Tupper Lake), and two unsubstantiated claims related to drugs and liquor, which Mortimer, who dealt in these commodities, continued to pursue.[18]

Part of the genius of Mortimer's stories, then as later, was that he made Forbes sound like a small-town crook—a man tempted to fraud by easy access to drugs, materials, and contracts, as if he could pull them with his own hands from a corner-grocery shelf or take a cut from a deal on the street.

Mortimer portrayed him as if he were a bootlegger, a familiar stereotype in 1923, rather than the head of a major government bureaucracy with layers of administration between the executive office and the "goods." He ignored the fact that Forbes would need aides to carry off a heist and that the aides Mortimer got to know on the western trip (Merle Sweet and John Milliken) were models of propriety—by casting himself as Forbes's accomplice. Compared with the vagueness or inconsequence of rumors circulating at the time, Mortimer's characterization, though of dubious authenticity, was refreshingly clear. Mortimer's Forbes was a man who stole a wife from an adoring husband, borrowed large sums of money without giving a receipt while laughing aloud, and drank excessively at riotous parties: someone to be deplored because of who he was—a rogue.

Representative Larsen's call for an investigating committee was quickly replaced by a call in the Senate for a joint House-Senate committee, driven by forceful Democratic Senator David I. Walsh of Massachusetts. Instead, two days before the end of the Sixty-Seventh Congress in early March 1923, the Senate voted for an investigation by a select three-person Senate investigating committee with Walsh as one of the committee members. The allocated budget was $20,000. Walsh gave five reasons for moving ahead: reports of "waste, extravagance, irregularities and mismanagement" circulating in the press and in Congress; reports of "general dissatisfaction" inside the bureau; loss of staff because of the prevailing chaos; burdens thus placed on veterans as beneficiaries; and lastly, if the alleged conditions were substantiated, impairment of the bureau's morale. The first three were based largely on hearsay. Walsh had been furious with Forbes for not solving problems in New England, but none of these accusations suggested personal scandal or criminality.[19]

Republican Senators Tasker Oddie of Nevada and David A. Reed of Pennsylvania joined Walsh as committee members, with Reed as chair. Their goal was to look at Veterans Bureau leases and contracts, supplies, and other matters, to "send for persons and papers" as needed, and administer oaths to witnesses. The three senators met for the first time as a committee on the first day of the Sixty-Eighth Congress, March 4, 1923, less than a week after Forbes left his position. They spent little or no time discussing Forbes—none, according to the minutes. With General Hines newly in charge of the Veterans Bureau, the emphasis was on the future. Chairman Reed emphasized the need to improve administrative processes and reduce political pressures on the workings of the bureau. Director Hines, in his first week in office, identified four issues: (1) possible delays in hospital construction; (2) criticism of the handling of supplies at Perryville, Maryland; (3) some criticism of overhead costs of personnel; and (4) whether the bureau had taken decentralization too far. (He thought it had.) Hines promised full cooperation with the committee and appointed a staff member as liaison. Initially, the committee expected to begin public hearings in the spring of 1923. In that case, the discovery of problems and recommendations for their resolution would flow out of the hearings, as they usually did at congressional investigations.

However, the Veterans Bureau was a special case. Fact-finding was essential. None of the three senators wanted to run what was, in effect, a management study of a large, decentralized national conglomerate. The answer was to contract out—and here lies the single most-fascinating element of the Senate investigation of the US Veterans Bureau. An extraordinary individual, Major-General John Francis O'Ryan, quickly took over the investigation, becoming the fourth, and the most influential, member of the team. Republican Senator James W. Wadsworth of New York, who was chair of the Senate Committee on Military Affairs, recommended O'Ryan and asked him to consider becoming committee counsel. After making some high-level inquiries about whether he should accept, O'Ryan met with Chairman Reed, who said he would have entire charge of the investigation under the committee, that "no politics were involved," and there was "no desire to prosecute anyone criminally," and on these understandings, he accepted. General John F. O'Ryan of New York was a Democrat whose well-earned national visibility as a military leader and commitment to ex-servicemen meshed with his aspirations for a nationally prominent civilian position.[20]

The hearings were delayed to allow for data collection; the buy-in of groups of lawyers, physicians, and others around the country; the results of interviews and written reports; the chance to observe beneficial reforms undertaken by Director Hines in cooperation with the committee; and the identification of an appropriate slate of witnesses. The result was that the hearings began in the fall of 1923, rather than in the spring, after the shock of Harding's unexpected death.

In the months between the beginning of the Senate investigating committee in March and Harding's death in August, two other deaths occurred that
are significant to Forbes's story, and there were changes in other lives associated with him. The death by his own hand of forty-five-year-old Charles F.
Cramer, former chief counsel of the Veterans Bureau, was reported little
more than a week after the Senate committee began, on March 14. Cramer's
body was found on the bathroom floor of his home, shot in the head, a gun
by his side. Police ruled the death a clear-cut suicide. He was discovered by
the cook when he did not appear for breakfast. The evening before, apparently in good spirits, he had taken his wife Lila to the railroad station to
board a train for a twenty-four hour trip. Newspaper clippings about the
Senate investigation of the Veterans Bureau were on a table in the bedroom,
suggesting some connection to the death, and rumors abounded about incriminating suicide letters. According to Mrs. Cramer's lawyer, Charles Cramer did leave some letters, but these related purely to "personal matters,"
and as such were not revealed to the public. His widow received one of
the letters (and kept it private), but there is no solid information about any
others.[21]

The suicide of a newly separated senior official was bound to stir up questions about Forbes's conduct, as well as Cramer's at the Veterans Bureau,
with particular focus on hospital building contracts, which went through
Cramer's office for review. Forbes said he did not know why Cramer committed suicide, but he made some private inquiries and came up with "domestic
difficulties, and financial difficulties and some oil lands." He had heard rumors about Cramer's involvement in irregularities in the bureau, but there
were never enough facts to be able to take these seriously. He sent a wreath
to the house, "and that was all." Lila Cramer pulled herself together after her
husband's death and auctioned off the contents of their house. She attended
the auction wearing a "big willowy hat" and complained about the low prices the auctioneer obtained: $3.50 for a small Wilton rug. Having wrapped up
the estate, she went to Europe, out of the fray, returning early in September
from France.[22]

There was no clear explanation for why Cramer killed himself. The *New
York Times* considered Cramer a "victim of worry" but stressed the prevailing criticism of the Veterans Bureau as a confounding factor, plus Cramer's
hope to become an assistant secretary of war, which had been blocked by

the American Legion and other opponents, including some members of Congress. The *Los Angeles Times* described Cramer's death, reportedly the nineteenth recorded suicide of the year in Washington, DC, as symptomatic of the self-destructive character of the nation's capital: a city in which illicit liquor flowed, there was "drunken roystering" [*sic*] in some congressional offices, police protected gaming houses, and "dope" circulated, much of it from government stocks. Cramer was presented to his fellow Californians, Hollywood style, as a not-very-smart, socially ambitious man who got rich quick in the oil business in San Francisco, had poor eyesight, a crippled arm, a young and beautiful wife, and was lost in the "terrifying maze" of the Veterans Bureau, bewildered by the job, never able to "grasp it all." He had been "bitterly assailed" at the American Legion meeting in Indianapolis and forced to resign from a job that was too much for him. Like Mortimer's stories, this account had a pleasing cohesiveness to it.[23]

After he left office, Forbes was shunned by the Washington establishment. He had little to do in the spring and early summer of 1923 except wait (vainly) to be called to help the new director, General Hines or the emerging Senate investigation, and plan for a new career. He stayed for a spell in the country, near Staunton, Virginia, where his friend Sidney Bieber had some property in trust. Katherine Mortimer was there, too. They both attended the Staunton wedding of Mrs. Mortimer's younger brother George Tullidge to Anne Archer Hogshead in March, with Charles Forbes as best man and Katherine Mortimer matron-of-honor. The Tullidge family was there in force, without, of course, their in-law Elias Mortimer. Dr. George B. Tullidge was finally back from his sojourn in Mexico, and so—for a visit—was his convicted older son, Dr. Edward Tullidge.

Edward Tullidge was the focal point of his family's concerns. While rumors swirled in the United States that oil interests were stirring up rebellion in Mexico, he moved across the US-Mexican border at will, representing the Royal Mexican Petroleum Company and speaking on Mexican oil politics. After returning to Mexico from a speech in Los Angeles in April, he was arrested in Mexico City on President Obregon's orders and escorted across the US border near Laredo, Texas, thus becoming an illegal presence in two nations. Recaptured in the United States in June, after his parents had successfully used their influence to have the hard-labor/state prison requirement of his sentence changed, Edward Kilbourne Tullidge, MD, aged thirty-three, entered the federal penitentiary at Leavenworth in mid-July to serve a five-year term. He was escorted there by three US Marines. He expected to work as a doctor in the prison hospital at Leavenworth and help prison authorities control the use and circulation of drugs among the inmates. To his outrage and dismay, he was assigned to menial work and soon became a "regular nuisance and quite troublesome," according to the warden. Among other things, he was smuggling out letters that he did not think would be approved for mailing.[24]

Forbes needed rest and recuperation and to plan for the next step in his career. He did not return to the construction industry. Kate and Marcia Forbes were still abroad. It was not even clear where he would next be based. In Washington, the Harding administration continued on without him. Director Hines was well regarded, and in the spirit of reform, the Senate committee was gathering information from all Veterans Bureau districts. The Veterans Bureau was recognized as a problem being addressed. Its former administration was not (yet) equated with a "scandal." Similarly, there was no sign that anything momentous would come out of a probe of Teapot Dome (the oil leases case).

Attorney General Daugherty was touched by tragedy when Jesse W. "Jess" Smith, his close friend and associate, killed himself by a bullet to the head on May 30, after President Harding learned of shady deals done by Smith and talked to him in no uncertain terms. Smith died at Daugherty's apartment at the Wardman Park Hotel when Daugherty was staying at the White House. His corpse was lying on a bed with his upper body hanging over the edge and his head in a metal wastebasket, presumably to contain the mess. There was an inevitable but fruitless rumor: Was he killed because he knew too much? Daugherty was not in good shape. He was sick in the early months of the year. Criticisms of the Justice Department continued, including some from members of Congress. His son Draper, named in connection with a murder in New York in March, was committed to a Connecticut sanitarium as an "inebriate" in April. In June, Draper escaped from the sanitarium with the help of an accomplice and "fled in a fast roadster." He was sought by police and found in July, working for a coal company in Chicago.[25]

President Harding regained energy with the promise of better health and some strong support from the press. The congressional system was not working well, rent by self-interest, rings, and coteries. A *New York Times* article summarized the problem: "What seems to be the futility of our President is in reality the futility of our governmental system.... 'Normalcy' is a mirage that hovers over the desert of Congressional recalcitrance.... The eye of Congress differs from the human eye in that it closes completely against light.... The great mass of voters are sullen, vindictive."[26]

Harding decided to take his message to the country at large. On June 20, 1923, he left Washington by special train for the West Coast and then on to Alaska, accompanied by more than sixty people, on a so-called voyage of understanding that was designed to restore faith in the Harding administration. Three cabinet members were in the group: Albert Fall's successor, the effective Dr. Hubert Work; Secretary of Agriculture Henry C. Wallace; and Secretary of Commerce Herbert Hoover (who joined the party on the West Coast). At key locations along the route, Harding made speeches from the rear platform of the train, his voice amplified by a powerful sound system; the group included an acoustical engineer. In St. Louis, he made an extensive speech on trying "to get this great country of ours on the right track again," and supported American participation in the World Court as an issue separate from joining the League of Nations. In Kansas City, he reviewed the problems of railroad transportation and pushed for a consolidated, nationwide system of transportation. At different locations, he spoke of farm aid and on other topics. He spoke to veterans. In the trip as a whole, he made more than eighty speeches. This was not remotely a restful trip. In Alaska, he fell sick but reportedly recovered and went on.[27]

Forbes left Washington for the West Coast in July. By then he had met his two oldest children several times. Mildred Forbes was married to Carlos Sands, and they had a baby. Colonel Forbes was now a grandfather. After two decades of neglect, he wanted to be treated as a father, but his hope was greater than his ability to mend fences—if they could be mended at all. Russell passed up the opportunity to see his father just before he left for San Francisco. "My dear Russell," the father wrote to the son from the Hotel Pennsylvania in New York:

> I tried to get in touch with you but I become so blue at times I am beside myself but when this investigation is over I know that the public will get the true side of the Bureau and understand the effort I made to build up a big honest and

efficient force . . . I shall keep you informed what I do and where I locate in the meantime keep your good spirits be a big strong man, shun bad company and I hope that with gods help we will all get out of life some true happiness. I love you both so much and I am sorry for much but your affection will help me. . . . Kiss the baby for me.[28]

Travel was always a pleasure for Forbes, especially by sea. Journalist Will Irwin reported that Forbes visited Cuba. Merle Sweet received a postcard from Forbes from Panama City; he was traveling west "by water" via the Panama Canal. With no way to get in touch with him, Sweet wrote Charles Hurley, Forbes's old boss on the West Coast, to ask him to tell Forbes when he saw him that Sweet had some things he should see. The August premium on Forbes's life insurance was due, and Sweet did not want to pay it in case Forbes's bank balance was low. Forbes should wire him. The hospitals under construction at Northampton, Tupper Lake, and American Lake (which Forbes had fought for, but for which he would get no credit) were all progressing. Hurley's firm was building American Lake. Sweet, who by then worked for Director Hines, reminded Hurley that he was a little behind schedule.[29]

Sweet wanted to talk with Forbes about his sister Marie Forbes Judkins, who was fighting with other nursing staff at the Veterans Bureau district office in Boston. A male nurse, Haywood C. R. Mott, wanted her job and was colluding with other nurses and American Legion officials to get it. Judkins was also fighting with nurse Mary Bannon, who had her own faction of supporters and resented that she had not been appointed chief nurse instead of Judkins. The new district manager suspended all three of them in April, after urging them, to no avail, to "bury the hatchet on the spot." Judkins was reassigned in May to the lesser job of head nurse at the vocational school on Commonwealth Avenue. In the weeks that followed, she sent missives to Veterans Bureau director Frank Hines, asking for reinstatement as chief nurse and complaining about her new assignment. An investigation was largely favorable to her, except that she was "irritable." Hines suggested she transfer out of Boston if she did not like her new assignment. Marie was given the same underlying message as her brother Bob: Your time has passed.[30]

For the next step in his life, Forbes planned to launch an import-export business headquartered in San Francisco. He had told Merle Sweet there might be employment in it for him. Sweet met with a Mr. Dejohng for this purpose on a trip to California accompanying General Hines and told his wife "the proposition looked good." Forbes also expected to involve young George Tullidge, whom he had employed at the bureau to survey equipment in hospitals and clinics throughout the system. On his last day in office, Forbes had sent Tullidge off on a ninety-day inspection tour in six Veterans Bureau districts. Young George's absence from the bureau caused alarm and confusion when General Hines took over, raising suspicions—actually rumors—that Forbes had paid his protégé a generous salary to do nothing. Hines's directive "Find out where this man is" led to a flurry of telegrams before he was located and reined in as a member of the new regime. Tullidge stayed for a while, but a government job was not for him.[31]

And so the lives of all concerned might (or might not) have continued in mundane fashion with no major national scandal in view, except that on August 2, 1923, the picture changed abruptly. Warren G. Harding died of a "stroke of apoplexy" at 7:30 p.m. Pacific Time, at the Palace Hotel in San Francisco, after returning from his exhausting trip to Alaska. He was fifty-seven years old.

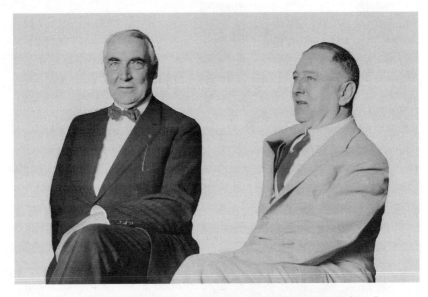

10. Harding with Attorney General designate Harry M. Daugherty, [1920].
Library of Congress, http://www.loc.gov/pictures/item/npc2007001905/.

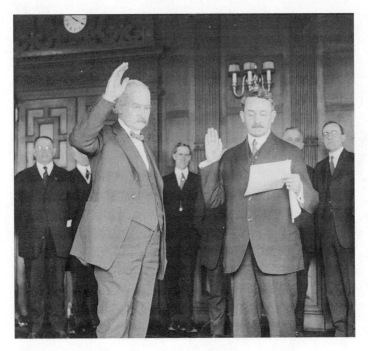

11. Secretary of the Interior Albert B. Fall is sworn in, 1921.
Library of Congress, http://www.loc.gov/pictures/item/npc2007003516/.

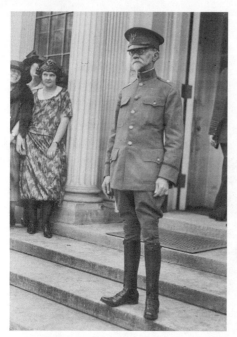

12. White House physician
Charles E. Sawyer with sightseers,
1921. Library of Congress, http://www
.loc.gov/pictures/item/hec2013001463/.

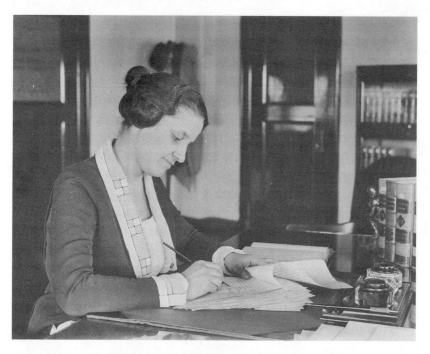

13. Assistant Attorney General Mabel Walker Willebrandt, 1921.
Library of Congress, http://www.loc.gov/pictures/item/hec2013002102/.

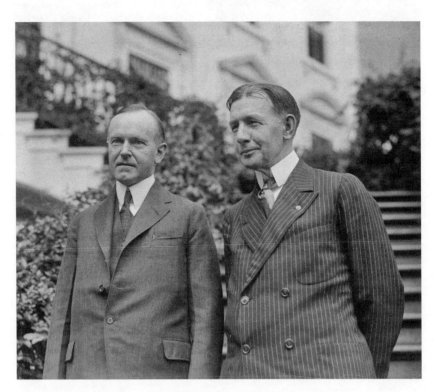

14. President Calvin Coolidge and his running mate, Charles G. Dawes, 1924.
Library of Congress, http://www.loc.gov/pictures/item/npc2007011637/.

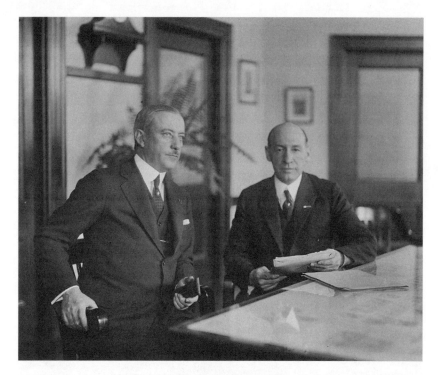

15. The two generals: John F. O'Ryan and Frank T. Hines, 1923.
Library of Congress, http://www.loc.gov/pictures/item/hec2013012887/.

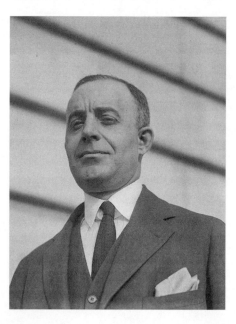

16. Elias H. Mortimer at the time
of the Senate Hearings, November
1923. Library of Congress, http://www
.loc.gov/pictures/item/npc2007009890/.

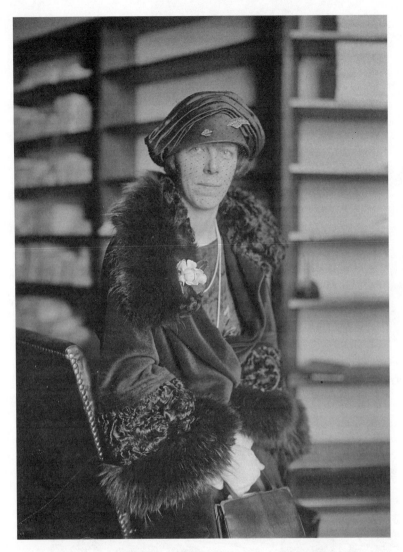

17. Katherine Tullidge Mortimer at the time of the Forbes trial, 1924.
Library of Congress, http://www.loc.gov/pictures/item/npc2008006052/.

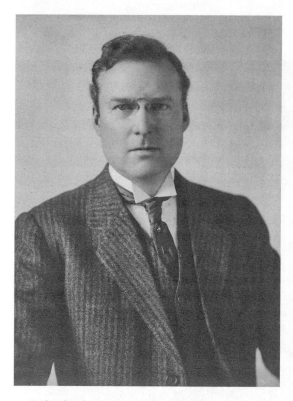

18. Federal Judge George A. Carpenter.
Library of Congress, http://www.loc.gov/pictures/item/2002695168/.

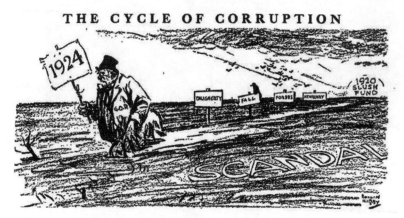

19. "The Cycle of Corruption [Daugherty, Fall, Forbes, Newberry]"
as perceived by Rollin Kirby with the 1924 elections in view.
By permission of the estate of Rollin Kirby Post.

PART

IV

SCANDAL TIME

10 COOLIDGE, COMMON CAUSE, AND THE POLITICS OF SCANDAL

Calvin Coolidge took the oath of office as the thirtieth president of the United States in Plymouth, Vermont, on August 3, 1923. He announced that he would follow Harding's policies. "The world has lost a great man," Coolidge said. In San Francisco, wild rumors circulated. Had Harding had an accident? Was he murdered? Brigadier General Charles E. Sawyer, Harding's physician and adviser, temporarily broke down. Harding's secretary, George B. Christian, Jr., expressed feelings shared by many: "I have lost the best friend I ever had, and so has every American." In Washington, newspaper reporters wept. The morning after Harding's death, his swiftly embalmed body lay in an open, flower-covered casket in the sunny drawing room of the presidential suite at the Palace Hotel. Callers were admitted to pay their respects. Harding's face had a "placid and unworried look." Black crepe hung over the hotel doorway. Businesses and banks were closed. At 5 p.m., there was a small private funeral service in the suite. At 7 p.m., the ceremonial funeral procession began from the hotel to the Southern Pacific Railway Station and then by special train to Washington, DC.[1]

As the funeral train traveled east across the United States, it was greeted by crowds along the route. Assistant Navy Secretary Theodore Roosevelt, Jr., and Senator James Wadsworth went to the White House to see the cortege arrive on the evening of August 7. "The night was breathlessly hot," Roosevelt wrote in his diary. "The streets were lined with people of all ages and all types. There was dead silence, with a hush you could almost hear." Then came the sound of horses' hooves, the "clatter of equipment," cavalry, the caisson covered in flowers. A unifying wave of sentiment (briefly) swept the country. Roosevelt had met with General John F. O'Ryan (director of the Senate investigation) earlier the same day, and O'Ryan had told him about "troubles in the Veterans Bureau"; the news was spreading.[2]

Harding's death had an unresolved, messy quality to it. How could a man who exuded such confidence, optimism, and health at his inauguration give up his life without apparent warning after less than three years in the job? Tragedy was overtaken by suspicion. If he was not murdered, was he mistreated by his doctors? Questions continued on the East Coast for weeks: Why was there no oxygen? Why did Harding take the trip? Had he foresworn alcohol and the shock had weakened his system? None of this speculation improved the dead president's reputation. In an age of stereotypes, dramas, and popular fictions, his public image, or "character," was open for definition. Theodore "Teddy" Roosevelt had projected a heroic, larger-than-life personality as president. Woodrow Wilson was an autocratic wartime leader who had been greeted like a king when he traveled to Europe for the Paris Peace Conference. Harding's attempts to humanize the White House and build a sense of normalcy depended on Congress acting positively on his political agenda to provide the necessary balance—ballast—to his symbolic role as a reassuring, down-to-earth occupant of the White House. He had been unable to count on this balance of powers in the time allotted to him, and his exercise of presidential forcefulness had piqued congressional confrontation.

Rumors of incipient government scandals added to doubts about his administration. Although, according to Herbert Hoover, Harding was not concerned about such rumors during the Alaska trip, they acquired major significance after his death, as we'll see. The "Harding scandals" acted as a clarifying and unifying force for public opinion during the Coolidge administration. Charles R. Forbes, Albert B. Fall, and Harry Daugherty (with others) were designated villains. Although Harding was not accused of being involved in scandal, he acquired a lasting reputation as a weak and foolish man who trusted corrupt, betraying friends.[3]

A contemporary described Calvin Coolidge as a "sallow, ginger-haired man of medium height, with pallid, cold blue eyes," a man of "granite reticence," and a "strict and somewhat grim enigma, inhumanly efficient and inhumanly silent." He was also a family man in his early fifties with an attractive wife and two healthy, vigorous teenage boys, Calvin Jr. and John. Coolidge did not need to establish a "character;" he was already master of his image. Like many successful politicians of the time, he moved into politics from the law, becoming an experienced politician in Massachusetts: former mayor of Northampton (site of Forbes's contested hospital construction contract), state senator, lieutenant governor, and then governor of Massachusetts. To break the Boston police strike of 1919, he fired the strikers and called in the National Guard, emerging with the reputation for law and order that propelled him into the vice presidency. He was quiet, with a dry wit, austere, viewed as the quintessential New Englander who, with a lineage going back to the seventeenth century, embodied the old puritan virtues. His primary public duty as president was to keep the country going after the death of his predecessor. A prime political goal was to make sure he became the Republican nominee and the winner of the 1924 presidential election (which he did with great success).[4]

Coolidge challenged Congress to deal with the problems they saw in the operation of executive departments, as well as changes in the law. He stood above the fray as an astute observer, letting congressional investigations run without attempts to influence them. When he was asked to comment on the emerging scandals, his reaction revealed the art of taciturnity at its best, mixed with deflection, and talking but saying nothing. The Senate's ongoing investigation of the Veterans Bureau was Congress's action, he explained in November 1923: "It is not to be made by me. The Committee will make their investigation, and after they have heard all the evidence, they will make a report. When that report comes in, I suppose it may call for some action. Sometimes reports do. From the evidence that appears to be coming out, I suppose this report will call for action. But when it is finally made, then such action as the Committee determines, and such facts as they develop will be taken under consideration, and appropriate action will be taken."[5]

As Harding's vice president, Coolidge had attended cabinet meetings. It was tacitly agreed that he would not be held responsible for any scandals in the Harding years. There was nothing to be gained by associating him too closely with the previous administration. When blame came, it would not be on him.

Calvin and Grace Coolidge gave Florence Harding the time she needed to move out of the White House. There, besides packing up clothes and other personal effects, she went into a frenzy of sorting and disposing of papers in the residential quarters and, with George Christian's help, the Oval Office. Rejected documents went into the fireplace to burn for each of five nights. Harding's papers from the executive office were put in crates that she took with her in a convoy of vehicles to Friendship, the estate of her friend Evalyn Walsh McLean. There she worked on into September, consigning chosen files and letters to a bonfire on the grounds. The remaining papers were packed up and sent back to Marion, Ohio, where she worked on them again, burning papers in the pot-bellied stove in Harding's private office at his old newspaper, the *Marion Star*. If she was spurred on, as she intimated, by the desire to preserve her husband's memory, her actions were counterproductive. Many of Harding's personal files are missing from the surviving archive, including correspondence with Charles R. Forbes and others, making it impossible to construct a full picture of their relationship. It was as if the widow was expunging her emotions on a funeral pyre. Laddie Boy, President Harding's dog, she gave away.

Florence Harding's biographer, Carl Sferrazza Anthony, has estimated that about half of all the letters were destroyed. It was probably during these burnings that the personal correspondence between Harding and Forbes and between Mrs. Harding and Mrs. (Kate) Forbes were destroyed. The absence of correspondence between Harding and Forbes makes Harding's relationship with Forbes in the last months of Forbes's tenure hazy and ambiguous and leaves unanswerable questions. For example, was Harding expecting to see Forbes in San Francisco after his Alaska trip, as Forbes would claim? An early analyst of Harding's personality wrote that he "so hates to be driven himself that he will never try to drive others." Yet, as has been shown, Harding made strong decisions when he was convinced they were necessary. With the destruction of documents, his description as a weak president emerged in the absence of a mass of countering evidence.[6]

Public opinion formed with surprising speed. Less than a week after the return of Harding's body to Washington, a review in the journal *Outlook* reported an emerging consensus in the press: Warren G. Harding was a fine man, but he chose his friends poorly and trusted them too much. Among the virtues assigned to him were humility, lack of vanity, and the ability to listen. Failures in his administration, including the Veterans Bureau—"perhaps the most costly failure of all, because it must be reckoned directly in human life and human happiness"—were credited to the "confusion and unsettlement of the times," to conflicts within the Republican Party, and to Harding's belief in the morality and goodwill of his associates. Harding had not neglected the veterans, the journal proclaimed; rather, he had placed too much confidence in its director. Colonel Forbes was the first to be blamed. Other major "disloyal friends" would hit the headlines within months: former Interior Secretary Albert B. Fall in the oil reserve scandals (Teapot Dome) and Attorney General Harry M. Daugherty, who remained in his position until March 1924. The image of Harding as a man whose friends exploited him appealed to diverse political groups—and continued as a shorthand explanation of the scandals. For Republicans, the scenario conveniently isolated the scandals into specific areas of the Harding administration and provided, in each case, an individual other than Harding to blame: Forbes, Daugherty, and Fall.[7]

The death of the old administration and its rebirth under a new leader created new political opportunities. Scandal provided an unexpected boost for party politics with an eye to the 1924 elections: Democrats versus Republicans. Progressive versus "regular" Republicans. Schism against schism. Scandalous revelations allowed Congress as a collective body to show its strength through congressional investigations, as well as in legislation. Historian Robert Ferrell put this nicely when he described the Harding scandals as "congressional object lessons" for Coolidge, showing who was in charge of the federal government. Coolidge played the scandals with skill by detaching the new Coolidge from the old Harding administration, even though their policies were virtually the same. The oil scandal, showcasing the figure of Fall as a rabid anticonservationist, was helpful in resurrecting the Progressive Party under the leadership of Senator Robert La Follette, Sr., who ran as a third-party candidate in 1924. The scandals could be used to unify splintered, disunited Democrats in moral cause against Republicans. Democrats had Republican scandals to condemn. Republicans thrived by recognizing dangers that lurked in the heart of government and the need for ruthless vigilance in rooting out suspected evildoers.

Having begun work in the spring of 1923, the Senate investigation of the Veterans Bureau had a head start over other purported scandals of the Harding administration. By the time of Harding's death, O'Ryan's staff had amassed a library of information about "the troubles in the Veterans' Bureau," as he saw them, and reforms in the bureau were well under way under General Hines. The three committee members, Senators David Walsh, David Reed, and Tasker Oddie, had been committed to the cause of reform from the start. The evidence produced by their strong investigating team suggested, further, that there had been administrative malfeasance and possible crime in the bureau during the Harding administration.

Each of the senators blamed Forbes without meeting with him. The situation seemed self-evident. Forbes had run the bureau; the bureau had problems; the director was at fault. The force in setting up the investigation, Democrat David Ignatius Walsh, was an energetic, able, outspoken, public-spirited lawyer of Irish heritage and Jesuit education who was a champion of labor, committed to helping the poor and oppressed, and a seasoned politician with progressive views. He had served as lieutenant governor and then governor of Massachusetts. (He was the forty-eighth governor of that state, Coolidge the fiftieth.) Walsh had been in the US Senate since 1919 and remained there through World War II. He dedicated himself to the needs of war veterans, particularly those in New England, who were served by the bureau's fractious Boston office during Forbes's tenure and was exasperated with continuing deficiencies in service.[8]

The committee chair, David Aiken Reed, Republican, had served in the World War as a major in the Seventy-Ninth Division, 311th Field Artillery, held the Distinguished Service Medal, and was a member of the American Legion. Reed had chaired the influential Pennsylvania Industrial Accidents Commission for five years before the war, while practicing law. (He was appointed to the Senate in August 1922 to fill the seat of Republican Senator William E. Crow after Crow's death.) Reed graduated from Princeton and the University of Pittsburgh School of Law and joined a Pittsburgh law firm that was the successor to the one founded by his father, Judge James Hay Reed, which had long served the Mellon interests. Not surprisingly, Senator Reed was a close associate of Treasury Secretary Andrew W. Mellon, an influential cabinet member in both the Harding and the Coolidge administrations. The senior senator from Pennsylvania, George Wharton Pepper, wrote of Dave Reed that his mind was "the most alert I have ever seen in action." He collected rare books and manuscripts, had a special interest in the history of printing, was a skilled marksman, and played the mandolin.

Chairing the Veterans Bureau investigation provided him with an early, visible chance for leadership. (A second chance was soon to come. His name appears on the restrictive Johnson-Reed Act of 1924, which established strict national quotas to control the mix of immigrants, with a very strong bias toward northern Europeans.)[9]

The third member of the committee, representing the western states, Tasker Lowndes Oddie, was not a particularly visible member of the Senate. His biographer describes him as "more of a follower than a leader." Diverted from a conventional career by poor eyesight as a boy, this son of a successful New York / New Jersey stockbroker was sent to Nebraska to be a cowboy. He later returned to New York for law school and admission to the bar. Interest in real estate took him to Nevada, where, brawny, prematurely bald, and six feet tall, he became a spade-digging prospector and with extraordinary luck (unfortunately not to be repeated) was one of the original locators of the rich Tonopah silver field. For part of his life, he was wealthy, but the money trickled away through his hands. He spent two years as district attorney of sparsely populated Nye County, moved up in Republican politics, served as governor of Nevada, and was elected to the US Senate in 1920. The committee dispatched him back west over the summer of 1923 to visit California and Arizona to study veterans hospitals.[10]

The fourth significant figure, committee counsel John F. O'Ryan, was a military strategist who had built the New York National Guard into an admired, highly disciplined fighting force in the years before World War I. He was the only National Guard Commander to take his unit into the war under his command: the Twenty-Seventh Division of the American Expeditionary Force. He did not always play by the rules; the term used in the army was "unorthodox." According to General Bullard, his biographer, in O'Ryan's final military review General Pershing "indulgently passed over a lot of 27th Division customs which had been in conflict with army regulations." Critics considered him unnecessarily Spartan. He drilled his men mercilessly under conditions as near as possible to actual warfare; required pristine uniforms even in conditions of heat, dust, dirt, and danger; treated alcohol as an unmitigated evil, forbade visits to brothels, and had no tolerance for fools or weaklings. His troops adored him. Those who did not conform were transferred. His personal style ranged from self-deprecating charm to ruthless intimidation. He was trim, dignified, and well dressed: "supple, springy and energetic in his movements," Bullard wrote. In 1923, he was a member of the New York Transit Commission with a salary of $15,000 a year ($210,000 in twenty-first-century terms), discussing such matters as the New York City subway system, and he continued in that position while supervising the Senate investigation on an unpaid basis. O'Ryan's father was a classicist who taught Latin and Greek at Seton Hall and inspired his son with interest in military psychology and strategy, from classical times onward. Young O'Ryan trained in the law and had a law office in New York City, but it was in the military that he excelled. He assumed high moral and social authority. John F. O'Ryan shaped the Senate committee's investigative agenda, selected and organized witnesses, sifted evidence, and posed almost all the questions at the hearings in the fall. The senators acted as a tribunal. O'Ryan was the director and impresario of events.[11]

General O'Ryan's first job for the investigation in the spring of 1923 was a preliminary survey of charges made against the Veterans Bureau by American Legion officials and others. His second was to create a plan of action. Chairman Reed left him to it and departed on vacation to Bermuda. In the absence of needed information, it was clear that there would not be hearings for months. To do the legwork, O'Ryan appointed a very able aide, Major Davis G. Arnold, who had been finding private practice an uphill battle after working for relief agencies in France and in the Near East. Arnold became the anchor for information for the team and a Veterans Bureau employee. (He was also temporarily assigned in 1924 as a special assistant to the attorney general in the Forbes case.) O'Ryan designated two National Guard officers to work for him in New York. Lieutenant Colonel Edward Olmstead, O'Ryan's former executive officer, served in this capacity for the investigation, and Captain James A. Walsh was assistant executive officer. In addition, a Veterans Bureau staff assistant, R. C. Routsong, was designated as bureau liaison to the investigation.

This was a high-powered team. During the next six or seven months, up through the period of Harding's death, its members reviewed masses of documents from inside and outside the Veterans Bureau and located and interviewed scores of potential witnesses. (Sixty were to testify at the hearings in the fall.) O'Ryan took the materials gathered under his direction, which his staff duly organized and synthesized for him, then assessed the main points and ran with his conclusions, as a good general would. Just as he would judge a new military recruit, his assessment of the character of the witness was an important ingredient for him in interpreting the evidence: important in "determining the credibility of the witnesses based not only on what they said, but their appearance and the manner of giving their testimony."[12]

Letters went out to every senator and member of Congress on O'Ryan's letterhead (49 Lafayette Street, New York City), asking for volunteer service from leading attorneys, preferably veterans, and seeking examples of "dereliction on the part of the Government service" and suggestions for improvement. Letters went to national and state commanders and district rehabilitation committee chairs of the American Legion, Disabled American Veterans, and Veterans of Foreign Wars. The American Legion extended the cooperation of all its branches, appointing its political representative, the ebullient John Thomas Taylor, as liaison, and related organizations such as the American Hospital Association offered their cooperation. Letters went to presidents of Chambers of Commerce in cities with Veterans Bureau activities (almost 500 cities), asking for investigators in vocational training (136 were produced), and to Kiwanis clubs. Bar associations of each state were asked to produce pro bono lawyers, "men of the highest character and preferably veterans of the war," to conduct local investigations. The letter to medical associations noted that already a corps of about 300 lawyers had been established throughout the country and asked for medical cooperation. Finally, requests were made through the War Department (Judge Advocate General's Corps and Medical Corps). Over the summer of 1923, O'Ryan and his staff established a national network of 596 lawyers and 541 physician volunteers, most of them World War I veterans. Thus staffed, O'Ryan embarked on a patriotic quest, an efficiency sweep, and incomparable national and regional buy-in for the investigation. In parallel, the three senators developed proposals for reforming veterans' legislation.[13]

General O'Ryan became the de facto arbiter of past behavior in the US Veterans Bureau. On the assumption that a fighting unit was only as good as its chief, and conversely that a badly functioning, slack, possibly immoral organization reflected grossly inadequate leadership, he turned his gaze on Colonel Forbes—specifically, to Forbes as a problem—as part of his organizational assessment. Initial statements that administrative derelictions that suggested criminality were not to be part of the agenda went by the board.

In March 1923, O'Ryan announced that his initial investigation would be followed by an "investigation to ascertain the facts in relation to the waste and extravagance which are said to exist," and in April that based on his preliminary survey he would uncover "dishonesty on a pretty big scale here and there." Veterans Bureau Director Frank Hines worked with O'Ryan to reduce staff and fix problems as they were identified. Organizational improvements were made quickly. The job that had worn out Charles R. Forbes, a mere lieutenant colonel in the Signal Corps, had been taken over by the combined efforts of two prominent generals, a Senate committee, a high-level investigative staff, and a national network of volunteer lawyers, doctors, American Legion members, and others. The O'Ryan blitz was a successful public relations coup and a highly effective political exercise—based on the premise that the bureau had been riddled with graft and inefficiency. By these moves, the team sent a strong message to Republicans and Democrats alike that the Veterans Bureau was being systematically, expertly, and visibly cleansed.[14]

Most complaints to O'Ryan's office were about benefits and vocational training. Of 1,083 complaints, only 33 concerned hospitals. O'Ryan wrote Senator Walsh in early October: "I think we have collected enough reliable data to enable the Committee to form accurate judgments concerning the subject of hospitalization. A great many criticisms and sinister rumors were investigated, but most of them turned out to be gross exaggerations. Others related to past circumstances that it was impossible to verify because of the inability to ascertain the names and present location of witnesses." Apart from "outright graft," a topic he did not explain or expand on, the "real abuses which exist . . . can be traced to poor judgment and inexperience on the part of Government officials charged with making decisions. Really very few complaints have come from veterans alleging bad treatment in hospitals. . . . As to costs, poor locations, incompetent plans of Veterans Bureau hospitals, etc., we will be prepared to go into these matters quite fully."[15]

There was no overt suggestion at the time of Harding's death in August that Forbes was the root of the bureau's problems or that he was a bad man. O'Ryan said he tried to keep Forbes out of the investigation and did so for the first couple of months (that would be through May) but was forced by circumstances to bring him into it: "It was unavoidable." He did not explain what those forces were, but by then, criticism about Forbes was coming from various sources, including General Sawyer's probing of supplies at the Perry-ville supplies depot and continuing complaints about the decisions made for the Livermore hospital in California.[16]

Brigadier General Charles E. Sawyer, coordinator of the Federal Board of Hospitalization, lost favor in the new administration. President Coolidge reappointed him and his colleague Dr. Boone as White House physicians, but in late September, it was announced that Sawyer would retire from government service to direct the Harding Memorial Association. Boone described Sawyer as a man who was not easy to work with, and was at times resentful, and Coolidge did not like him. At the same time, Sawyer had been complaining for months about the disposition of supplies at Per-ryville, Maryland, and these complaints were taken very seriously. In May 1923, O'Ryan asked James A. Drain, a brigadier general in the Washington State National Guard, to act as an unpaid assistant to him to investigate the Perryville sale.[17]

"Both the Veterans' Bureau and the purchasers were shooting in the dark," Drain observed in his report. No inventory had been made for at least two years before the materials were transferred from assorted military depots to the Veterans Bureau (much going to the Public Health Service first, again without inventory), and there were no receipts made at the time of trans-fer. Drain concluded that the sale was "unwise and unjustifiable" and that public servants should use "more than ordinary business care in disposing of public property," but he found the pricing of goods reasonable. George W. Morgan of Wilmerding, Morris and Mitchell, auctioneers and commission merchants, New York, valued the unsold property received by the buyers, Thompson and Kelly of Boston, Massachusetts, and found that some items were sold for less than they were worth and some for more. General Drain's conclusion was that the Perryville sale "involved either cupidity or stupidi-ty," and of the two, "I am inclined to think, in the absence of evidence to the contrary, that it was a case of stupidity." This was not the desired conclusion for the investigating team, who expected evidence of graft. O'Ryan ignored Drain's assessments and tried to exclude the report from the published hear-ings. "I have not even read the report," he said. But for once, O'Ryan was overruled. Senator Walsh, also of Massachusetts, pointed out later in the investigation that Thompson and Kelly had requested the report after they had been publicly accused in the hearings of being party to a questionable transaction with the government, and the committee could be accused of withholding evidence if they suppressed it.

By the end of the hearings (in November 1923), O'Ryan believed the Perryville sale was the "most unconscionable transaction I have ever heard of in connection with the disposal of Government interests." That was because, superseding Drain's report in his view, his staff had found that someone in the Veterans Bureau had been buying new sheets and towels by the thousands, together with other goods, including floor wax, and this stuff was placed at Perryville at the very time the bureau was disposing of its supplies—and here the purchase evidence was clear. Bills for the delivery of new sheets—more than 5,000 at a time—were produced at the Senate hearings from Veterans Bureau records for dates in August, September, October, November, and December 1922. At the very least, this was a horrifying example of administrative ineptitude.[18]

In contrast to the Drain report, a report from California Judge Adolphus E. Graupner received serious consideration. Graupner wrote a clear, twenty-eight-page brief for O'Ryan and the Senate investigating committee, dated October 20, 1923, on the facts of the purchase of the hospital site at Livermore as he saw them, adding in salient but unsubstantiated rumors that the committee staff might wish to investigate. The main points were that the Livermore property transactions smelled of graft, that the bureau's chief lawyer, the late Charles F. Cramer (here referred to in passing as "Charlie Cramer") engaged in suspect dealings, and that Forbes was administratively inept and morally suspect. Graupner's Forbes, according to the mix of facts and rumors conveyed to Washington, grossly overpaid for the Livermore site; hired a pathetically inadequate California architect Matthew O'Brien for no good reason and at great expense—and did not turn him off when it was clear he was producing nothing useful; involved the US district attorney in San Francisco in his schemes; told the owner of the Livermore site he could harvest his wine "if he acted right and kept his mouth shut"; had the Federal Board of Hospitalization approve the site when General Sawyer was not at the meeting; upset the manager of District 12, an engineer who had not been consulted; upset the bureau's tuberculosis head (Dr. Stanley Rinehart); made unwanted advances to female nurses; and on at least one occasion hosted an orgy. Graupner also accused Forbes of hiring an old friend, Francis Betts

"Dry Dock" Smith, to do little or nothing, and reported that Smith said he expected to get the Livermore contract instead of O'Brien: "Forbes owes me the job." O'Ryan accepted Graupner's statements, summarily stating of Forbes's appointment of Smith at the Senate hearings, "I am perfectly frank to say that I think it was simply giving the man a job." None of the above individuals was called as a witness at the hearings, and nothing was made of Forbes's claim that President Harding made the key decisions at Livermore. Criticism of Harding by name was off the table at the hearings.

O'Ryan took Graupner's report seriously as a depiction of Forbes's feckless, even scandalous, behavior. Sawyer greeted the Graupner report with appreciation. "My dear friend," he wrote Graupner on reading the copy the judge personally inscribed to him. "My heart and soul are with you in your efforts to present facts for consideration and in your efforts to point a way for improvement. May success attend you all."[19]

With Coolidge as president, both Sawyer and the experienced con man Elias H. Mortimer were ready to appear when needed as valuable witnesses in the Veterans Bureau hearings. Mortimer had long been adept in inserting himself into events by introducing himself to people, claiming he had relevant materials, and setting off influential rumors. Congressman Larsen had been convinced that he had written an affidavit to President Harding damning Forbes. Congressmen Langley and Zihlman had borrowed money from him. Corporate chiefs had believed his lying claims of connections to the White House and, not least, Mortimer had sanitized his reputation by working as an informer for the Department of Justice. Mortimer would appear when the time was propitious and produce his list of accusations against Forbes. It is not clear when Mortimer first connected with the Senate investigation, but his first claimed meeting was with General Drain on the Perryville case at the Manufacturers Club in Philadelphia in the late summer of 1923, soon after Harding's death.

Mortimer's account of that meeting was as follows: "General Drain did not interrogate me in order to ascertain so far as I could tell from his questions everything that I knew about any corrupt practices in the Veterans Bureau. He asked me to tell him the story as Mr. [James] Williams, Mrs. Mortimer's uncle, had told him." That story centered on a meeting at the Williams house in Philadelphia, where allegedly Forbes had talked with Williams about the illegal disposition of drugs from Perryville. Mortimer: "I recited everything to him in a couple of hours in a general way producing no documents of any kind." Assuming this meeting occurred as claimed, Drain ignored Mortimer's contribution. In response to a question from Senator Reed at the hearings, Mortimer said that Drain was "the first man that examined me," that O'Ryan's aide Major Arnold talked with him in Philadelphia about the same time, and shortly after that Arnold and O'Ryan visited him in his "other office in the Real Estate Trust Building in Philadelphia." He did not answer the part of Senator Reed's question that encompassed any earlier contacts with aides to O'Ryan outside of the definition of "examined me." The critical point here is that Mortimer came to O'Ryan's attention in time to get his evidence into the investigators' information system and to emerge as a truly brilliant, formidable witness at the hearings. His evidence was so polished it sounded as if he had been prepared for months.[20]

Separate pieces were coming together. Forbes's two major foes were to be witnesses at the Senate hearings: Sawyer (his "nemesis") on the Perryville case and Mortimer (whom he underrated) on hospital contracts, the Colombia development proposition and other issues, including Forbes's activities and demeanor on the western trip.

Charles R. Forbes reached San Francisco in late July or the first two days of August 1923, after sailing through the Panama Canal. About the same time, the Harding party arrived there from the other direction after visiting Alaska. Forbes wrote later that he had expected to meet and talk with Warren Harding on this visit: "I was there to meet him by appointment," but instead, "I last saw him in death as he lay in his casket, his strong face and magnificent features reflecting the life of this nobleman." It is unlikely that Forbes saw Harding's body. Theoretically, he could have attended the open viewing at the Palace Hotel on August 3, 1923, when members of the presidential party were in a state of shock, but surely someone (such as a Secret Service agent) would have recognized him and noted his presence. More likely this was a false memory stemming from wishful thinking, or poetic license, designed for the audience he was then writing for: fellow inmates at the Leavenworth Penitentiary. Nevertheless, the coincidence of his arrival and Harding's death was traumatic. Forbes had lost a man he revered and his future. He clung to the belief that "my personal destiny would have been different had he lived." Once again, he succumbed to stress with illness. On August 7, the day the funeral party reached Washington, he was admitted to the Stanford Hospital on Clay Street, San Francisco, with chills and fevers, remaining there through September 19. One report referred to his illness as an attack of encephalitis. The *Washington Post* reported Forbes's initial condition as serious, due to an infection contracted during military service, but toward the end of his stay, he was "very much improved." His new career in import-export was on hold. Later he was hospitalized in Seattle, near to his and his wife's home on Vashon Island.[21]

His life was in tatters. Sick in Seattle, he was served divorce papers. Kate Marcia Forbes, back in the United States from Europe, filed for divorce on October 6. She had raised the question of divorce before—on three occasions, Forbes recalled—and he had objected, as he did again, but this time she outmaneuvered him. She had spent fifteen months as an independent woman free to choose where to travel and what to do. Her former married life had literally made her sick, and she had medical evidence to support her. He had shown "cruel and inhuman treatment" toward her so that her health was physically impaired, and she was now a "very sick woman." Forbes was not a suitable person for custody of their daughter, she claimed. He hired a lawyer, denied the charge of cruel and inhuman treatment, and obtained visitation rights. Her lawyer countered with a plea to the court to expedite matters, as her health was such that she could not "safely await the outcome of a long continued litigation." Kate Forbes kept the three lots she owned in her own right on Vashon Island, providing her with the family home. With admirable speed, the divorce was approved on October 11, eleven days before the Senate investigative hearings on the Veterans Bureau opened, on October 22. "Divorces are rather frequent in Seattle," an official of Seattle's law department explained to skeptical questioners on the East Coast. Bob and Kate had been married fourteen years.[22]

A wide-awake Seattle reporter transmitted the news east. Much was made of the fact that they divorced under the names under which they had married, which excluded their middle initials, and that his signature was oddly messed up. In the divorce proceedings, Kate recorded his name as Charles Forbes, no initial. Similarly she, who had married as Kate M. Goodwin and wrote under the name Kate Marcia Forbes, was plain Kate Forbes. He signed the verification document for the divorce with his usual signature, Charles R. Forbes, but then the "R" was scratched out and "F" written over it. Forbes said later that he had no recollection of doing this: "I was very sick at the time." To say all of this looked peculiar is an understatement. However, this would not have come to light had the divorce not coincided with the Senate investigation of the Veterans Bureau, the assiduousness of its director, and the start of public hearings critical of his personality and character. O'Ryan suggested that Forbes was trying to hide his divorce, but probably wondered about the legitimacy of the marriage; that is, whether Forbes was guilty of bigamy, as an anonymous letter suggested (see chapter 9). According to suspicious minds, Colonel Charles R. Forbes of Washington, DC, was trying to hide his identity. "The suit was handled with the utmost secrecy," the *Washington Post* reported, "and efforts were made to conceal both the action and the granting of the divorce."[23]

Forbes's cascade of troubles between early August and mid-October 1923 included loss of Harding, loss of health, loss of wife and child to divorce, loss of his home, and inability to pursue his business interests. Other troubles were just beginning. As he accepted his divorce, Forbes heard from friends that charges were being made against him in Washington and that the public hearings of the Senate investigation of the Veterans Bureau were soon to begin. Potential loss of reputation joined the list.

Characteristically, and unwisely in retrospect, he chose action rather than waiting for the outcome. He pulled himself together to travel back east, hoping his son Russell (the possible writer of anonymous letters against him) would meet him and perhaps give him comfort. Father sent son a series of telegrams along the way: October 14, 1923: "Several days before I arrive will wire train." October 15: "Been in hospital here [Seattle]. Will start east slowly tomorrow." October 20: "Arrived Wentworth Hotel [New York]. Please come over as early as you can both." October 21: "Please be careful any one coming to house you know nothing. Love." And finally from Washington, DC, after the first day of the hearings, October 22: "They are attempting to frame me will stick it out if able have not been able to see Smith yet love C R Forbes." James S. Easby-Smith was an attorney and a friend.

Charles R. Forbes—an unwanted participant as far as the investigators were concerned—checked into the Hotel Washington under the care of a physician the day before the hearings began.[24]

By then, investigators had been working behind the scenes for months, and none of the members of the investigating team thought highly of him. Committee chair David Reed had told his friend Senator James Wadsworth in the early months of the investigation, "We are on a dirty trail leading straight to this man Forbes." Tasker Oddie, fresh from his travels to investigate veterans hospitals in the west, relied on Judge Graupner's severe criticisms of Forbes; and David Walsh despised Forbes for his slow and ineffective responses to veterans' problems in New England. For John F. O'Ryan, Charles R. Forbes was an officer who fell way below O'Ryan's military standards: a slacker, a drinker, a man of loose morals, a cheat, and, courtesy of Mortimer's claims, a crook.[25]

With much of the detailed investigation under way or completed, the committee's hearings were not so much investigation as revelation. O'Ryan had a smooth opening lined up: a brief welcome by the committee chair, followed by an explanation by O'Ryan of what he and his team had accomplished, to be followed by Director Frank Hines on problems found and improvements made in the Veterans Bureau; and then on the third day, O'Ryan's back-and-forth interrogation of Elias H. Mortimer, who would describe Forbes's character with persuasive vignettes and build evidence against him of taking bribes and conspiring to commit fraud. The Veterans Bureau hearings were nicely packaged, wrapped up like a play whose conclusion has been written.

The oil lease hearings, which began on October 23 and ran concurrently, were a fishing-for-facts investigation at this point. Compared with the Veterans Bureau case, movement was slow. Back in April 1922, Senator Robert M. La Follette, Sr., had sponsored a resolution for the Committee on Public Lands to investigate the transfer of the oil leases from the Navy Department to the Interior Department, followed by the granting of drilling leases to major oil corporations. The first investigative task, to review a mass of documents from the Department of the Interior, devolved on subcommittee chair Senator Thomas J. Walsh, a Democrat and lawyer from Helena, Montana, who had fought against the copper interests and against collusion between politics and big business in that state. Walsh worked deliberately and doggedly over the next eighteen months to tease out relevant matters of law, history, and fact without the extraordinary resources of a General

O'Ryan—or, for that matter, the need to reform a major government enterprise. Secretary Albert Fall's successor, Secretary Hubert Work, had reform of the Interior Department under way. There were rumors of illegal doings in the oil lease transactions but nothing concrete. Former Secretary Fall, the first witness at the October hearings, described his actions on the leases as desirable and correct. Two days later Navy Secretary Edwin Denby testified that he signed the papers transferring the naval oil reserve leases to Interior but could not add much to that. Experts on oil drilling and others came and went. Teapot Dome historian Burl Noggle describes the opening of these hearings as "lusterless." Unlike the Veterans Bureau hearings, there was as yet no satisfactory scenario or plot. Those were to come in the New Year.[26]

The two sets of hearings, for the Veterans Bureau in room 410 of the Senate Office Building and the oil leases in room 210, provided consecutive chapters in the larger, merging narrative of the Harding scandals, though in fact each case was distinct. The Veterans Bureau took the prize in the fall, the oil hearings in the spring. The former produced a scandal based on one man, Forbes; the latter followed with a scandal based on Fall. These two investigations were joined by the investigation of Attorney General Harry M. Daugherty in March—and a further array of witnesses. For a southern reporter who covered all three hearings, the overall impression was one of confusion, a "blurred nightmare" in retrospect. There were "missing links" in all of them and accusations left dangling—"not pursued to the end." What was memorable was a parade of characters, "smelling, some of them, of the bar and the poolroom," who appeared in a serialized melodrama: "The Scandals of the Harding Administration."[27]

Scandal had become a common theme, a common cause. Congressional action on the Harding scandals began visibly on October 22, 1923, when hearings opened on the US Veterans Bureau. Warren Harding had been gone for little more than eleven weeks.

There was a dramatic, unexpected addition to O'Ryan's prepared script. Charles R. Forbes, risen from his bed, entered the committee room leaning on a cane, gaunt and pale, like the ghost of times past or an unwanted visitor at a feast.

RUSH TO JUDGMENT
Senate Hearings Target Forbes

On Monday morning, October 22, 1923, the three members of the committee investigating the US Veterans Bureau—Senators David Reed (chair), David Walsh, and Tasker Oddie—sat on the long side of a rectangular table in room 410 of the Senate Office Building facing the audience and prepared to begin their long-awaited hearings. A great gilt-framed mirror hung over the tall mantle behind the senators, reflecting the room's ornate cut-glass chandelier. A separate table and chair awaited the first witness. The director of the investigation, General John F. O'Ryan, backed by his staff, commanded a third table, piled with documents. Significantly, for the ensuing spate of scandals, members of the Washington-based press were present, eager to write front-page stories and send them out across the nation.

When Colonel Charles R. Forbes planted himself down conspicuously—pugnaciously—at the end of the senators' table, an opportunity occurred immediately. He had come to be heard, and when he tried to do so (as he did several times), he was quashed. "He appeared to have gone through severe illness," wrote a reporter for the *New York Times*: "His face was tightly drawn and his vigorous figure appeared to have suffered under a long nervous strain." His appearance was disastrous for any image he might wish to project as a responsible government official. Senator Ashurst of Arizona described him in his diary as a "man with disheveled hair, loose lips, and trembling hands."[1]

O'Ryan reported in his opening statement that the Veterans Bureau had not functioned effectively in 1922 and early 1923 (that is, under Forbes) and that its expenditures of $467 million in fiscal 1923 were unprecedented. Thus, he set the stage for potent themes of malpractice, temptation, and the likelihood of fraud. Forbes interrupted him midsentence. O'Ryan halted. "Colonel Forbes," said Chairman Reed, in a belated acknowledgment of his presence.

Forbes said he wanted to make a statement. Reed said he might produce a written statement for the committee but not interrupt the proceedings "for the sake of order and rapid progress." Forbes considered this "a bit unfair to me": he had traveled 3,000 miles from his sickbed, wanted to be of help but also protect his reputation, "which is being attacked in this hearing," and have the opportunity to challenge what was said and not have press reports across the country describe him as "sitting here mute." Reed was both firm and denigrating. This was "not a trial of Colonel Forbes or any other particular individual," he said. Objections would not be tolerated from anyone "who may consider he is reflected on." O'Ryan continued with his statement. Forbes stayed put. After another interruption, O'Ryan was heard to tell Reed off the record, "You will have to shut him down."[2]

The first witness, General Frank Hines, testified with grace, authority, and gentlemanly restraint, listing progress at the Veterans Bureau under his management and illustrating his talk with detailed charts. By the end of the first morning, it had been established that a man who knew what he was doing was effectively and rapidly transforming a previously malfunctioning organization. In the afternoon, Hines gave an upbeat report on the construction of veterans hospitals. He singled out Hospital 81 in the Bronx (chosen by the White Committee and criticized by Forbes) as poorly sited, which it was, and American Lake (chosen by Forbes and built by Forbes's old boss Charles B. Hurley) as "splendidly located for an ideal hospital." Hines told the committee he was expanding the bed supply, from about 25,000 to more than 30,000 hospital beds, of which 46 percent were slated for tuberculosis and 32 percent for neuropsychiatric patients (in contrast to prior criticism of Forbes for adding too many hospital beds) and lambasted dentistry (as Forbes had before him), noting that papers on fraud had been turned over to the Department of Justice "at one time" (under Forbes). Hines tried to explain to the committee that some difficulties were inherent in the organization of the Veterans Bureau: "The bureau is a large machine. It has taken a long time to become effective. . . . You can readily understand that we are bound to make some slips." O'Ryan quickly changed the subject. In the first two days of the hearings, his systematic review of the bureau's programs made it clear that Hines had brought needed skills and energy to the bureau and that constructive reform was under way, whereas Forbes had made decisions according to cronyism and political pull, paid individuals who were incompetent or did nothing, and (relying on the report O'Ryan had received from Judge Graupner) participated in circumstances "surrounded by graft," illustrated by his decisions for the hospital at Livermore.

Positive results from Forbes's tenure were attributed to Hines or disregarded, including a report by an expert accountant and auditor, Fred W. Lindars from New York, selected by O'Ryan, and mentioned later in the hearings, which commented "very favorably upon the methods in vogue here," though there might be too much "checking and rechecking." The role assigned to Forbes was as a failed, possibly corrupt, leader, such as a deposed king in a drama. His greeting by the committee showed him to be a man without status—a rude interloper into civilized proceedings.[3]

Forbes did not appear the next two days. By the end of the third day (October 24), General O'Ryan had established fundamental themes for the hearings based on his perception of Forbes's low moral character, and Elias H. Mortimer had become a star witness. Mortimer's answers to O'Ryan's rapid-fire questions quickly associated Forbes with corruption, immoral behavior, and membership in a "ring" of conspirators, evoking images of money-driven racketeers in prohibition cases. It was hard not to make this connection when the *New York Times* headlined the first day of the hearings as "General Hines Charges Fraud and Waste in Veterans' Relief" on the same front page as "Means, Liquor Plot Exposer, Indicted in Big Conspiracy." (That was the flamboyant, corrupt special investigator Gaston Means, who was under indictment for supplying the New York bootlegging trade with the "finest quality liquors" from bonded warehouses, with an alleged profit for the New York ring of more than $100,000.) O'Ryan: "Well now, did any of the members of this ring, this group, such as Thompson or Black, ever tell you how much they had paid Forbes up to any particular time?" Mortimer produced the highly questionable figure of $30,000, which he said he had heard as "hearsay" from the late contractor James Black, who mentioned this as an impression Black got from contractor John Thompson. There was no confirmation; Black had died in February after four months of illness, and Thompson was not called as a witness.[4]

Mortimer was in his element, poised and confident, illuminating his testimony with a fine sense of detail. He inserted innuendo about Forbes and Mrs. Mortimer, added colorful observations, and skated nonchalantly over circumstantial and absent evidence. He acknowledged his role as a fellow conspirator, knowing he would not be charged. O'Ryan took Forbes's lack of worth for granted and treated Mortimer courteously. They were an effective team. Newspapers generally agreed. Forbes's "former chum" gave his shocking testimony under oath, one remarked, "and we must assume it to be true unless disproved."[5]

General O'Ryan's opening strategy paid off. Dramatic excerpts from the hearings were reported far and wide: "Forbes Allowed Fee of $64,000—Paid for Useless Hospital Plan." "Forbes Grafted on Vet Bureau Job, Is Charge." "Accuses Forbes of Plotting Big Graft—Witness Describes Booze Parties and Wild Times—Says Veteran Bureau Head Tried to Sell Liquor and Drugs." Subheadings in the *Atlanta Constitution* included "Drinking Party Trail from Coast to Coast" and "Embarrassed in Hotel." Chairman Reed was convinced that there had been a conspiracy in which both Forbes and Mortimer were involved: "It is my judgment that having established a conspiracy that anything said by any of the conspirators is evidence against them, and if the committee agrees with that, I think we can hear conversations, even if Colonel Forbes was not present when they took place." Reed also announced (and the other senators concurred) that because of Mortimer's "very extraordinary testimony" and Forbes's "rather dramatic appearance" on the first day, Forbes should be called as a witness. O'Ryan agreed to "give him the opportunity to come if he cares to" but stipulated that he would be subject to cross-examination, and his role should be limited. Scheduling Forbes's testimony was a matter of tactics: O'Ryan left Forbes in limbo until the hearings were winding down and called Mortimer back to reestablish the basic themes at the end.[6]

Forbes issued a statement to the Associated Press that Mortimer's testimony was "utterly and absolutely false." He called the story of the "recent receipt by me of a $5000 bribe" false and "so absurd as to be ridiculous." Businessman John W. Thompson made a statement in St. Louis that he knew Mortimer only slightly and that Mortimer had never represented his company. Washington State builder Charles B. Hurley strongly denied Mortimer's charges of his role in a byline from Seattle:

> Any suggestion of Mortimer that either I or the Hurley-Mason Company secured the American Lake Hospital contract through understanding with Colonel Forbes, Mortimer, or anybody else, that Forbes or anybody else was to share with

us in the profits of the contract, is absolutely false and never had any foundation in fact. . . . The [Army] Quartermaster General's Office not only drew the plans for the buildings but it analyzed the bids and recommended that the contract be awarded to the Hurley-Mason Company, which was the lowest bidder. . . . Colonel Forbes had nothing to do with it except to sign the contract we submitted to him, which he was compelled to do under the law.

None of these statements made any difference. At the end of the first week of the hearings, Senator Reed made his position clear. Evidence showing conspiracy and corruption would be turned over to the Department of Justice for criminal prosecution. Reed said the committee had so far "only scratched the surface" and referred to the "scandal" in the Veterans Bureau. On October 26, Attorney General Daugherty announced that he had had a conference with President Coolidge and was preparing to present evidence of the alleged frauds in the Veterans Bureau to a special grand jury. On October 27, Senator Oddie called at the White House as a member of the investigating committee to report on the hearings to President Coolidge, who steered a fine course, upholding the separation of powers while taking a firm line. He wanted a full probe, it was reported, and hoped the Senate would go sufficiently far to see whether action by the Department of Justice was justified. According to a White House statement, "none of those guilty in the frauds will escape."[7]

Belatedly, after the first day, Forbes consulted his lawyer. James S. Easby-Smith was a civilized Alabama gentleman, writer, scholar, and classicist, who knew Bob and Kate Forbes from their Washington days. A trim, intellectually curious man in his early fifties, he held a graduate degree in classics from Georgetown University, where he taught law for many years while in private practice. He had also served as attorney in charge of pardons at the Department of Justice and as a US attorney and published a history of the Department of Justice and translations of the songs of Sappho into English poetry (both available at the time of writing via the Internet). During World War I, he administered the selective service system (the military draft), for which he received a Distinguished Service Medal. Afterward, he dropped his military title, Colonel. He was well known and respected in Washington as a man of intrinsic fairness. Easby-Smith stood by Forbes as his counsel through the hearings, trial, and thankless appeals in a case stacked against his client, supporting him unconditionally and without full payment. As a first step, he worked with Forbes on the statement of innocence he was determined to present at the hearings, if and when he was called to do so. Meanwhile, October ended, November moved in, and O'Ryan strengthened his case.[8]

Easby-Smith and his client had a herculean task. It is not easy, often impossible, to prove a negative. Mortimer had to be shown not to be the truth-teller happily accepted by the investigators and the populace but, rather, a fantastic liar. Forbes had to show he had not received money as loans, paybacks, or bribes; had not engaged in conversations about spoils, as had been vividly reported; and had not used a coded message system to advance the conspiracy's goals; indeed, he had to show he was not part of a conspiracy at all. Forbes also had to demonstrate that he had been justifiably upset when he made interruptions on the first day of the hearings and was not fundamentally an uncivilized, out-of-control wild man, which is how the story was characterized in Washington's gossip networks.

The use of a code for communicating via coded telegrams was the easiest topic to address, because Mortimer could not confirm that Forbes had a copy of the codebook, only that "I know he was supposed to have one." (Later he changed his tune and said he did.) Other challenges were difficult because significant pieces of evidence to support Mortimer's statements were missing, if indeed they ever existed. He had no receipt for the $5,000 in cash he allegedly gave Forbes (privately, in a bathroom) in Chicago. Other documents had been stolen from Mortimer's apartment at the Wardman Park Hotel in three separate burglaries, or so he said. (He hinted at the hearings that at least one of these was conducted by someone connected with the Veterans Bureau and that Forbes was trying to get into his bank vault.) Among the missing papers were an old checkbook, which would supposedly document a sum of $1,000 or $1,500 Mortimer said he had given to Forbes by check; a copy of the putative advance list of veterans hospitals to give Mortimer's clients an advantage in bidding for construction contracts; and examples of coded letters and telegrams between Mortimer and Forbes. Mortimer made both the documents and the thefts real by descriptions that became more vivid when he was called back at the end of the hearings. The lost papers included a "great many of the telegrams that I had submitted to Colonel Forbes that he had made notations on; a great many letters that were sent to me, of a confidential nature, from Mr. Black and Mr. Thompson [fellow conspirators], and telegrams, all relating to veteran hospitals." Although he did not call the police, after the third burglary of his apartment he had a steel plate and two new snap locks installed in his apartment, number 508-B, and the steel plate was still there when he moved out on March 1. "And, Senator [Reed], I had this special Yale lock put on, and they had to cut a hole out of the door to put the thing on." Easby-Smith could show (as he did at the trial) that Mortimer lied when he said he reported the thefts to the security officer at the Wardman Park. However, by that time, concern about a burglary or two seemed trivial compared with the central, serious issue at hand: namely, that a senior government official had conspired against the federal government.[9]

Forbes and Easby-Smith waited, but the Senate hearings moved ahead without them being heard. During the middle sessions, October 29 through November 12, creamery purveyor and Mortimer-acolyte James M. Williams, Katherine Mortimer's uncle, evoked fanciful images of broken packages of narcotics being spirited out of government warehouses at Perryville in milk trucks under Forbes's direction. According to Williams, Forbes said he would have Mortimer arrested by "strong-arm" men and "flog him and turn him loose with the promise that he would leave Washington." Forbes sat in the audience making notes while Easby-Smith kept him from interrupting. O'Ryan, an acknowledged expert on supply trains and logistics, spent a good part of three days focusing on Perryville: it was a "perfect outrage," and "almost inconceivable" that the Perryville depot should harbor 84,000 new sheets and more than 1.1 million towels when sheets were being offered for sale at a fire-sale price; new sheets came in and "went out the other side" to waiting boxcars. Witnesses attempted to explain the purchases of sheets as the result of a time lag between ordering and delivery, with old orders still being filled while policies were switched to closing down the depot. Such explanations were thrust aside. As for the purchase of more than 30,000 gallons of cleaner and wax and more than 19,000 gallons of liquid stain, as a train of witnesses demonstrated, it was not clear who had been responsible for these purchases.[10]

Forbes was absent when his admitted nemesis, Brigadier General Charles E. Sawyer, testified on November 7. An erect, earnest-looking white-haired elderly gentleman, tiny and trim, Sawyer stood rather than sat at the witness table "to have advantage of better light" as he read the statement he had written that morning. The crux of it was that Sawyer ordered materials unloaded from loaded train cars at Perryville on President Harding's authority, but Forbes was "insubordinate" and Harding asked him to resign. The charge of insubordination was front-page news. The *New York Times* headlined this point as "Tells How Harding Ousted Col. Forbes for Defying Him." (In his testimony later, Forbes said he followed Harding's directions.)

Sawyer laid out towels and blankets on the table like a small-town salesman, some in their original wrappings, samples he had collected from Perryville to show President Harding. An olive-drab army blanket was "good enough to be used in any private home, anywhere in the country," while a gray blanket was "perhaps not so good" but "would at least keep men warm on cold winter nights." O'Ryan examined the sheets as if he were a customer and asked whether they were of the type known as "Pequot," which a witness had described as "de luxe, high-grade, first-class sheets." Sawyer thought they were. He suggested that Forbes's supplies chief, Commander O'Leary, might have selected his own sample of goods to show the president "with the intention of showing how bad they are." Chairman Reed asked Sawyer his views on the Veterans Bureau. Sawyer claimed that the "autocratic power . . . to a single individual" [Forbes] was the "cause of a great deal of trouble." Reed and Sawyer discussed veterans' medical services. Reed: "You would not put a dement of filthy habits in the next bed to a mild case of melancholia?" Sawyer: "No sir." The mentally ill patient was no longer an outcast. Sawyer: "Today we know that many of his troubles are due to physical derangements and from infections from tonsils, from sinuses, from absorptions from the intestines, from kidneys, from livers and so on." Having gained valuable evidence against Forbes on the Perryville case, O'Ryan invited Sawyer to produce a document to describe his ideal leaders in neuropsychiatry.[11]

Elias Mortimer was riding high. He was providing essential facts to an eminent major-general and three US senators—and winning points for them! He was famous. He could not afford to make any slips. Outside the hearing room, he put direct and indirect pressure on his wife, not yet divorced, who could support his otherwise uncorroborated statements, by lies if necessary, if she could be made to do so. Notably, she had been present in the suite at the Drake Hotel at the time Mortimer claimed he handed $5,000 in cash to Forbes.

In a letter to his father-in-law, Dr. George Tullidge, he made the unbelievable claim that he, Mort, could get General O'Ryan to look at Dr. Edward Tullidge's case for release from incarceration in the federal penitentiary at Leavenworth and act on it. O'Ryan "told me to bring all of the papers down to him personally," Mortimer wrote Dr. George, but say nothing to anybody about it. A postscript to the letter suggested the quid pro quo. Put bluntly: Give me your convicted son's insalubrious record (which could be held for blackmail), and I will be nice about your daughter at the hearings. His actual words: "I will protect (Katherine) in every way." The answer from Dr. George was no. A few weeks later Mortimer tried a direct deal with Dr. Edward Tullidge, this time promising to have his case for a pardon taken up with the navy via "prominent personal friends" of Assistant Secretary of the Navy Theodore Roosevelt, Jr. The deal here was that Edward had to get his sister Katherine to stop divorce proceedings, because if not, Mort's friends would halt their efforts. Edward broke with Mortimer at this point. Mortimer continued to play his games with his wife: harassment interspersed with loving letters.[12]

Katherine Tullidge Mortimer was ready to expose Mortimer for brutality and for lying business practices. She testified to the Senate committee at her own request, but the testimony was given in private. She asked for the release of the testimony and asked to testify publicly to "vindicate her character and good name" after a number of "very grave and serious, if insinuating attacks" had been made against her. Senator Reed criticized her in the process of denying her requests: "Because Mrs. Mortimer was a woman we permitted her in her statement to cover matters that she wanted to bring up, that, in our judgment, had nothing to do with the purpose of our appointment. . . . We were not appointed to investigate the domestic affairs of Mr. and Mrs. Mortimer." She could have gone directly to the press but her lawyer, former Judge Daniel Thew Wright, persuaded her not to do so. A woman's character was "a very fragile thing," he said, "as delicate as the frost upon the morning window, which a breath dispels, and it is forever gone." He called on the senators for fair play. However, since insinuations had already been made, it was not clear what he thought "fair play" was. Mrs. Mortimer's private testimony was not released and appears no longer to exist.[13]

Background investigations continued while the hearings were in session. Finding a stash of money hidden by Forbes would strongly support Mortimer's claims of bribery and corruption. Major Arnold, O'Ryan's key staff member, instructed a former naval intelligence officer, Lieutenant Commander C. V. Cusachs, to see whether Forbes had hidden money in property near Staunton, Virginia, and to find out what he was up to as he waited to be called to testify. Cusachs had been awarded the Navy Cross for analyzing German submarine movements when posted to Madrid but proved sadly unskilled at pavement-pounding detective work. On October 30, he visited Staunton, where someone told him the plan was to develop the property at Augusta Springs as a business to market mineral water and suggested a search warrant for the "merry parties" that went on there. But that was all. On November 5, in Washington, he heard through the club grapevine that a cargo of wine had once been shipped to Veterans Bureau lawyer Charles Cramer, with Attorney General Daugherty acting as the middleman and also that Forbes had "deposits in many banks."

On November 7 and 9, he conducted surveillance on Forbes, who was staying at the Hamilton Hotel, where the hotel manager, Mr. W. H. Barse, told him Forbes was ill. Forbes, however, had his own detectives, and knew he was under surveillance. Somewhat rashly, he fed messages through Barse, with Barse's help, via Cusachs to the Senate investigating team. Forbes had a number of letters from President Harding endorsing everything he had done as Veterans Bureau director, Cusachs reported. O'Ryan "had always shown great animosity to him." Forbes said that he had "never touched a cent of government money, and that if he had he would be worth millions today instead of being a poor man." Forbes was "on a fight to a finish." Unless he was allowed to appear on the stand on Monday, November 12, Forbes told Barse, who told Cusachs, who told Major Arnold, he would call a press conference and tell a "story which would be more startling to the public than anything they had yet received." It was "criminal" that "that Dirty Hound Sawyer" had not been cross-examined, in view of his "lowdown immoral character" (which included picking up young girls, according to Forbes).[14]

Colonel Forbes, fists clenched to fight, had not paid attention to the fact that General O'Ryan had built his career as a master in tactics and that he was expert in interpreting enemy information and using it to his advantage. His team received the information that Forbes was set up for intemperate confrontation—and could be provoked into foolhardiness when raging about General Sawyer. O'Ryan scheduled him for November 13.

An unusually large crowd of spectators packed the room on Tuesday, November 13, 1923, to listen to what Colonel Charles R. Forbes had to say. Some had waited in line for hours, but the wait was worth it. One observer described him as a "man who had broken down under the strain of his work and the defamation which had been heaped upon him." Nonetheless, far from broken in spirit, he proclaimed a "general, sweeping, and absolute denial of every charge, statement, innuendo, and insinuation which in any matter whatsoever reflects upon the honesty and integrity of my official or personal conduct while I occupied the office of Director of War Risk Insurance or Director of the Veterans Bureau." The charges of "official and personal neglect, dishonesty, graft, liquor drinking, loose conduct, and any and every other dereliction of duty, official or personal, which have been ascribed to me either by the witness Mortimer and Williams and others, or charged against me by the counsel of this committee," were "utterly false and groundless."

So far, so good, but then, however valiantly, he courted trouble. First, he accused General O'Ryan for misleading the Senate committee and the committee for being taken in. Second, he countered the charge that he was part of a conspiracy to commit fraud against the government by claiming that the opposite was true: "A conspiracy has been on foot, the purpose of which is to encompass my destruction by means of perjury, subornation of perjury, attempted subornation of perjury, and the suppression of material facts and documents bearing not only upon my personal conduct as Director of the Veterans' Bureau, but also upon the official conduct of the affairs of the bureau by myself and my subordinates." Among these, he made multiple criticisms of General Sawyer (and thus implicitly of Harding, whom Sawyer reportedly represented) for impeding his work at the bureau.[15]

Leaving senators, investigators, and audience to ruminate on these accusations, Forbes's lawyer, James Easby-Smith, then began a list of prepared questions for him to answer calmly, one by one. The two men completed this in a workmanlike fashion in the midafternoon the next day, marked by some emotional lapses by Forbes.

This was the only time Charles R. Forbes gave public testimony on his role as director of the US Veterans Bureau. The gist of his testimony follows:

On hospitals. The structure of decision making for new veterans hospitals went beyond the Veterans Bureau. Forbes was not the sole decision maker. He was responsible for veterans hospitals for only ten months, and no new hospitals were constructed start to finish during his tenure. He felt obliged to go along with Sawyer's directives because Sawyer claimed presidential authority, and President Harding never clarified their relative responsibilities. The engineering departments of the army and navy (not Forbes) drew up plans and specifications.

Speed of construction was needed at the hospital at Northampton, thus the contract that promised construction in the shortest time was a matter of common sense, and the decision saved forty or fifty days. Forbes's old firm, Hurley-Mason, received a contract for almost $1.4 million for construction work on the hospital at American Lake in Washington State, but it was the lowest bidder, and Forbes had no financial interest in the firm. Each new hospital was discussed with President Harding, and it was Harding who suggested getting a local architect for Livermore.

Mortimer's testimony that he had received a confidential list of hospital sites before others was false. There never was such a list, "and he knows it." ("Don't get excited," said Easby-Smith.) Sites were advertised in the newspapers eight days in advance of bidding. If Mortimer stated he had earlier information on hospital sites than anyone else, Forbes said, "he states it as a lie." (Mortimer, present in the room, smiled at this point, leading Forbes to exclaim, "You laugh!" Again Easby-Smith advised him, "Do not get excited, Colonel.")[16]

On selling surplus supplies at Perryville. The Perryville depot was "one of the best junk piles the Government had," with stuff "just thrown around," it cost $700,000 a year to maintain, and Forbes was for closing it down, but there was political pressure in Maryland to keep it open. The government had sold other war surplus for less than Forbes had authorized for Perryville.

Forbes had little firsthand knowledge of the Perryville supplies; he was "unfamiliar with this stuff, because I was not at Perryville." Three bidders were considered for the Perryville contract. (At this point, Forbes became unsuitably colloquial, damaging his cause—Easby-Smith had difficulty moving him off the topic. One would-be bidder was a "little fellow" called Mr. Silberman, who came into his office and "threw out a handful of cancelled checks on my desk. And I told him to get out." Then the next day, "in walks this hombre sitting right over here [indicating a Mr. Anchester, who was present at the hearings], swinging a gold-headed cane like a drum major." Anchester said, "I am a friend of W.J. Burns of the Department of Justice, and I want to figure on this surplus property, and I am going to get some of it." Forbes asked Burns about Anchester and what Burns said "would not do to put on that paper there." The third, successful, bidder was Thompson and Kelly.)

Forbes obeyed Harding's two orders to stop the sales and had heard no charge of "insubordination" until Sawyer used the word at these hearings: "I would never commit insubordination to the President. I wouldn't do it if I was a corporal, to a sergeant. I wouldn't do it to the President of the United States."[17]

On Forbes's relationship with Elias H. Mortimer. Forbes was under the impression that Mortimer's business was arranging contracts for medical supplies and that he worked for Mulford & Company of Philadelphia, a pharmaceutical company. He fell out with Mortimer after learning he was "the social and professional bootlegger of Washington."[18]

Forbes never discussed Veterans Bureau liquor or narcotics supplies with Mortimer, and he had nothing to do with liquor or narcotics, for which the medical and supply divisions were responsible. Mortimer had talked with him about construction of veterans hospitals, "but I never gave him any encouragement." Mortimer's testimony that he had spoken with Forbes about hospital contracts at Atlantic City was "absurd" and "false," including the assertion that the contracts would be let on a cost-plus basis: "I have always been opposed to cost-plus contracts, always." (He was on record for arguing strongly against them at congressional appropriations committees.)[19]

Elias and Katherine Mortimer accompanied Forbes on the western trip in the summer of 1922 because Mortimer "suggested that he had never been to the Pacific Coast, and would like to go," and Forbes saw no reason not to invite them. There was "no carousing or anything wrong" on the trip, and Mortimer was the only person who got drunk. Forbes described Mortimer's heavy drinking, his "repeated and habitual getting full," and his abuse of his wife during the western trip: "He would usually meet some men around town and come back to his quarters very much intoxicated."[20]

Forbes had never allowed Mortimer to pay his expenses on an official trip and never asked Mortimer for a loan of $5,000. "I never accepted a penny from him in my life." Again, "He never loaned me a bean, nor did I ever ask him for any."[21]

Forbes had not said he expected to become secretary of the Interior, succeeding Albert Fall, as Mortimer had testified: "I had given up long before that any figuring on anything in the Government service."[22]

He denied all knowledge of a communications code. On learning that his code name was "McAdoo," Forbes surprised Easby-Smith by responding, "Thank you!" (Former Treasury Secretary, and President Wilson's son-in-law, William Gibbs McAdoo was then a leading candidate for the Democratic nomination for president.) The code, Forbes said, was "perfectly ridiculous."[23]

Repeatedly, in response to quotes from Mortimer's testimony, Forbes accused Mortimer of lying. Easby-Smith read out O'Ryan's prompting of Mortimer when he asked Mortimer to agree that Forbes had told him, "We fixed things so that no one lost any money." Forbes: "Again Mortimer lies." Easby-Smith: "Colonel, try to restrain yourself, won't you?" Forbes: "I am restraining myself."[24]

On Forbes's relationship with building contractor John W. Thompson. Forbes met Thompson in Washington about a month before the western trip and saw him in Chicago but had made no plans to meet him there. He did not know anything about Thompson's subsidiary companies and had never met him, as Mortimer had testified, in Walter Content's apartment in New York, where there was allegedly much drinking.

On the testimony of James Williams. Forbes did not talk about narcotics with Williams at any time, as Williams had testified. The last time he visited them "the house was full of company." Forbes had no private conversation with Mr. Williams in the kitchen, as claimed. Williams, who was in the dairy business, sat on a chair in the middle of the living room and "began talking about cheese. He talked cheese for about four hours and a half."[25]

On criticisms of Forbes's integrity. Forbes never took a decision without being advised by experts. He objected to the "charge or insinuation of dishonesty. . . . I want to tell you honestly and truthfully from the bottom of my heart. I have nothing to conceal, and I think it is—excuse me please." Again, he was overcome by emotion.[26]

After Easby-Smith exhausted his set of questions (there were many more than noted here), O'Ryan attacked the charges Forbes made in his opening statement: "You thought originally that this investigation was of the bureau and not of you. . . . You believe it is an investigation of you?" Forbes, "I do." Who were the conspirators? Forbes named Mortimer, Williams, and "others." O'Ryan, with a supercilious edge: "And all those who have testified against you?" No, Forbes replied, only those who had been "induced to testify" against him: "Those who have perjured themselves, and have been so browbeaten that they were afraid to do otherwise." Here Easby-Smith backed up Forbes by saying they had proof of this. O'Ryan's interrogation suggested subtly, without actually saying so, that Forbes was delusional.[27]

O'Ryan characterized Forbes's relationship with General Sawyer, quite fairly, as "strained," tied him up in verbal knots, and provoked him to say that Sawyer had lied in his testimony. O'Ryan: "Had the doctor any improper motives in giving the testimony that he did, or do you believe him to be simply mistaken?" Forbes: "No: he is not mistaken: he just told a lie." Forbes tried to get O'Ryan to understand that Sawyer had impeded his actions, to no avail. O'Ryan ignored him. With consummate skill, he presented Forbes as an administrator who was inadequate, untrustworthy, and confused.[28]

Next, O'Ryan made a frontal attack on Forbes's professional expertise, beginning with his qualifications. Forbes had referred to himself as an engineer. "What kind of an engineer?" Civil engineer. "What college did you graduate from?" Forbes: "I took my work privately and special work at Columbia." "Do you hold a degree?" No. "How are you a civil engineer, if you do not hold a degree?" He cast doubt on Forbes's assertion that he could get a state license if he needed one, and then walked Forbes rapidly through a confusing array of topics, asserting dominance. The session on November 14 ended with O'Ryan in full flow at 4:30 p.m., ready to begin again on the morrow. He appeared to be enjoying himself.[29]

The following day, Thursday, November 15, 1923, O'Ryan went all out to bring Forbes down: "It is a well-known recourse of embarrassed witnesses to distract attention from themselves by attacking others. Colonel Forbes

I regard as irresponsible. I expect, however, to prove much more than irresponsibility in his conduct of office and in his lack of care of the disabled. I expect to prove convincingly the whole truth of Mortimer's charge that Colonel Forbes was one of a gang of conspirators who were tied together neck and jowl to defraud the Government. I expect to show further that this criminal conduct was in consonance with his previous life record."[30]

Front-page news carried the following headlines: "Says He Will Prove Forbes a Grafter." "Forbes Led Gang of Conspirators, Declares O'Ryan." Forbes's personal history and character were now fair game. Senator Reed protested, as he had before, that this "is not an investigation of Colonel Forbes," but then waffled: "But the charge has been made that witnesses have been suborned, and that testimony has been suppressed; and if those charges are true, it is important that the committee should know them." O'Ryan interrogated Forbes about his family background. "Are you a native-born citizen, or naturalized?" (In other words, are you a real American?) Forbes explained he was a citizen through his father's naturalization papers, which was true. O'Ryan jumped to what he was paid when he worked at the Hurley-Mason Company. Forbes says he had a $6,000 "drawing account." O'Ryan seemed to be suggesting that Forbes was a $6,000 man, not worth his $10,000 salary at the bureau. Peppering him with questions, O'Ryan completely unsettled Forbes.[31]

Leading questions made the interrogation move fast. Why did Forbes permit unacceptable conditions in Veterans Bureau hospitals? When Forbes tried to explain, O'Ryan turned to Reed: "I would prefer, Mr. Chairman, that this witness, who was allowed full rein yesterday to make stump speeches, be required now to answer questions categorically."

O'Ryan asked Forbes about giving a highly paid job to Mortimer's brother-in-law (Katherine Mortimer's younger brother George Tullidge, who is misidentified in the hearings as "Ralph"). "Now, Colonel Forbes, do you swear before this committee that that appointment was not made to please Mrs. Mortimer?" Forbes seemed mesmerized, then solemnly replied, "I swear." The hammering continued. Did Colonel Forbes "recall that on October 6, this year, an action was commenced against you in Seattle?" The question forced Forbes to say that the case was a divorce action brought by his wife. Easby-Smith objected to questions about the divorce. Reed ruled the question acceptable if O'Ryan could show evidence of "moral turpitude" with respect to any government authority, past or present. O'Ryan produced a copy of the divorce papers and suggested that Forbes used the name Charles Forbes without his middle initial in the divorce papers to avoid publicity. The questions had come a long way from an investigation of the Veterans Bureau.[32]

O'Ryan: Why did Forbes consider Elias Mortimer an attractive companion? "Well he seemed to be plausible" is the best Forbes could do. O'Ryan gave the impression that he, John Francis O'Ryan, would never have been taken in by Mortimer and that, by saying Mortimer was "plausible," Forbes was either lying or a fool. Nothing was made of the fact that Mortimer was plausible enough to be the star witness at the hearings, but that was not the issue. Mortimer was a tool O'Ryan was exploiting as he would any valuable informer in a war. In turn, Forbes was apparently Mortimer's tool.[33]

The committee members wanted to speed up proceedings and get back to their other work. After the lunch recess on Thursday, Reed came out with a statement that the committee strongly supported General O'Ryan and praised him for "carry[ing] out the purposes of his appointment with zeal that does him credit." Forbes drew on a hidden reserve of energy. Confusing attempts to say what trip happened when, as O'Ryan kept producing new copies of hotel bills, provoked him: "What kind of a badger game is this?" Reed rebuked Forbes. The battering continued. Did Forbes expect the committee to believe that Mortimer had no business purpose in making the western trip? Forbes: "Absolutely." Did he by then not think Mortimer had some ulterior purpose in mind? Forbes: "I do not know what he had in mind." Though invited to do so, Forbes refused to involve the bureau's former legal counsel, the late Charles Cramer, in possible crime. He seemed more relaxed, even excessively so, veering toward flippancy. The best we can say of his performance is that he survived O'Ryan's ruthless, well-honed cross-examination.[34]

By the end of Thursday, Forbes had been giving testimony for three days, but O'Ryan had not finished with him and Easby-Smith had further questions. Forbes reconfirmed to O'Ryan that he had known nothing about the code: "Absolutely: never saw it in my life until you put it on the desk here the other day." He confirmed that he reviewed a contract document for the Colombian project and had Milliken of the bureau's legal department look at it from the legal perspective but said he did not discuss the project with Mortimer and did not consider further involvement. O'Ryan leaned on Forbes's personal weaknesses and Forbes did not see the trap. How was it that he carried around with him on the western trip a man (Mortimer) who was, according to Forbes, a drunkard? Forbes: "He would have his little souse parties, and I would tell him unless he cut it out he would have to leave the party. He would always apologize and say, 'I am perfectly all right, and I won't do it again.'" O'Ryan: "And you believed it?" Forbes: "I believed it." O'Ryan: "Continuously?" Forbes: "Yes; I did."[35]

O'Ryan petitioned the committee to introduce further materials about Forbes's past. "Oh, I do not intend to say what those records are," said O'Ryan ingenuously, when Easby-Smith objected; he merely thought it his "duty" to show Forbes's record, "good, bad, or indifferent, whatever it may be." Reed refused the petition, but the denial helped substantiate descriptions of Forbes as outlandish or picaresque, a man with a disreputable background.[36]

Everyone was tired. Fortuitously, brief testimony from veterans' representatives sparked new energy when they complained that the hearings were irrelevant to veterans' needs. Leaders of Disabled American Veterans (DAV) were outraged at the direction the hearings had taken, not because they were unfair to Forbes but because they had gone off-track: "The men want to know what is hoped to be gathered from all these charges, denials, and countercharges which at best read like a newspaper account of a dog fight." Two of the senators rushed to defend themselves. Republican Reed lectured DAV Commander James A. McFarland on the importance of listening to the "defense" being made "by an official who is charged by very grave crimes" in his administration of the Veterans Bureau, thus portraying Forbes as an accused criminal in need of a defense. Democrat Walsh: "We never again can have in charge of this bureau a man who allows politics to control his action, or who allows incompetents to serve under him." He declared that the president (Harding) should be held responsible.[37]

Easby-Smith regained the floor on Friday afternoon. His points included (among others): Forbes did have his suspicions of Cramer, but it was "so much hearsay." There was nothing concrete to substantiate the many rumors. Forbes regretted firing his chief medical adviser, Dr. Haven Emerson. Kate Forbes had some (minimal) involvement with the Mortimers. Katherine Mortimer had telephoned Forbes at the Wardman Park to go up to the Mortimer apartment where he found her injured (by Mortimer). Forbes was reluctant to get "mixed up in family rows," and so on. Each little piece of evidence was useful, but there was no effect large enough to overcome received perceptions of Mortimer and Forbes.[38]

The proceedings were becoming more and more like a trial. O'Ryan cross-examined Forbes, pushing at his "moral character." First, sex: The name of the actress Forbes met in Atlantic City was "Teddie." (This was actually the name of the racy flapper Francine Larrimore played on stage.) Ms. Larrimore had asked Forbes to meet her in Europe for a "good time," but he declined. Then liquor: "You are quite sure about this drinking on your part in the bureau, are you?" (He meant lack of drinking, to which Forbes had testified.) Marital behavior: O'Ryan tried to shake Forbes over his divorce record (without asking Forbes whether he had been divorced from his first wife).

Finally, Forbes was excused as a witness. His face was flushed, his voice weak. His physician gave him a sedative. The Associated Press, reaching across many of the nation's smaller papers, summed up the past few days: "The sharp plowshare of the senate veterans' committee driven forward again Friday through the affairs of Director Charles R. Forbes, turned up another collection of charges, denials and counter charges."[39]

Easby-Smith's remaining efforts backfired. His first witness, Stephen Davis Timberlake, the smart, long-winded lawyer from Staunton, Virginia, who had counseled Katherine Mortimer about her divorce, launched into long and convoluted testimony against James and Margaret Williams and Mortimer. O'Ryan would have cut him off, but O'Ryan was away for a change, and Major Arnold was in control. Walsh claimed they might have to strike Timberlake's testimony from the record. Reed said Timberlake had called Mortimer "an unrepeatable and filthy name" during the recess the previous day. Timberlake said he called Mortimer a "very opprobrious name" because "he had the effrontery to speak to me while I was addressing Mr. Hogshead," his friend from Staunton. When Mortimer hid behind Major Arnold, Timberlake said, he invited both of them outside. He did not say, as Arnold alleged, that he would knock Arnold's head off. Timberlake referred them to the Capitol police to confirm what he said. It was time for a change of direction.[40]

On Saturday, November 17, the Senate investigating committee made a declarative statement: no more attempts would be allowed to impeach Elias H. Mortimer. Shorn of the possibility of shaking Mortimer's testimony, Easby-Smith focused his string of witnesses on pro-Forbes testimony: hospital contracting procedures were not in Forbes's hands, sobriety existed at work, Forbes had not seen coded messages, Forbes's staff had seen no evidence of favoritism or corruption, and so forth. Such facts were dull stuff for audience and reporters, not good theater. But, then, on Saturday evening, O'Ryan and Mortimer came back onstage and regained control of the production. O'Ryan strengthened his stated belief in a conspiracy. Mortimer dropped more sexual innuendoes and sharpened up his role as a cruelly deceived husband: "I had never had any trouble in my life before until I met this fellow Forbes."[41]

Most usefully for the accusations, Mortimer gave a brilliant new description of the secret handover of $5,000 he said he had made to Forbes at the Drake Hotel, Chicago, when they were on the western trip:

Forbes was in with Mrs. Mortimer when Thompson and I were in this bathroom. I got the money. [Here the audience could imagine a fistful of crisp 500-dollar bills changing hands, $15,000 in all.] Thompson came out and went in with me into our room, and I said, "Forbes, I want to see you." He said, "All right, Mort." He came out and we went in there and I counted them out. [Fingering and crackle of $5,000 worth of banknotes.] He put them in his pocket and didn't do anything more, only just laughed and went back into the room and started shooting craps. After that we dressed for dinner, and Thompson took us out to a club, one of the country clubs there.[42]

It mattered not in the crafting of public opinion that Mortimer's account varied from other claims he made, or whether the transaction happened. The public was familiar with similar stories about bootleggers and others passing ill-gotten gains to one another. Such stories could be found in the press, in fiction, and on the ubiquitous movie screen. His account was, in a word, believable. In it, Mortimer and Forbes were cronies, equally complicit. The gem in this telling is the laugh.

Thus, the early themes of the hearings survived. By the end of the hearings there were two strikingly different versions of Forbes as a "character": the Forbes who had put the Veterans Bureau together (a thankless job), had started the US national veterans hospital system, and was defended by

Easby-Smith and the Forbes described by O'Ryan and Mortimer as a crook in league with other crooks. Press accounts portrayed the character of Colonel Forbes not as he and his supporting witnesses presented it, but as he was described by the investigators: soaked in the forces of corruption and its attendants—graft, sex, booze, and greed.

James Easby-Smith said his formal goodbye to the Senate investigating committee on Monday, November 19, submitting additional materials to the committee later in the week. The transcript of the hearings supports his contention that the positive case for Forbes was not made, but this was an investigation, not a court of law, and not the first or last congressional hearing to be biased. The committee had investigated and concluded. Charles Sawyer was a believable witness on the Perryville supplies. Elias Mortimer dropped his stories into willing ears. John F. O'Ryan seemed convinced of fraud from the beginning. He told Easby-Smith his purpose was to bring out "the complete story of this conspiracy" and that he was not interested in hearing about discrepancies in testimony. The senators did not object. If there was fraud in government, it was their duty to detect it.[43]

Privately, James Easby-Smith held strong views. The hearings "were unfair in the extreme," he wrote Kate Forbes. "After consuming several weeks with hearing utterly inadmissible and incompetent testimony, most of which was pure hearsay and plain perjury, Colonel Forbes took the stand and was examined by me, and then cross-examined by the committee and its counsel, for three days . . . and after proceedings for one single day the committee cut me off and refused to permit me any further time to present evidence. It is simply impossible for me to find language to express my feeling concerning the conduct of this committee and its so-called counsel." He ended with a message of characteristic graciousness to Kate, who remained affectionately attached to the husband she was divorcing: "It may not be necessary but it may be of some consolation to you for me to say that I have investigated Colonel Forbes's life and conduct with extreme care and in the most minute detail, and I do not hesitate to express the opinion that he is absolutely innocent of any official or personal wrongdoing and that the attacks made on him before and during the Senate investigation constituted one of the most unjust and unjustified persecutions of a faithful official that has ever come under my notice."[44]

SCANDAL WEAVERS

Scripting a Story of Rogues, Graft, and Greed

At the end of November 1923, when the Veterans Bureau hearings were over and the Senate committee and John F. O'Ryan were writing their reports, the oil hearings came into their own. Witnesses revealed that while serving as interior secretary, Albert B. Fall had spent a suspiciously large amount of money on his ranch properties in New Mexico and paid long-overdue back taxes. Soon it was revealed that in 1922 he had quietly approved leases to oil millionaires and their corporations to drill for oil on government lands: notably, the lease of Naval Reserve No. 3 (Teapot Dome, Wyoming) to Mammoth Oil Company (Harry F. Sinclair), and Naval Reserve No. 1 (Elk Hills, California) to Edward L. Doheny.

Democratic, Progressive, and Republican senators seized on the conclusions of the Veterans Bureau hearings as proof of pervasive evils in the Harding administration, with the oil hearings promising more proof. The two Republicans on the Senate investigating committee, David Reed and Tasker Oddie, visited President Coolidge at the White House on December 1, 1923, accompanied by Frank Hines, the director of the Veterans Bureau. Attorney General Daugherty announced that criminal prosecutions would be brought and that he had lined up one of the "most vigorous prosecutors in the country," Assistant Attorney General John W. H. Crim, a hard-driving legal crusader in his midforties with a reputation for fighting graft and corruption in antitrust cases, war frauds, and liquor and bootlegging conspiracies. In the summer of 1922, Crim had investigated allegations of fraud in the office of the Alien Property Custodian, Harding-appointee Thomas W. Miller, a former director of the Republican Campaign Committee. Crim had submitted his resignation from the Justice Department effective December 15 to return to private practice but agreed to take on the Forbes case at a "personal sacrifice." General John F. O'Ryan and Major Davis Arnold of the

Senate investigating team would work with him, providing a seamless transition from hearings to indictments.[1]

Crim saw his new assignment as a call to arms against a rabid band of nation-threatening monsters. He wanted the "most aggressive, personal cooperation at the very outset of the President and yourself," he wrote Daugherty in a long memo, and expected to need the "aggressive cooperation" of other members of the cabinet: "The Reed Committee . . . saw such a disgusting situation, the entire gamut of the conduct of the lowest, commonest crooks imaginable. Grafting was relatively the most respectable thing they did. This rascality is not confined to the Veterans Bureau. . . . It is a much bigger thing than the rascality of Forbes. While his picturesqueness made him a conspicuous member of the ring, there are others not connected with the Veterans Bureau involved. Major Arnold feels that perhaps there will be 200 cases grow out of this." Daugherty tried to moderate Crim's saber-waving by reminding him that the entire resources of the Justice Department would not be his for the taking—"we must remember that there are other persons in the Department besides you and me"—but he clearly knew that under Crim no stone would be unturned.[2]

At the Department of Justice, Crim worked closely with Assistant Attorney General Mabel Walker Willebrandt, who supervised the turncoat bootlegger Elias H. Mortimer, who was ready to reprise his role as star witness at the expected trial of Charles R. Forbes. Willebrandt was canny in selecting key targets and using informers, as well as getting good press. "She doesn't give a hang for publicity yet gets it all the time," a City Police Court defender wrote admiringly from Los Angeles, where she had worked. In a well-publicized raid against the "Savannah Rings" in Savannah, Georgia, in August 1923, eighty-four men had been arrested under the Volstead Act. Willebrandt supplemented inadequate resources at the Justice Department by getting help in the field wherever she could. Elias Mortimer, embedded in the illegal liquor business, was worth his weight in gold—both to her and to Crim. Mortimer's prominence at the Senate hearings showed that he possessed skills that went beyond prohibition cases, though these continued to be his base, and that he was a believable, first-rate witness.[3]

Mortimer's informal relationship with the Department of Justice was soon regularized. He became officially "on call" for the department on February 1, 1924. Soon he was acting openly as a paid government "agent." In March, Willebrandt wrote to the commissioner of Internal Revenue asking for an extension for him in filing his federal tax return: "For several weeks, Mr. Mortimer has been continuously engaged in appearing before the grand juries at Chicago and Washington, DC, in connection with criminal prosecutions being handled by this Department." Mortimer was assigned a federal agent, Gaspare J. "Mike" Allegra, ostensibly to protect him and keep him out of trouble, though from the record they seemed to function like partners. Allegra had come with his family from Sicily as a child. In 1924, Mortimer was living in New York, and Allegra was working as an undercover agent out of the FBI's New York office.[4]

The well-publicized oil hearings, coming soon after the Veterans Bureau hearings, fed speculation that corruption in government departments was widespread during the Harding administration and that something had to be done. In the New Year of 1924, besides Fall, Sinclair, and Doheny, the hearings involved Secretary of the Navy Edwin Denby, Assistant Navy Secretary, former Sinclair Oil director Theodore Roosevelt, Jr., and Attorney General Harry M. Daugherty, who had allegedly "smoothed" legal action in order to allow government oil leases to be transferred to private corporations. The scandalous news in late January was that Fall had lied to Congress about accepting a loan of $100,000 from millionaire oilman Doheny—in cash, delivered in a black satchel by his son. President Coolidge informed the press that the Department of Justice had advised him to employ high-ranked special counsel to prosecute the oil cases. Congress passed a joint resolution that the president should appoint an investigating committee independent of that department—a slam against Attorney General Daugherty. In mid-February, Secretary Denby resigned under pressure from both Republicans and Democrats for his role in transferring naval oil leases to the Department of Interior. Daugherty kept his job until March 28, when he too resigned. Albert Fall was on a seven-year cavalcade of pain. In 1931, he became the first cabinet member convicted of a felony who went to prison.

"The shadow of a great scandal has fallen on the Republican administration," wrote Arthur Sears Henning for the *Chicago Tribune* in January 1924. Congress was staking out the high ground against a corruption-ridden administrative bureaucracy. Self-righteous men howled for revenge. Journalist Mark Sullivan passed two gems along in February. First: "No propaganda coming out of Russia had done as much to undermine public confidence in government and big business as has the oil scandal." Second, President Harding had been a man of integrity whose administration would be remembered for the betrayal of public trust by his friends, as indicated by this headline: "Harding's Old Friends Seen as a Blight . . . Fall and Forbes Only Two in Point."[5]

The Senate Committee on Investigation of the United States Veterans Bureau issued three separate "preliminary" reports and no final report. The first, introduced by Senator Reed and published at the end of January 1924, addressed needed changes in the laws dealing with veterans' benefits and their administration, which were scattered across different pieces of legislation. The committee introduced a bill as a basis for immediate codification of the statutes and recommended twenty-two other changes. Codification was achieved under the World War Veterans' Act, June 1924, together with extensions in veterans' services. Senator David Walsh, the Democratic member of the committee, introduced the third preliminary report, which focused on improvements in hospital care. The hearings had positive aspects for the Veterans Bureau in stimulating revisions in the law, expanding services, and providing better management tools (and a higher salary, $12,000) for the director.[6]

The second report, from General John F. O'Ryan, focused on the manifold failures of Charles R. Forbes. News that the Veterans Bureau district offices were generally working satisfactorily was tucked away in small print in the appendix. Far-seeing recommendations for the "Betterment of Conditions" were included in the O'Ryan report. Its message, however, was one of condemnation: Forbes was "neither able nor honorable in the conduct of his office." In O'Ryan's view, changes in the laws were not enough: "No statute can supply character where character is lacking, or ability where it does not exist." Among Forbes's reported weaknesses was engagement in a "continuing round of social pleasure," with "lavish entertainment." O'Ryan presented Forbes's criminality as proved, and Mortimer's story of the $5,000 loan as fact: Ten $500 bills "were actually delivered to Forbes by Mortimer in the bathroom of Forbes' suite at the Drake Hotel in Chicago, June 22,

1922." It had been "conclusively established by the testimony of witnesses, by documentary evidence, and by the corroborative effect of numerous tell-tale circumstances that were brought out, that fraud and corruption existed in the bureau and that Director Forbes was a leading actor in the established conspiracy to defraud the Government." O'Ryan made handwritten changes on a draft of the report to make his critique more powerful. The Perryville transaction became "more the work of buccaneers in the looting and scut-tling of a ship than the mere negligence of trusted Government officials"; while new sheets "were run through and out the other side to the waiting cars of the contractor who carried them off as part of the booty."[7]

In annihilating the reputation of a lieutenant colonel who had not come up to scratch, the general acted as judge and jury. There was a word for his method: "debunking." As defined by a serious writer on public opinion and propaganda, Will Irwin (soon to be introduced): "The art of debunking, as old as the human race, consists mostly of massing the flaws, weaknesses, faults of your victim and telling them without recording his strengths, powers and virtues. Any mere man who ever lived could be deflated to a rag by this process." Forbes was deflated to a rag.[8]

Initially, the three senators distanced themselves from the O'Ryan report, referring to it as "General O'Ryan's report" and to his findings and recommendations as "his own" and "not those of the committee." They endorsed his view of "the wretched incompetence, waste and dishonesty of the administration of the bureau under Director Forbes" but avoided naming Forbes as the sole culprit or as an out-and-out crook. But they soon fell into line. The public mood was to condemn. Senator Reed declared that the committee's "non-partisan, unbiased policy" had been followed, and he had that in mind in appointing a "representative Democrat of New York" (O'Ryan) as counsel. Reed received the congratulations of his senatorial colleagues for a job well done. According to the *New York Times*, the Veterans Bureau scandal was more abhorrent and disheartening than the oil scandals. Teapot Dome had its princely oil millionaires—Doheny with his palatial estate in Pasadena; Sinclair with his Manhattan mansion and opulent railroad car. The Veterans Bureau scandal was an American morality tale in which officials cheated America's distressed and wounded heroes, a story replete with influence peddling, drunken parties, dirty deals.[9]

An impressive amount of talent was focused on a dramatic "character" named Charles R. Forbes in the early months of 1924, over and above the considerable talent available to the Senate committee and Justice Department. Loring Pickering of the Northern American Newspaper Alliance, a syndicated feature service of the Associated Press, launched an important literary project when he asked fifty-year-old writer William Henry "Will" Irwin to create an exciting, readable narrative of the case out of the confusing transcripts of the Senate hearings. Pickering thought the Forbes case had more juice to squeeze out of it as a story. Irwin remembered his initial doubts. He was apparently being asked to do "muckraking" (digging up dirt), which was then out of style ("the novelists were assuming the task," Irwin wrote). Also, the time to complete the expected series of articles was short, because the offer required the articles to be published before the grand jury handed down its indictments, and the Justice Department was steaming ahead. However, the timing would give the series thrilling relevance. Irwin had spent considerable time overseas during and after the war, national publicity would be welcome and the money was (presumably) good, and Pickering would provide him with two assistants. General O'Ryan would also be helpful. In January, O'Ryan sent a telegram to Senator Reed for photostatic copies of the committee's original exhibits and then made them available to Irwin to copy as he wished.

Will Irwin was one of a new, twentieth-century breed of professional journalists. He majored in English at Stanford University, where he became a lasting friend of Herbert Hoover. Outgoing, well read, a jokester, he became a member of the "artistic bunch" of painters, poets, novelists, actors, and stage directors in San Francisco, where he worked as a reporter for the *San Francisco Chronicle* before moving east to work for the *New York Sun*. During World War I, he worked for the US government's war propaganda machine, the Committee on Public Information, as did many writers of the time. Hence, his interest in the making of public opinion. He accepted Pickering's offer and agreed to review the Senate hearings to take a look at the case, "and, if the facts were as he understood it, to stir it up." And stir it up he did. He described his contribution later, writing about himself in the third person: "This man brought to light no unpublished facts. After a few interviews by way of getting the atmosphere, he buckled down to four large volumes of committee reports, already in print. From them and them alone he wrote a running story of the scandal in the Veterans Bureau. And for the first time the public understood the situation, felt the proper righteous indignation; and Forbes went to trial." Irwin's articles provided an accessible, racy narrative of the hearings, as seen from the O'Ryan and Mortimer points of view.[10]

Forbes's perspective was noticeably absent from the series. For much of 1924, he was ill in the Brighton district of Boston, where he had sought comfort from the two women who had known and loved him longest: his widowed mother, Christina Forbes, and his married older sister, nurse Marie Forbes Judkins, with whom their mother lived. In New York, where Irwin lived, Elias H. Mortimer, however, was very much present. He spent "whole afternoons at my house, spilling what seemed elaborate romances," Irwin wrote. Soon Mortimer found the key to Irwin's imagination in the powerful narrative of love, betrayal, and revenge: Mortimer had an attractive wife, a "pretty and smart young woman very popular in one of several presidential sets." Forbes had cheated him and wrecked his life, and Mortimer was after retribution at any cost. Years later Irwin wrote of Mortimer, "Whenever I pass a rosewood sofa in our living room, I seem to see him yet—a slight, youngish man, his dress correct to the last detail, his dark hair always in perfect order, his face handsome almost to prettiness, yet hard." Suffering, he wrote, "had tied a permanent knot between his brows and in repose his dark eyes were somber." He "followed one star—revenge." After days and nights of agony, he had resolved to come clean—"'even if I have to spend the rest of my life in jail.'" This was a great dramatic performance. Mortimer knew that as a vital witness for the prosecution he would not go to trial. According to Irwin's friend Samuel Hopkins Adams, Irwin remembered Mortimer saying, "I'm going to get that bastard if I go up for life."[11]

Negative descriptions of Forbes intermeshed with the competence of a well-oiled machine. Federal Judge George A. Carpenter summoned a special grand jury in Chicago on February 6, 1924, with Mortimer as a key witness. O'Ryan's report for the Senate committee was officially published on February 7. Irwin's seven-day series ran in major newspapers beginning February 11, with multipage episodes, photos, and exhibits. The grand jury handed down indictments against Forbes and Thompson on February 29. In short order, O'Ryan lambasted Forbes as a crook, Crim associated him with Mortimer's account of crimes, and Irwin stirred up public opinion. Distinctive pictures of Forbes wove together. Crim used the words "rascality" and "picturesqueness" in his memo to Attorney General Daugherty. O'Ryan effectively called Forbes an immoral predator. Irwin described him as the "most picaresque figure in recent American life." His Forbes had a mythical quality. He was a man imbued with disconcerting charm, the ability to make speeches, and sexually charged charisma. Crim's Forbes was a criminal whose acts threatened the very fabric of democracy. O'Ryan's Forbes was a military man who unscrupulously pilfered supplies and deserved court martial, but Irwin's Forbes was a wayward rogue, with a bit of hucksterism thrown in: "Lively, vital, witty in a rough way, his mouth full of good stories and harmless gossip of the day, he had above everything the trick of personality." Mortimer told Irwin that Forbes "could stand up before a thousand people and make 'em laugh and cry as he wanted."[12]

Irwin retold Mortimer's story that he had given Forbes a bribe of $5,000, described a conspiracy to rig hospital contracts, and emphasized the Senate investigating team's finding that $225 million was thrown away in graft and waste (mostly attributed to the "waste which always accompanies graft") in the Veterans Bureau in its first two years. Each of these became a lasting factoid of the "Forbes scandal." The series came out under headlines that represented each paper's editorial view. Samples from the Atlanta Constitution: "Forbes Pours Lives of Crippled Heroes into Pot of Graft . . . U.S. Army Deserter Betrays High Trust" (February 11, 1924); "Mortimer Fiddles His Golden Violin for Forbes's Dance . . . Mortimer Pays All Bills after Forbes Promises Much Profit to Former's Employers" (February 12); "'Scotch Generals' [Bottles of Scotch] Meet Col. Forbes on Pacific Coast . . . Grape Crop [at Livermore] Fails to Worry Forbes. 'We'll Get All the Wine We Want'" (February 13); "Frolic of Forbes Lands Juicy Plum in Lap of Builder . . . Chief of Vets' Bureau with Lady Friend Leap Fully Clothed into Lake by Way of Prank" (February 14); "Delirium of Graft at Perryville Sale Seals Forbes' Fate . . . Open Looting Draws Unwarranted Attention" (February 15); "Written Promise of Charles Forbes Only Paper Scrap. General Sawyer Gives President Harding First Intimation of Friend's Betrayal of Trust" (February 16); "Mystery Shrouds Closing Chapter of Forbes's Case . . . Sawyer Says Harding Demands Resignation. All Graft Not Money; Much of It Used as Political Trading Stock for Republicans" (February 17). The series fizzled out toward the end. In Atlanta, the first five articles began on page 1, and the last two on inside pages. But by then the job was done. With the momentum of a freight train gaining speed, the O'Ryan report, Irwin's newspaper stories, the grand jury, and the indictments convicted Forbes in the court of public opinion before a trial date was set.[13]

Forbes waited in Washington while the grand jury was sitting in Chicago, expecting the worst. In poignant letters to his ex-wife, Kate (who was waiting for their divorce to be finalized), he described his ordeal as "awful and heartbreaking. . . . I have been framed and they are constantly trying to bring about more disgrace upon me" (February 15). "I am so tired and so sick of it all that I could just eat nails . . . the scoundrel behind it is that low hound Mortimer"; and fate had brought him to Washington to be a "[scape] goat" (February 21). "I have this awful stigma to live down. . . . It's the worst thing that could happen to any man's life"; nevertheless, he would "fight to the last ditch." Under no circumstance, he wrote, would he betray his buddies in the war: "I loved those boys and gave everything in the world to help them and hold their comradeship, I was loyal to their cause and their interests" (February 25). Four days later the grand jury handed down its indictments. There were four indictments against Forbes and wealthy St. Louis businessman John W. Thompson, the two of the five alleged conspirators named by Mortimer who were still available for prosecution. (Cramer and Black were dead, and Mortimer had been granted immunity.) Forbes and Thompson were named jointly in two of the indictments: conspiracy (with "others unknown") to commit bribery and offenses against the government and conspiracy to defraud the United States. In the third, Forbes was indicted for accepting a bribe (the $5,000 allegedly given to him by Mortimer), and in the fourth, Thompson was indicted for bribing Forbes.[14]

　　After his indictment, Forbes spent a day with James Easby-Smith, his attorney, preparing a statement for the press. Its main points were as follows: his acquaintance with John W. Thompson was slight and purely social; Thompson was "as completely innocent as myself"; he had been framed ("I am convinced that for the want of a more convenient political goat I was selected as a victim and a sacrifice"); a "puppeteer" pulled the strings (presumably O'Ryan), whose name his lawyer would not let him mention; and the three senators knew all the time that "the charges against me are as false as hell's own brood." Saying he welcomed a fair trial, with an implied emphasis on the word "fair," on March 6 he pleaded "not guilty" before the United States commissioner in Washington to the charges handed down by the grand jury and posted a $10,000 bond.[15]

Well before a trial was scheduled, the public image of Charles R. Forbes (by this time often called "Charlie Forbes") meshed into the larger narrative of corruption in the Harding administration. From the spring of 1924, one article after another across the country described Harding as the pawn of an "Ohio Gang" of whiskey-drinking, poker-playing, decadent, sordid, anti-American and treacherous cronies who surrounded a naïve but honest president. One critique compared Forbes with "jackals in human form who sneak across a battlefield after dark robbing the wounded." Crim, the government prosecutor, hoped for an early resolution of the Forbes case with an expected trial date in April, before the national political conventions. Forbes and Easby-Smith took an express train to Chicago to confer with lawyers at the Chicago firm Sims, Welch, Godman and Stransky and to prepare for the trial. Forbes made a statement in mid-March: "I am confident of demonstrating the utter falsity of all the charges made by Mortimer, upon whose testimony, I believe, the government's case is founded. . . . My opinion is that Mortimer is a character assassin of the worst type." When asked what he thought about the Senate investigating committee, Forbes's eyes flashed: "If I told you that, you couldn't print it."[16]

John W. H. Crim, however, had made a serious procedural error. Hot on the trail, he had contracted with a firm of private stenographers, Satterlee and Binns, to take notes at the grand jury proceedings, thereby breaching the theory of secrecy of the grand jury. The presence of the stenographers undermined the legitimacy of the proceedings. Another grand jury would have to be appointed and the process started again, with new indictments. Parallel pressures in February and March 1924 to push out Harry Daugherty as attorney general further complicated Crim's life by threatening to remove the man who had appointed him. The next attorney general might take Crim off the case. Forbes and his attorneys would have to wait for months, as it turned out.

Crim was rescued from a potentially ruinous situation by a brilliant exercise of diversion and misdirection: Elias Mortimer and Mabel Walker Willebrandt, Crim's former colleague at the Department of Justice (who supervised Mortimer), suddenly introduced a powerful but extraneous set of accusations that swamped press coverage of the Forbes case. Out of the blue, or so it seemed, Mortimer made startling charges of corruption against two unnamed members of Congress for crimes committed under the Volstead Act—charges that were unrelated to the Veterans Bureau, or to Forbes. Crim rushed to Washington, where he conferred with members of the Senate and House without giving the names of the two suspects. President Coolidge was said to be determined to get to the bottom of these "mysterious allusions of wrongdoing." Stories ran "like wildfire" in congressional cloakrooms in Washington, rivaling the "choicest whispered stories of the oil scandal." Seen from afar, as in Billings, Montana, the alarms were overdone: "Its sensibilities already overtaxed by the kaleidoscopic career of the oil scandal, the national capital is about to witness the further ordeal of a grand jury investigation into astonishing charges against several important public officials." They were good copy. Crim and Mortimer were in the headlines.[17]

One of the accused was Congressman Frederick N. Zihlman of Maryland. Mortimer had cultivated Zihlman in his usual way and lent him and his wife money, and then allegedly tried to bribe him. Zihlman reportedly told Mortimer: "If you are that kind of a man, I want nothing more to do with you." A federal grand jury looked into charges against the congressman but ignored Mortimer's testimony referring to Zihlman and thus effectively exonerated him. The second, Congressman John Wesley Langley, sponsor of the Langley bills for veterans hospital construction, to whom Mortimer had lent a large amount of money, was not so fortunate (and may well have been guilty). Langley was indicted in Kentucky, his home state, on March 27, 1924, with Mortimer as star witness, and subsequently tried, convicted, and imprisoned. Assistant Attorney General Willebrandt took direct charge of this case. Mortimer had been part of a plan to remove a large quantity of whiskey from the Belle of Anderson distillery in Kentucky (which could be done legally with appropriate permits for medical use) without paying the necessary tax, and Langley was implicated. As noted (in chapter 6), Langley resigned from Congress in January 1926 after the Supreme Court declined to review his case.[18]

In the process, in the months between Forbes's first indictment and his trial, Crim saved face thanks to Mortimer, Mortimer accumulated credit, and Crim accorded him respect. Crim was to describe Mortimer at the

Forbes-Thompson trial as an "undercover man" employed by the Justice Department to "ferret out just such details as Forbes is alleged to have conspired in." Elsewhere, Crim said Mortimer was a "paid informer of the government," with a salary of $4,000 a year. In August 1924 (while Forbes was still awaiting a trial date), Willebrandt wrote US Attorney William Hayward in New York about the New York case in which Mortimer was still involved as a defendant, *United States v. Clifton, Codina, Mortimer et al.*, suggesting he downplay Mortimer's role and protect his participation as a witness in the Forbes case. In the Langley case, she argued, Mortimer's accuracy "was a matter of astonishment to all of us with whom he worked." Crim, too, was "outspoken in belief in his dependability in every dealing they have had." Hayward reviewed the evidence, decided that Mortimer was "at best a passive conspirator," and agreed that the case against him should not be pressed.[19]

Crim still had the prospect of new leadership at the Justice Department to face. On February 20, 1924, freshman Senator Burton K. Wheeler of Montana, a feisty and ambitious Democrat, had introduced a resolution in the Senate to a create a select committee to investigate Harry M. Daugherty for alleged failure to prosecute those accused in the oil scandal, among other issues; and the Senate approved, 66–1. Wheeler, not averse to what he called "bare-knuckle fights," began to probe, and soon heard reports that Daugherty was "up to his neck in massive graft." This was a promising agenda for Democrats as they geared up for the 1924 elections, but for Republicans, too, Daugherty, the supposed kingpin of the Ohio Gang, had become an unwanted burden. In mid-March, President Coolidge decided on Harlan Fiske Stone, a respected legal scholar, dean of Columbia University Law School, as Daugherty's replacement, and, finally, after investigative hearings had begun, Daugherty resigned. On the stand and in newspaper reports on the hearings was Roxy Stinson, the ex-wife and widow of Daugherty's associate Jess Smith, who had died by his own hand—her eyes soulful, ambitions large, bangles clinking as she gesticulated. There, too, was the infamous, overweight Gaston Means, an old-style detective of large presence and cocksure grin, who, by his own account, broke the law regularly and without compunction on special assignment for the government. While the Forbes case was on hold, the Daugherty scandal and the oil lease scandal were entertainments for the masses. Magazine writer Arthur Ruhl compared the Justice Department hearings to a small-town matinee or vaudeville transported to the capital: an "ironic comedy in disillusion." Bands of sightseers crowded the chamber "to suffocation," while many others overcrowded the "oil matinee" in another hearings room.[20]

Attorney General Stone reviewed Crim's position, but after Stone questioned Crim he kept him on as prosecutor for the Forbes trial—and was eventually pleased with the result. In June 1924, a second grand jury took place quietly, out of the headlines, and returned new indictments. The trial was delayed until late November, after the national elections.

In a second case, in April 1924, a federal grand jury indicted Forbes in Baltimore, Maryland, for conspiracy to defraud the United States in disposing of government supplies at Perryville. The accused coconspirators were Naval Commander Charles O'Leary, former chief of supplies for the Veterans Bureau, and Nathan Thompson, president of the Boston firm Thompson and Kelly, to whom supplies were sold. Brigadier General Charles E. Sawyer testified before this grand jury. On April 25, Colonel Forbes appeared voluntarily at the Federal District Court in Baltimore to plead not guilty. Bail was set at $10,000. Forbes's lawyer, Easby-Smith, pushed to keep to the initial trial date in November, but the government was granted extra time to collect evidence. General Sawyer, standing erect and projecting moral rectitude in court, might (or might not) have swayed a jury against Forbes, but had no chance to see. Sawyer died of a cerebral hemorrhage in Marion, Ohio, on September 23. The Maryland case was eventually dropped, partly because of Sawyer's absence, partly because investigators were failing to find clear evidence of fraud, and partly because Forbes was convicted in Chicago and that seemed to be enough.[21]

Jostling candidates for the national political party conventions in 1924 (three of them, including Senator Robert La Follette's Progressive Party) took spring and summer headlines. By early April, preelection speeches marked Forbes as a political target. In any review for or against Coolidge's reappointment, somebody was sure to shout, "How about Forbes?" and "How about Daugherty?" In July, the sudden tragic death of President Coolidge's younger son, Calvin, from sepsis caused by an infected blister on his foot after a tennis game, generated a wave of sympathy for the bereaved parents.

Back on the stump in August, Coolidge formally accepted the Republican Party's nomination for the presidency in the forthcoming elections. "The chief issue of this campaign," he said, "is honest government." The people of the United States "hate corruption." Individuals charged with wrongdoing were being prosecuted. Coolidge won the election, keeping the presidency he had acquired through Harding's death. Charles G. Dawes was elected vice president.[22]

Crim, the prosecuting attorney in the Forbes case, was a witness at the Brookhart-Wheeler hearings on the Department of Justice, testifying as an expert on the future organization of the department. He spoke up for Harry Daugherty, his former boss, attesting to his integrity. "He had his faults," Crim said, "but I'll have to judge the evidence myself before I'll believe he prostituted his office. To me he never faltered." Mortimer was subpoenaed to appear before the committee for his alleged role in whiskey deals and attempts to get a pardon for convicted bootlegger Charles Vincenti in return for $50,000 (the equivalent of $700,000 in twentieth-first-century terms). He was not put on the stand. His estranged wife Katherine Mortimer was called but only to testify that, yes, it was Mr. Mortimer's signature on the contract for the Vincenti deal.[23]

As attorney general, Harlan Fiske Stone brought university-based professionalism and belief in bureaucracy to a job previously held by a political deal-maker. Stone sought to modernize the Justice Department, as, in their different ways, Frank Hines was doing at the Veterans Bureau and Hubert Work at the Department of Interior. Stone fired old-style detective William J. Burns as head of the Bureau of Investigation in May, making J. Edgar Hoover the acting director. (Hoover became director of the bureau—the FBI—in December 1924 and held that position until his death in 1972.) Human relations within the organization needed improvement. Assistant to the Attorney General William J. "Wild Bill" Donovan wrestled with both Crim and J. Edgar Hoover, who controlled the work of special agents and the files they produced. Stone called a special meeting in Washington in September to iron out the various relationships and to address an altercation Crim had with Hoover on the number of special agents assigned to him—too few, Crim complained. Donovan ceded responsibility for prosecuting the criminal aspects of the Forbes case to Crim and agreed to help him in those efforts but retained responsibility for prosecution under civil law. Meanwhile, Hoover professionalized the FBI with admirable skill, holding his agents to required standards and procedures. Some basic animus remained: Donovan felt free to challenge Hoover's decisions, while Hoover considered Donovan an "unimaginative civil servant" who engaged in meddling. Each kept files on the other.[24]

For Crim, putting together the Forbes-Thompson case in Chicago, Attorney General Stone's questions about what he was doing and how he was doing it was unfair criticism. Crim needed sympathy, for facts were sparse and rumors roared. The cases are "essentially those of conspiracy," he told Stone, but "two of the four conspirators are dead." (Mortimer, the fifth, had done a deal with the prosecution.) After Crim offered his resignation, Stone backed down, promising to "do everything possible to hold up your hands so that the government's case may proceed to a successful conclusion." Whatever their doubts about each other, all concerned at the Department of Justice agreed that Forbes was guilty and should be indicted and convicted as a national example of government corruption. Crim referred to the "Forbes case," not the Thompson-Forbes or Forbes-Thompson case, and left Thompson in the background as a prop: a shadowy figure whose role as a conspirator was simply assumed. John W. Thompson, up until then a successful, reputable businessman, did not testify in public at any point in the case, including the Senate hearings and the trial. Though well served by lawyers, he comes down through time as a wraithlike presence.[25]

Crim's imperial orders were not appreciated by the long-suffering, quietly hostile Bureau of Investigation (FBI), as he mobilized agents around the country to drop everything, find people and evidence and send him immediate results. These orders continued even as the trial was taking place. Finding the witnesses was problem enough. Lila Cramer, the young widow of Veterans Bureau lawyer Charles Cramer, proved particularly elusive, even though the US Post Office was checking her mail in Washington, DC, and her father's mail in Kansas City. Agents were still hoping (in vain) that she would produce a suicide letter that would incriminate the conspiracy as a whole. Forbes's former government aide, Merle L. Sweet, was hard to find because after the Senate hearings ended in December 1923, he left the country on behalf of Forbes's fledgling San Francisco business, Charles R. Forbes and

Company, Exporters and Importers, for Soerabaja, Java, in what was then the Dutch East Indies, where he expected to stay for two or three years. Marguerite Sweet, Merle's wife, had sold their furniture and was waiting for instructions to sail when she received an alarming telegram commanding her to appear before the first grand jury. "What does this mean?" she wrote Crim. Her husband returned in haste to the United States, arriving May 10, only to hear rumors that he had been bribed to leave the country, was a material witness against Forbes (when he was actually a strong supporter), and had fled the country without filing a tax return. (He had had to wait for the US tax forms to arrive in Java.) Sweet wrote wryly to the American consul in Soerabaja: "Who knows but that this suggestion of my being an important contributor to the Department of Infernal [sic] Revenue may prove to be a big ad for Yours truly M.L.S." Humor was a necessary commodity. Forbes and Company was destroyed.[26]

Katherine Mortimer's uncle, James Williams, and his wife were important prosecution witnesses. Mr. Williams was expected to testify that Forbes had discussed illegally transporting narcotics held by the Veterans Bureau via the Williams fleet of milk trucks, and Mrs. Williams was expected to agree with him. (Forbes said no such discussion took place.) Williams could also attest to the employment of his nephew, young George Tullidge, as a low-wage truck driver for his creamery company before Forbes employed him in an overpaid engineering job in the Veterans Bureau. Federal agents found Mr. Williams at home in Philadelphia, duly served him a subpoena, and ordered him to appear with his wife in Chicago. Mrs. Williams refused to go. She had been in Florida for six weeks and saw no reason to accompany her husband to a cold and windy city in February. Crim send an urgent telegram to the FBI office in Miami, causing Special Agent Leon Howe to check her presence "under the pretext of wishing to buy the house." A separate subpoena was served on her; she demanded money for the trip, and the agent made her a train reservation to Chicago.[27]

False leads wasted the time of federal agents, such as a report to the FBI from Mortimer associate Henry Anchester that a Mrs. Forbes, supposedly a second cousin of Charles R. Forbes, lived in the Majestic Hotel in Philadelphia and knew that Forbes had "large sums of money in his possession . . . and that she knew of sums of money that he had received for 'crooked deals that he had pulled while in Washington.'" Special agent E. E. Conroy took time out from his inquiries about the sales of surplus supplies at Perryville to interview her in Philadelphia. This Mrs. Forbes quite emphatically stated that she was not Forbes's relative, had never seen him, never been employed by the Veterans Bureau, and knew nothing about him "except that she had heard Mortimer, who lived in a room opposite to hers in the Rittenhouse Hotel [in Philadelphia], make derogatory statements in regard to him; and that she had no knowledge of Forbes having any money or having received any for 'crooked deals.'" Agent Conroy noted in his report that Anchester's previous information had not proved reliable and concluded that this claim was also unreliable. Crim viewed the FBI as obstructive.[28]

At times, federal agents practically fell over one another. For example, Special Agent Y. O. Wilson embarked on an investigation for Assistant Attorney General Donovan of how Director Forbes paid for the impressive automobile he bought after his return from his western trip (during which Mortimer allegedly handed him $5,000), only to learn from a vice president of sales for the Hoffman Motor Company that numerous Department of Justice agents had been there seeking the same information. None of them came up with anything concrete. The car was expensive, a six-passenger vehicle selling for $3,585, plus extras. Forbes was allowed $1,400 as the trade-in price for his Cole automobile, paid $1,000 in cash, and signed a sixty-day note for the rest. None of this money (nor any deposits in Forbes's bank accounts) could be traced back to Mortimer.[29]

The Baltimore indictment set off a parallel rush to find evidence, this time for phony contracts, kickbacks, and rigged bids in selling government supplies to a private corporation for twenty cents of their imputed dollar value. FBI agents were soon bogged down in hopelessly inadequate detail. How did you compare the cost of one bolt of blue Melton cloth with another, when they had come from different depots, from different suppliers, at different dates without accompanying paperwork? Thompson and Kelly, the firm that bought the Perryville consignment, was a reputable business in Boston, set up to buy surplus materials in large quantities and sell them at a small profit to firms such as Montgomery Ward for retail. There was no evidence that Forbes had profited in this, nor anyone else. Neither Forbes nor O'Leary (his accused coconspirator) had suspicious deposits in their bank accounts. FBI agents and special accountants started painstaking investigative work on the Perryville case in April 1924 and were still at it in June 1925, working through a scorching, un-air-conditioned summer and dismal winter days. Special Agent Conroy worked on the Boston end in April and May, accompanied by an agent from the Boston office. They could find no dirt on Nathan Thompson of Thompson and Kelly. Born in Covna, Russia, he became a naturalized US citizen, moved up from small enterprise to big, and prospered. Thompson and Kelly had been charged with improperly offering for sale pajama lots bearing the Red Cross insignia, but the firm stated they did not realize this was illegal and had vowed to remove such patches in the future; the investigation closed. Detail after detail piled up in Conroy's report of more than forty pages, but nothing jumped out as incriminating with respect to the Perryville sale.[30]

The sick man at the center of all these efforts, Charles R. Forbes, endured. In Boston, in the middle of May 1924, Dr. John H. Cauley visited him every day for problems of vomiting and inability to sleep. Forbes continued to be confined to bed and unable to travel, "very much upset," Cauley wrote Easby-Smith (Forbes's lawyer), lest anyone should feel that he was feigning illness, and "is most anxious to be in court when necessary." Forbes sounded desperate and despondent, threatening to "rip the innermost circles of Washington wide open." He compared himself to "poor old Jess Smith," who had also been framed, he said—and now "they're trying to murder me." Cauley rated Forbes's ability to travel as "conservative" in mid-June. A consultant, Dr. John T. Bottomley of 165 Beacon Street, stated that it "would be entirely unsafe even to leave the hospital, not to speak of undertaking a railroad journey." Crim reviewed Forbes's case for Attorney General Stone at the beginning of July: "I am convinced from facts before me that he has been for several weeks in a dangerous physical condition, a great part of the time in a hospital. It may be several weeks before he will be physically able to go to Chicago to plead, and it is more than possible that he will never be tried for the reason that he is likely to linger a few months and die."[31]

Katherine Mortimer was also in poor health in 1924. She had a heavy load to bear: Mortimer's persecution of her, the dragging out of her divorce proceedings, the possibility that she might have to testify (and be roundly criticized) at a trial of national significance, and the absence and serious illness of Bob Forbes, whom she could not openly visit for fear of further scandal. Still in her twenties, she was wasting away. From Leavenworth, her incarcerated brother, Dr. Edward Tullidge, advised intravenous iron and mercurochrome by mouth. "Dearest Sweetheart," he wrote "Kay" to cheer her up after the first grand jury in Chicago, "... you are all I have left ... you know that you're very ill and breakdown makes it harder for me knowing that you are so far away and so I cannot go to you." Her parents recognized Mortimer as the prime cause of Katherine's condition. Dr. George Tullidge, his eyes opened, hoped his son-in-law would overreach: "The dirty skunk has tried to put over something else which would astonish you if I could tell it to you," he wrote Edward, whose mail was censored. "But he will shut up before long. In the latest scandal in Washington, of which he is the author, he has probably hung himself. I refer to the accusation against two congressmen which Crim so foolishly trumpeted over the country as a wonderful result of his genius for investigation and finding out frauds." Katherine's mother put the sentiment more graphically, pecking imperfectly on a manual typewriter: "can one Wicked person upset the world as this Mortim [sic] has well he will com [sic] to his end before long." They were overoptimistic.[32]

In May 1924, Katherine Mortimer regained her health, only to be involved in a bizarre episode in Philadelphia. A certain Caesar Tata, a well-dressed tailor in his thirties, telephoned to tell her he had valuable information to impart if she would come down to the train station. Katherine persuaded him to meet her instead at her parents' home in Overbrook and called the police. Detective Brannon and a policeman hurried to the house and hid behind a door with Katherine's mother to listen in. Tata was oddly precise in his report: He had met Mortimer on October 13, 1922, in a restaurant at Eighth and Christian Streets in Philadelphia with three other men, "Codina," "Fletcher," and an unnamed elderly man. The group talked about liquor deals, a Philadelphia enforcement agent who had been "fixed," and Mortimer's plans to be the next prohibition agent in Philadelphia. The men offered Tata money to "hire men to do away with Forbes," employing as many men as he wanted and paying any amount. Tata said he attended three other meetings in a hotel on Broad Street. At the last one, Mortimer was drunk, "the night of the Army-Navy game in this city." Tata claimed he strung them along but never agreed. When he finished talking, the police revealed themselves and arrested him as a suspicious person. A preliminary hearing was held before Magistrate O'Brien the following day, at which Katherine Mortimer testified that Tata had been offered money to "do away with Forbes." Almost immediately, Tata recanted: There was no murder plot, he said. The deal was only to get some "dope" on Mrs. Mortimer and Forbes, not to kill him, and Katherine misheard: "she in her excitement colored it to suit her own self." Alternatively, Tata said: "Mrs. Mortimer is trying to make a mountain out of a mole hill." Charges against Tata were dropped.[33]

This charade reads, even now, as almost unbelievable, but less so if one assumes Mortimer was its director, for the incident accomplished several goals: (1) It sent his wife a message of his control. (2) It fueled newspaper publicity of a love triangle. At least one newspaper published a triple photo of Colonel Forbes, Mr. Mortimer, and Mrs. Mortimer on its front page, headlined, "Three Involved in Alleged Murder Plot." (3) Mortimer ended up with continuing FBI protection and government income that might otherwise have been lost. Crim had been considering relaxing his "close control" of Mortimer, including the need for continuing his assigned federal agent Mike Allegra, in favor of having Mortimer call in each day by telephone. The day of the incident, Allegra sent a wire to Crim in Chicago, citing the report in the *Philadelphia Evening Bulletin*. Allegra then "delivered" Mortimer to Assistant Attorney General Willebrandt in Washington. By a magnificent bending of the facts, Allegra told Willebrandt that the Tata story was *Forbes's* propaganda and that Mortimer was scared and wanted continuing protection. Willebrandt agreed: the news from Philadelphia was a "frame-up" hostile to Mortimer. Other attempts on him might be made; he was in danger; he should not travel alone. The Justice Department needed him.[34]

Willebrandt warned her valuable asset to keep clean. His "frankness" to a jury was convincing, she told him, but he must not be discredited before the trial or make "wild and inconsistent statements." Avoid the "personal things concerning your wife, which are naturally fraught with so much emotional stress for you," and build up a "reliable and conservative business standing." Her advice came with a sting: "Of course you know my word is at stake in the New York bond matter, but if you keep Mr. Allegra advised of your plans I shall be satisfied that I can keep my word in court." Willebrandt reported all this to Crim. "I am watching the outcome of the Forbes case in Chicago with tremendous interest," she wrote. "I certainly hope there will be a trial soon and a conviction. The man is guilty if anyone ever was." The ends would justify the means.[35]

The components of the trial were coming together. Charles R. Forbes revived sufficiently to be on his feet in mid-October 1924. He had been ill more or less constantly, with short periods of recovery, since President Harding's death. He was not in the best of health in November, when the trial finally began in Chicago. Nevertheless, Easby-Smith was optimistic that the facts were on their side. Neither of them fully appreciated—how could they?—that it was the fictional, devil-may-care, amoral "Charlie," member of the Harding Gang, who was on trial, not the shattered, factual "Bob."

13 THE TRIAL OF CHARLES R. FORBES

The trial began in Chicago on Monday, November 24, 1924, three days before Thanksgiving. Fall and winter of 1924 were warmer than average, but that was little consolation for outsiders arriving in the Windy City; it was chilly. The imposing courtroom of federal judge George A. Carpenter, Northern District of Illinois, Eastern Division, was in the massive Roman-inspired Beaux-Arts federal building (since demolished) in the Chicago Loop. Over the jury box loomed an image of the biblical Moses on his knees before God, receiving the tablets on which the Ten Commandments were inscribed. Among them: Thou shalt not steal. Thou shalt not bear false witness. Thou shalt not covet thy neighbor's wife. In the public's eye, the focus of the trial was clear. Newspapers referred to it as the "Forbes trial," and reported that the government prosecutor, John W. H. Crim, had accused Forbes of causing $225 million of taxpayers' money to go into "private pockets."[1]

The staunchly Republican Judge Carpenter was a six-feet-tall, athletic-looking, bespectacled Harvard man in his fifties with sandy-gray hair, who had served on the federal court since 1910. Having run for election and re-election as a Cook County circuit judge, he was well aware of the importance of public opinion. The judge, like many Americans of the time, saw the country as in danger of falling apart. American democracy and social order were precious jewels that must be guarded vigilantly against the evils of corruption. The Thompson-Forbes case was "one of the most important cases in the last 100 years because it strikes right at the foundation rock of our government," he proclaimed in his charge to the first grand jury. "If the officers of this government, the men who occupy high or low positions under the government are false to their trust, if it can be passed by lightly by the people the whole foundation wall of our government is going to crumble." Carpenter and Prosecutor John W. H. Crim approached the case from a similar point of view.[2]

After months of preparation, Crim was as ready as he could be. He had a brilliant, well-rehearsed star witness, Elias H. Mortimer, whose straightforward story the two of them would present. Namely, that the defendants, John W. Thompson and Charles R. Forbes, were guilty of engaging in a conspiracy with the late James W. Black, the late Charles F. Cramer, and the unindicted Elias H. Mortimer to commit fraud against the government of the United States under section 37 of the US Criminal Code (offenses against the operations of government). The goal of this conspiracy, Crim planned to prove, was to arrange lucrative government contracts for Veterans Bureau hospital construction with eventual profit for all concerned. Thompson and Black were multistate building contractors, Director Forbes of the Veterans Bureau was officially in charge of hospital contracts, Cramer was the bureau's legal counsel, and Mortimer was the fixer and middleman.

Crim's victories in corruption cases, conspiracies, and liquor deals had polished his role as the representative of good over evil. His commanding, grandstanding presence before a jury included a piercing legal look—bushy eyebrows drawn together, eyes narrowed darkly under jutting brows. In court, he planted himself on the floor as if he was a force of nature, tipping his head forward a little, not too much, pugnaciously. He was the accuser. He was federal power personified.

Crim built his prosecution on the following six claims: First, there was circumstantial evidence of a conspiracy, proved by an impressive series of dates and places of meetings, backed by hotel records, where two or more of the five accused conspirators had met, and there were also letters and telegrams among members of the group. Mortimer's specificity on incidents and dates, embellished with striking details and flourishes, gave the ring of truth to his evidence, true or false. His account of one meeting with Forbes went like this: "The conversation with Col. Forbes was in the Portland Hotel, Portland, Oregon, in the morning shortly after we arrived there, I would say about 8:00 to 9:00 o'clock. I cannot give the date exactly, it was approximately the 10th to 12th of July, 1922."

Second, there was evidence that the conspirators worked together on projects other than those connected with the Veterans Bureau: notably, the development project in Colombia (in which Thompson and Black were principals), which was described at the Senate hearings, and Thompson's quest to get full payment for the German oil tanker he had revamped for wartime use, which was commandeered by the US Navy. Crim argued (on the basis of Mortimer's evidence) that Thompson was prepared to give $100,000 to Mortimer for expediting his claim. According to Mortimer, Forbes said, "Sure, it can be done," and that he wanted Cramer to be involved. Mortimer would then split the fee three ways between himself, Forbes, and Cramer, knowing this was a "corrupt proposition." Crim, ably backed by Mortimer, held that both the Colombia proposition and the ship propositions were lures to convince Forbes to grant Mortimer's clients government contracts for hospital construction.

Crim's third and fourth claims as prosecutor were central to the government's case, because if proved they would show Forbes and Thompson conspiring with each other, plus Mortimer and others, in corrupt deals within or via the Veterans Bureau: namely, that Forbes had granted a contract for hospital construction at Northampton, Massachusetts, to the Pontiac Construction Company, a Thompson-Black subsidiary, by rigging the bids and that Elias H. Mortimer had bribed Forbes on several occasions, most notably with $5,000 in cash at the Drake Hotel in Chicago on June 20, 1922.

A fifth, and implicit, claim was that Forbes had the personality and motive to do the things he was accused of doing. The motivations assigned to the key players followed themes established at the Senate hearings, in General O'Ryan's report, in Will Irwin's persuasive articles, and in more recent descriptions of Harding's "Ohio Gang": Forbes was a crook, and Mortimer was both a paid government undercover agent and a betrayed husband who was motivated by vengeance when Katherine Mortimer left him for Forbes. Mortimer played the role of a husband tricked by a blackguard brilliantly. In turn, Crim presented Mortimer as a man whose evidence, though distasteful, was credible.

Finally, federal money was available. In his dramatic opening statement, Crim explained to judge and jury that the second Langley Act appropriated $17 million (more than $230 million in twenty-first-century terms) for hospitals to be constructed under the aegis of the Veterans Bureau. Crim stated bluntly that the conspirators planned to siphon off $1 million. He pictured Mortimer and Forbes studying the Langley bill for the money they could make from it. Contractors Thompson and Black agreed to give 35 percent of their net profits to Mortimer, Crim reported, and Mortimer would hand over half of that to Forbes.

But that was only one instance. The trial proceedings are scattered with Mortimer's statements about unrealized plans that involved large sums of money. It is fair to say that Mortimer's evidence was the case. As the press noted at the time, to make these accusations stick, the prosecution had to substantiate Mortimer's testimony, and the defense to make a strong counterattack on Mortimer. Elias Mortimer represented both the strengths and weaknesses of the case. If he were believed, the prosecution would win. If the jury had substantial doubts about him, it would fail.[3]

The defense's task was to show that the key government witness was an out-and-out liar, that there was insufficient evidence to substantiate the prosecution's claims, and that there was no evidence that crimes had been committed.

Crim's legal team included two lawyers from the US Department of Justice, Earl Morrissey and Oliver E. Pagan, who had been working for him over the intervening months, and private-practice Chicago lawyer, Ralph F. Potter, whom he had persuaded Attorney General Stone to let him hire. Forbes had the loyal James S. Easby-Smith as his lawyer plus Chicago lawyer, Elwood Godman. Thompson's high-priced defense team was headed by former Senator James Hamilton Lewis (Democrat), known for his "fire" and "silky persuasiveness" in court. His role was to provide gravitas and strategy for Thompson's defense team and, if necessary, influence decisions in favor of his client when there were conflicts in the interests of Thompson and Forbes. Thompson's courtroom defense fell into the hands of Franklin J. Stransky of Chicago, and particularly to the fiery Randolph Laughlin of St. Louis, where Thompson lived.[4]

Despite this legal heft, Thompson was doomed to be a secondary figure at the trial. If Forbes was guilty of the conspiracy as defined, so was Thompson. Witnesses called in Thompson's defense testified to his longtime reputation for honesty and fair dealing in St. Louis, New Orleans, and Chicago, but in the end, this testimony carried little weight.

Jury selection for the Forbes-Thompson trial was completed on Tuesday, November 25, 1924, three weeks to the day after President Coolidge's triumph in the polls. As jury selection began, the room was packed with lawyers, including some from the Chicago District Attorney's Office. The jury included three farmers: the nicely named C. P. Fatland; Howard Thomas, a World War veteran; and Morris Kelly, who had one son killed and one wounded in the war. Two of the jurors were retired (Frank W. Hadlock and John Benjamin). The others were a justice of the peace (George F. Hay), a contractor (Ernest A. Clark), an engineer (Theodore Babcox), a man who worked in insurance (O. Dana Richardson), a salesman for cemetery lots (Herbert K. Saul), an employee of the Western Electric Company (William P. Randall), and a miner (Michael Finn). No women. Both sides clearly thought this was a reasonable set of jurors. They were selected with surprising speed given the number of lawyers involved. Only two of the twelve lived in Chicago, the rest lived elsewhere in northern Michigan. Would they be likely to see Forbes as a real person rather than as a personification of evil? Would they see a man who worked hard for his country or a hustler without conscience? The questions were open as proceedings began.[5]

Forbes appeared outwardly restored in health and confidence. His face and posture revealed signs of strain, but his complexion was ruddy, no longer gray. He was a quieter, older, less ebullient version of his old self. He sat at a table with his attorneys, concentrated and alert, taking copious notes. The *New York Times* reported that he "peered at the jurors through horn-rimmed spectacles and seemed very subdued." The *Chicago Tribune* noted his "remarkable poise," though he showed surprise and appeared "genuinely astonished" at some of Mortimer's stories. Mortimer sat with an escort of five "sharp-eyed men" (lawyers and federal agents assigned to Crim), who kept a watchful eye on Forbes—a nice example of courtroom stagecraft, suggesting Mortimer was valuable and Forbes a menace.[6]

Charles R. Forbes was almost forty-eight years old. His life had been marked by extraordinary stresses since he entered the army in 1917. Not least were the relentless judgments of his character and actions since the beginning of the Senate investigation. Questions that could count against him included his apparent lack of divorce from his first wife, his earlier desertion from the army in 1900, and his relationship with the wife of the chief witness. Easby-Smith's positive description of Forbes's life and career in his opening statement to the jury were reportedly "the first kind words Forbes had heard in many months in public." Nonetheless, Easby-Smith was optimistic about the defense. The best investigative efforts of FBI special agents had found no proof outside of Mortimer's word that Forbes had accepted $5,000 from Mortimer in a bathroom in a suite at the Drake Hotel, the most colorful of the stories at the trial. Nor was there evidence that Forbes had cashed or spent any five-hundred-dollar bills. Crim could (and did) prove that Mortimer had the money on hand as part of the $15,000 he had borrowed from Thompson and Black in Chicago, and the prosecution had the loan note Mortimer signed for the $15,000 at 6 percent interest, but the documentary trail stopped there. There was no documentary proof that Forbes had accepted any other amounts from Mortimer, as the latter charged and Forbes denied, and there was no documentary proof that Mortimer paid expenses for Forbes when they traveled together on Forbes's Veterans Bureau business. Forbes and other government employees used government vouchers for trains and transportation, which were scrupulously preapproved and documented by government bookkeepers and accountants, but for other expenses, Forbes and his aides were on a government per diem rate. There were no itemized receipts.[7]

Copies of numerous hotel bills were put in evidence at the trial, thanks to the indefatigable work of hotel clerks and federal agents, but they did not show who paid each bill. Mortimer could produce no canceled checks or even check stubs for the relevant period. Nor could Forbes, whose practice was to hand cash to his senior aide to pay expenses and let him calculate who owed what, over and above the per diem rate. Defense witness Louis T. Grant, who was then the manager of Veterans Bureau District 12 (California, Arizona, and Nevada), recalled that he saw Forbes's aide, Merle Sweet, pay a hotel bill for him, Forbes, and another bureau staff member, John Milliken, in San Francisco. (In contrast, Mortimer testified that he paid the hotel bills at the Fairmont Hotel in San Francisco for Forbes, Milliken, and Sweet, including laundry, valet, and phone.) There was no proof that Mortimer did *not* pay some expenses during the western trip. As in other instances, the fundamental question for the outcome of the trial was whether the jury found Mortimer believable.

Easby-Smith's plan was to shake Mortimer's credibility. In Mortimer's story, Forbes accepted $5,000 in a bathroom in a suite in the Drake Hotel, laughed, and called for a drink, and Mortimer did not insist on a receipt. Easby-Smith had a witness to show that it was physically impossible for Forbes to have met Mortimer at the Drake at 4:30 p.m. on June 20, 1922, because an experienced Veterans Bureau secretary, Edna Breese, was working in the hotel suite at the time, transcribing notes for letters and speeches that Forbes and his staff dictated, and she saw neither Mortimer nor Forbes. Fred E. Hamilton, the executive officer for the Chicago office of the Veterans Bureau, testified that he accompanied Forbes on visits to a boiler works and to the Speedway (Hines) Hospital on the morning of June 20, and returned with him to the Drake Hotel at about 2 p.m., where he saw Miss Breese, as well as Forbes's aide, Mr. Milliken, and Mrs. Mortimer, and then left. Breese testified that she saw Forbes briefly in the suite between 2 p.m. and 3 p.m. but not later. Between 4:30 p.m. and 5 p.m., she was with Katherine Mortimer in the Mortimer bedroom, looking at dresses Mrs. Mortimer had just bought. There was no sign of the dice game Mortimer had reported. Breese remained in the suite until 6 p.m. or 6:30 p.m. and did not see Mortimer at all during the day. Under cross-examination, she admitted that Forbes and Mortimer did not have to come into the reception room to get to their rooms, as there was another door to the corridor, but it is more than probable that they would have done so—Forbes to check on the secretarial work done for him, and Mortimer to see who else was around.[8]

For the Northampton case, Easby-Smith had witnesses lined up to testify that Forbes acted within legal and customary limits in making the decision to award the building contract for the hospital foundations to the Pontiac Company, and to show that army and navy architects and engineers were critical players in the processes of contract-setting and approval. Harold W. Breining, the assistant director of the Veterans Bureau in charge of fiscal matters, testified that Forbes told him he would use existing government construction agencies to supervise the work and that he insisted on competitive bids (which he did). R. C. Routsong, a member of Forbes's planning committee, testified that Forbes wanted the bids handled by the War and Navy Departments, and emphasized speed of construction. Colonel Edward S. Walton of the Army Quartermaster Corps, which handled the construction of the veterans hospital at Northampton, testified that Forbes was adamant for speed, "contracts for lump sums for the entire job, if possible," and contracts made through competitive bidding. Forbes suggested segregating the plans for Northampton into two parcels, one for the foundations and one for the superstructure, and though the army engineers initially "combated the idea" (because they did not think it would save time), Forbes won them over, and time was saved. Naval Commander Frederick W. Southworth of the Navy Bureau of Yards and Docks, which planned and constructed veterans hospitals at Tupper Lake and elsewhere, testified that the navy prepared the plans and Forbes examined them in detail: "Those plans were good plans and were used as a basis for some other stations." Easby-Smith had a good roster here. None of them criticized Forbes's methods or accused him of conspiracy or corruption. Breining made the important point that Forbes could not possibly have siphoned off any funds designated for construction projects because he had no authority to disburse money, and no funds were turned over to him. In other words, even if he had wanted to, Forbes would not have been able to get his hands on the money.[9]

Beyond specifics, Easby-Smith made a sweeping attempt to discredit Mortimer through the testimony of witnesses who had known him at different times and in different places. Thompson's lawyers had an equally strong motive for finding negative character witnesses, and greater resources. Ten defense witnesses testified that Mortimer's reputation was "bad" or "very bad," with six stating specifically, "I would not believe him under oath." Among the ten were the commander of the recently famous around-the-world flight (Major Frederick Martin), the editor of the *Stars and Stripes* (Sid Houston), and Mortimer's childhood friend and later his lawyer (Augustus Dowdall, whom Mortimer had tricked). Management witnesses at the Wardman Park Hotel testified that Mortimer had never reported papers stolen from his apartment and that he had not changed his lock on his apartment as he had claimed.[10]

Easby-Smith's most dramatic act was to call Katherine Mortimer's parents as witnesses to demonstrate that Elias Mortimer was determined to destroy Forbes—and thus further challenge Mortimer's bona fides as a witness. Dr. George Bowler Tullidge, suffering from a chronic heart condition from which he would die within three months, had come to damn the man who was still officially his son-in-law. His white-haired, sad-looking wife,

Katherine O'Donnell Tullidge, quite different from her normal appearance as a feisty, emotional woman, substantiated his account. Dr. Tullidge reported a conversation they both had with Elias Mortimer in the library of their house in Philadelphia in the autumn of 1923 when Mortimer threatened to bring Forbes down: "I will get even with Forbes even if I have to swear myself in jail with him. . . . I am going to get Forbes: if not in one way, I will get him in another." Why? "Because he could have made me a rich man by giving me contracts when he had the power, and did not do it." Tullidge testified that Mortimer had threatened their daughter, Katherine, who refused to confirm Mortimer's evidence. (Notably, Mortimer testified that Katherine was present in the suite at the Drake Hotel when he gave the $5,000 to Forbes. She could have backed him up by saying she had seen Mortimer go into the bathroom with Forbes, with Mortimer carrying money.) Mortimer reportedly said to Tullidge, "If you and Mrs. Tullidge do not make Katherine line up with me and against Forbes, I will drag her down into the mire." Easby-Smith obviously expected this poignant testimony, on top of other aspersions cast on Mortimer's character and intentions, to create a negative impression of him, leaving the case without adequate evidence—and thus Forbes would be acquitted.[11]

In a curious gap in the testimony, Easby-Smith did not confront the question of why Forbes had been attracted to Mortimer as a close friend and traveling buddy in the first place. When General O'Ryan had asked Forbes this pointed question at the Senate hearings, Forbes had remarked weakly that Mortimer was plausible. Thompson's lawyers did a better job here, arguing that Mortimer fooled and dazzled Thompson and Black. The two men thought he was a reputable agent and lent him $15,000 with a receipt and charging 6 percent interest as a simple commercial transaction. Thompson was presented as a simple soul, "big-hearted Jack Thompson," with a "generous Irish heart that could not refuse a friend, anything." Mortimer borrowed money from them and "wormed his way with consummate nerve into capitalist deals." No one explained how Mortimer managed to do this so frequently. The $15,000 was never seen again.[12]

The defense had reason to be optimistic on the basis of disputing alleged facts and seeding doubts about the veracity of a man referred to in the press as the "star witness." But was it enough? The answer, eventually, was no.

The charge of conspiracy strongly aided the prosecution. Allowing two or more conspirators to be tried together visibly suggested that the conspiracy was not hypothetical but real. Here before one's eyes were Forbes and Thompson linked like twins as codefendants, sitting in front of a jury before the first piece of evidence was produced. And there was Mortimer on the first day of testimony, speaking for the US government. Neither defendant spoke about conversations at which they were allegedly present, but Mortimer could and did. At one point, Thompson's lawyer, Randolph Laughlin, announced that he would put Forbes on the stand as a witness for his client. Judge Carpenter rebuked him for meddling in the Forbes side of the case.[13]

A conspiracy charge allowed for evidence about any two or more members of the conspiracy to be accepted even if other members were not present. Many of the meetings cited as part of the conspiracy did not include Forbes; yet, he was assumed to be an active participant. Eminent trial lawyer Clarence Darrow stated his concerns about a conspiracy charge elsewhere: A lawyer might introduce hearsay and promise the court to connect it up later, but even if such evidence was later stricken from the record, "it has entered the jurors' consciousness with a mass of other matter, and altogether it has made an impression on his mind. What particular thing made the impression, neither the juror nor anyone else can know." In the process, individual rights and legal protections might be ignored: "If there are still any citizens interested in protecting human liberty," Darrow wrote, "let them study the conspiracy laws of the United States."[14]

Judge Carpenter's legal philosophy was to protect the nation first. In his charge to the jury, he emphasized how insidious conspiracy could be; how dangerous to America; how evil when coiled around the very heart of government. The theory that made conspiracy punishable, Carpenter explained, was that it produced demoralization and danger to the public and to the peace and security of society. Legal rules were effectively relaxed, for in this broader social framework circumstantial evidence was to be expected: "The existence of an agreement may be shown in direct testimony of one of the conspirators or by the proof of circumstances from which it can be inferred or by both of these methods. . . . Conspirators, gentlemen, do not reduce their agreements to writing."[15]

The dates given for the Forbes-Thompson-Mortimer-Black-Cramer conspiracy were April 1, 1922, through January 1, 1923. Jurors had to decide not only whether there was a conspiracy during these nine months but also whether an overt act was done by one of the five conspirators that would "effect [demonstrate] the object of the conspiracy." The jury could include an act testified to by Mortimer, the unindicted coconspirator who was now the government's chief witness. Handing over the $5,000 in Chicago, as Mortimer alleged, was supremely important for showing, if proved, an overt act of the conspiracy that occurred in the jurisdiction of this Federal District Court. In sum, the prosecutor could describe meetings to engage in antisocial plotting and intrigue of any two or more members of the defined group of five (one unimpeachable and two dead); an individual could be damned by hearsay evidence before he had a chance to speak, and the jury could assume that a conspiracy was a social evil. Members of the jury could not possibly remember all the details in a complicated case such as this. The combined defense teams were counting on facts to swing the jury, rather than an intuitive, commonsense assessment of the characters and their stories. Mortimer's genius as a witness, drawn out skillfully by Crim, lay in embroidering his testimony, detail after detail, while firming up previously held views and manipulating opinions and appearances.

Jury selection and opening statements for prosecution and defense took up the first week of the trial. Mortimer commanded the stage in the second and third weeks, beginning Monday, December 1, 1924. *Chicago Tribune* reporter Philip Kinsley depicted him as a modern adventurer in Washington's "intricate byways," fighting a duel: "He was so cool and keen in his parries, so ready with resource, so backed, apparently, by the exhibits and documents presented by the grim prosecutor, John W. H. Crim, special assistant to the attorney general, who has had Mortimer under his wing for a year." In the *Chicago Herald*, Mortimer was "well-groomed, self-confident and voluble," nonchalantly outlining plots and schemes. The *Washington Post* was less admiring. Forty-year-old Mortimer spoke in "imprecise language, citing dates, places and person present without questioning by government counsel" and though he quoted "actual conversations," the judge overruled defense objections. All these views were prescient. Mortimer was at the top of his game, but flaws in his methods were discernible to those prepared to see them. The trial was all about perception.[16]

Prosecutor Crim and Judge Carpenter gave Mortimer considerable leeway.

He acted as though he were entitled to question and offend defense counsel. In one example, Easby-Smith read a passage from the printed testimony of the Senate hearings, in which Mortimer admitted he did not know whether Forbes had a copy of the communication code Mortimer had described for sending private telegrams, and then asked: "You so testified?" Mortimer: "If it is in the book I testified to it." Easby-Smith: "Is that the only recollection you have?" Mortimer: "Well I don't know if you are reading it or making it up, or what are you doing?" Easby-Smith reminded Mortimer that his counsel was there to protect him. The judge said nothing. Easby-Smith tried again: "Why didn't you tell that Committee that you gave Col. Forbes the dictionary and the code, as you have told this jury?" Mortimer: "Well, if they had asked me that question I would have told them. I gave him one and he knows I gave him one." Judge Carpenter stopped further development of this line of questioning: "The obvious answer is that nobody asked him the question." When Easby-Smith objected, Carpenter agreed that he could ask how Mortimer knew Forbes "knew it." The result was inconclusive.[17]

In another exchange, Mortimer refused to accept Easby-Smith's reading of his testimony at the Senate hearings with the words, "I don't know whether it is in the book, and I wouldn't take your word for it." Easby-Smith asked that this comment be stricken from the record, and Judge Carpenter agreed but ignored the further request to "caution the witness against his insolence." And so it went, with Mortimer tossing off phrases such as "It is none of your business." (About how he spent $5,000 that he retained from the $15,000 he had borrowed from the Thompson-Black loan.) Or, "I told you no ... don't know how many times a person would have to tell you that same thing." (On whether there was a bathtub in the bathroom where $5,000 was reportedly given to Forbes.) Or, referring to Easby-Smith: "He stands in front of me. Get him away from in front of me and then I will answer the questions so you can hear." (On Mortimer having changed his testimony from what he said at the Senate hearings, where he testified that Katherine Mortimer and Charles R. Forbes were not alone when they were playing craps at the Drake Hotel, and answering Easby-Smith in a very quiet voice.) It was difficult to make headway with such a stubborn witness. Mortimer was equally rude to Thompson's lawyers, but the defense kept at it. When Randolph Laughlin asked him what he did the day after he gave Forbes the money, Mortimer ducked the question, and Laughlin tried to bring him back. Mortimer: "Pardon me please, let me finish my answer before you start again." Laughlin: "I insist on an answer." Judge Carpenter: "Mr. Laughlin, you interrupted him in the middle of this answer. Now when the witness finishes the answer, then you may go on with the cross-examination." Mortimer was able to string out his answers, avoid answering straight yes-no questions, and add extraneous information with impunity. When he did answer Laughlin's question, he inserted his usual flair for detail: He left Thompson's office at 10:30–11 a.m.; went to the hotel to pick up his luggage; paid the bill for Thompson, Milliken, himself, and his wife (not apparently for Forbes, a notable omission); and took a taxi to the station. Thompson gave Mortimer two quarts of liquor. Then Thompson, Forbes, and Milliken talked on the platform. Milliken in his testimony (as a government witness) denied there was any platform discussion.[18]

The peculiarities of Elias Harvey Mortimer were glossed over by his ability to spin believable facts out of thin air and his brilliance in ducking questions, diverting attention, and injecting new information into his testimony. He obviously enjoyed himself and admired his own cleverness. A typical answer was the one he gave when questioned about the sum of $1,500 he said he gave to Forbes in August 1922 ($1,000 on one day, $500 the next) in the living room of his apartment at the Wardman Park Hotel as a kickback for the first foundation contract for a tuberculosis hospital at Tupper Lake, New York (which Mortimer was actually not involved with at all): "There was no one else in the apartment. I would not be foolish enough to pass any money to him in front of anybody, I realized it was a crooked transaction. So did he, but he was after all the money he could get." Few people can lie barefacedly and earnestly for days under questioning by high-powered lawyers. Mortimer could. Laughlin asked him, with a touch of sarcasm, if he had any prior experience in corruption before meeting Forbes, knowing that he did. Mortimer had no hesitation in saying no: "So far as I can remember this was the first embarkation I made on the sea of corruption." Forbes, he said, "helped him along." When Laughlin asked him about the money that he testified he gave Congressman Zihlman for bribery (in his former accusations against two congressmen), Mortimer ducked adroitly, claiming the bribery was nothing to do with him: "I was just to collect the money." Laughlin reminded Mortimer that during his evidence at the Senate hearings, covering more than a hundred pages, "you never once said, intimated or suggested one word about either Thompson or Black being present when any graft was discussed that was being given to Forbes." Mortimer said that wasn't true. Laughlin asked him to show where the evidence to substantiate his point was in the record. Judge Carpenter abruptly stopped this line of questioning: "We are not going through that Senate Committee record. We have our own troubles here." Nevertheless, Laughlin made some headway. The defense lawyers pressed hard and managed to confuse Mortimer sufficiently enough for a truly skeptical, tough-minded juror to question the evidence he gave.[19]

A plus for Crim's case was the constant insinuation throughout Mortimer's testimony that he was solely or predominantly motivated by the loss of his wife Katherine to Charles R. Forbes, the man she called "Bobbie." Mortimer's tragic story of love given and rejected and friendship traduced—propelling him into a smoldering jealous rage—had worked on writer Will Irwin and promised to work here, too. Even James Easby-Smith, Forbes's lawyer who, like Irwin, was steeped in classical literature, found this explanation compelling. At one point, Easby-Smith compared Mortimer to Othello, because of his "insane jealousy" and "method of vengeance." The romance of revenge played well. Mortimer lost no opportunity to denigrate Colonel Forbes, usurper. In one of his answers, Mortimer slipped in the tidbit that he told Frank A. Vanderlip, a prominent Republican, that Forbes was "a bigamist and a deserter from the United States Army." Judge Carpenter had references to Forbes's "private life" stricken out. However, they could not be unheard by members of the jury, nor could Mortimer's repeated references to Katherine Mortimer as an immoral, ungrateful spouse. Ably backed by his star witness, Crim played toward negative, fearful stereotypes of the fairer sex. Mortimer's latest story leading up to the $5,000 bribe reeked with innuendo: "We [Mortimer and Thompson] went into the living room, and then went into the bedroom, where we found Col. Forbes and Mrs. Mortimer shooting craps—and it cost me $220.00 that afternoon for his fun up there with her. They were shooting craps on the bed—he in his shirtsleeves, working hard." Eyewitness testimony from Edna Breese, a professional woman in her thirties, that Forbes was not in the suite at the Drake Hotel when this alleged transaction took place was dismissed on the ground that this "girl" could not have testified knowingly other than for the room in which she worked. American women had obtained the vote, could smoke, bob their hair, and shorten their skirts, but these and other aspects of the modern woman and how she should behave were only partly accepted. Male stereotypes of women were full of fear.[20]

Mortimer presented his wife as a chattel: "I am here against Forbes because he stole my wife!" Although he claimed he would have suppressed facts to "have protected that girl," and wanted her back, he could be crude: "I did not want to bring out certain things against Mrs. Mortimer's character, until it got to be common, public property over the entire United States, where he has had her at San Francisco last year and various other places." Forbes was "chasing around with Mrs. Mortimer, taking her to hotels, as he did in Reading Pa. on June 7." Or again, "I know Mrs. Mortimer used J.C. Martin [as an alias] on Col. Forbes's advice." She used the name Martin when she telephoned "her Bobbie" at his apartment in Washington and at the Plaza Hotel in New York, "where she met Col. Forbes on September 27, 1922; at the Rittenhouse Hotel in September, 1922 in Philadelphia, and at the Ritz-Carlton hotel in 1922." Unlike his many other references to hotel records, Mortimer gave no proof that any of these assignations occurred—maybe yes, maybe no. It did not matter; the jury heard the testimony.[21]

Katherine Mortimer, a spunky woman subjected to marital abuse, was willing to testify and was in Chicago during the trial. The defense was divided on whether to call her. Crim deflected her role as a potential witness by depicting her as an angry female, "trying to kill her ex-husband's story." She had appeared against him in a Department of Justice investigation in Washington, Crim said, where she "exhibited great hatred of the man who once supplied her with limousines, furs, and diamonds." In his final summation of the case for the jury, Crim criticized the defense for not calling her as a witness: "Why didn't I call her? Because her interests are on the other side. Her sympathies are on the other side, as I see them. She would be a hostile witness for the Government and a friendly witness for the defense. So let them call her and let me cross-examine her, and let her state who was in the Drake Hotel on June 19, 20th and 21st. Let her state where the money came from to pay the expenses of this western trip. She would know." Maybe yes, maybe no.[22]

Mortimer also hinted at an inappropriate relationship between Forbes and Carolyn Harding Votaw, testifying that her husband Heber Votaw had threatened to throw Forbes out of a tenth-floor window (no doubt the executive floor of the Veterans Bureau). This testimony was stricken from the record, but stricken from the record did not necessarily mean stricken from press reports. United Press International circulated Mortimer's tale that Mr. Votaw threatened to throw Forbes out of a ten-story window and that the testimony was stopped. The Votaws were noticeably absent from the roster of witnesses. Lila Cramer, widow of indicted conspirator Charles Cramer, was another potential witness, but was not called. The defense apparently was not sure what she might say. A reporter described her as an attractive woman who was "said to be a bitter enemy of Forbes." (Mrs. Cramer blamed Forbes for Charles Cramer's failure to become an assistant secretary of war, because Forbes declined to recommend him.) Each of the women behind the scenes had a mind of her own, but no one was interested in what any of them knew or thought.[23]

Elias H. Mortimer concluded his evidence and cross-examination on December 12, 1924, the end of the third week of the trial. Crim called fourteen additional witnesses for the government in quick progression the following week, without adding anything of significance. The defense began with its first witnesses on December 17, focusing on the legitimacy of the Northampton construction contract and the impossibility of Forbes receiving $5,000 from Mortimer at the Drake Hotel because Forbes was not there. Dr. and Mrs. Tullidge, Katherine Mortimer's parents, testified on December 19. The defense seemed to be going well. However, Christmas was rapidly approaching and judge and jurors (and others) were restless. After the first flurry of press interest, the trial moved along in a sparsely attended courtroom. Though reported nationwide through press networks, it was typically not front-page news—though there were some appealing headlines, such as "Steno Attacks Mortimer Yarn of Graft Toast—Saw Forbes That Day but No Scotch," and "Father-in-Law Smirches Star Foe of Forbes."[24]

On Monday, December 22, Judge Carpenter postponed the trial for a week, ordered to bed with a bad cold. This was convenient for those who lived in or near Chicago, but it completely disrupted the flow of the defense. According to a newspaper report, twenty defense witnesses were left hanging in Chicago, expecting to be called, among them Captain Leo Lannen, the former best man at Mortimer's wedding and now his sworn foe, and Merle L. Sweet, Forbes's former executive assistant and business associate. The defense let these two go. Lannen might have made an erratic witness, but Sweet's testimony could have been invaluable for adding detail, clarifying and correcting fact, and depicting Forbes as an effective leader and a good boss at the Veterans Bureau. Jurors had been told not to talk about the case, but they could not stop others from doing so at holiday parties, nor could they completely avoid the newspapers, where public opinion was solidly anti-Forbes, anti-Harding, and anticorruption—and conviction the expected outcome of the trial.

Newspaper reading was a particularly sore point for the defense. Forbes's Chicago lawyer, Elwood Godman, asked Judge Carpenter in the absence of the jury: "We feel in the interest of justice that Your Honor should instruct the jury not to read any articles in the papers or newspapers pertaining to this case." Carpenter: "Not to read them or not to believe them?" Godman: "Well, both." Carpenter was reluctant. He instructed the jury: "Gentlemen of the jury, the Court feels that it cannot ask any intelligent men not to read the newspapers." He adjured them, instead, to base their verdict on the facts elicited in the courtroom, "not from what is published in the newspapers" and flattered them with the thought that "you have all had experience enough to realize that there are certain things that influence stories in newspapers," which "want to catch the public." Jury members were thus asked merely to "disregard" newspaper accounts. During the week off, the *New York Times* ran two laudatory articles about Director Frank Hines's successes at the Veterans Bureau: the problem of too much red tape was being remedied, veterans were happier, services were good, and though the bureau was busy there was little waiting for attention in the Grand Palace Building in New York. Also, new funds made available by Congress would lead to additional hospitals and a training school for the blind near Baltimore.[25]

Mortimer's presence at the trial was no longer necessary. On December 23, he wrote a nonchalant letter on his Washington letterhead to "My Dear Mr. Crim," which represented Mortimer at his creative peak: "I am leaving for Winnipeg Canada tonight to spend Xmas with my Sisters and will be back in Minneapolis on Sunday morning Dec 28th." He gave Crim the address and offered advice on some of the witnesses who were expected to testify for the defense among other comments. Among them was Captain Lannen, the former army procurement officer whose career Mortimer destroyed. Mortimer described him to Crim as a crook who was "forced out of the army in Washington, as his record will show." Mortimer said he had never met two key defense witnesses for Forbes, who gave evidence about the day of the supposed $5,000 bribe on June 20, 1922, stenographer Edna Breese and manager Fred E. Hamilton from the Chicago office of the Veterans Bureau: "That is just a bluff about that girl being in our suite." Thompson and Forbes were "simply getting a bunch of people to try to discredit me." He did visit Dr. and Mrs. Tullidge in the fall of 1923, he wrote, but that was because they had asked him to get data to get Edward Tullidge out of prison. (An unlikely tale.) He never made any statements about trying to "get" Forbes. He had "never talked to Dr. Tullidge regarding Forbes at any time." He ended his letter with a flourish: "Wishing you a very Merry Xmas, I remain Very Truly Yours, E.H. Mortimer."[26]

What Forbes did over Christmas is unknown. During the week before, he had reportedly been robbed when someone entered his room at the Atlantic Hotel, though only pocket change was taken. He was comporting himself with remarkable restraint at the trial. No decision had been made about whether he would be called to the stand. The defense planned first to hear witnesses who would weaken or discredit Mortimer's testimony.

The trial resumed on Monday, December 29, 1924, six weeks after it began. (This was when the parade of defense witnesses testified against Mortimer's bad character and poor reputation, and then other witnesses testified about the assumptions and procedures for letting the contract at Northampton, and other matters.) The materials had become far less interesting to the press than stories happening elsewhere. A six-day recess in the eighth week slowed progress further. There was a rumor that Judge Carpenter had gone duck hunting. On resumption on January 19, Easby-Smith, eager to get at the facts, was reduced to reading from the minutes of the Federal Board of Hospitalization to establish that the board, not Forbes alone, had made hospital decisions. This was not a stimulating topic.[27]

On January 21, with all relevant facts in, as far as the defense could ascertain, the defense closed without calling Thompson or Forbes—to the apparent surprise of the prosecution. Elwood Godman, the Chicago lawyer representing Forbes, reported later that "peculiarly personal reasons" had influenced Thompson and Forbes not to testify. According to one report, Senator Lewis, the senior lawyer on Thompson's team, urged that the two men stand in their own defense, but he was overruled by other counsel. Defense counsel let it be known that they had enough evidence already; and leaving well enough alone can be good policy. If Thompson went on the stand, his papers, which had been impounded, could be released, and there may have been materials he did not wish to publicize. (Mortimer had hinted that there was some scandal that could be produced about Thompson.) Forbes would be open to questions about the specifics of his relationship with Katherine Mortimer, his military desertion, and even the "bigamy" charge Mortimer had tried to insert. Neither defendant was in the best of health or would necessarily be a good witness. Forbes had proved he wasn't when he testified at the Senate hearings. On the other hand, Forbes had declared not so long before, "All I ask is a fair chance to tell my side of the story to the jury and I will rest my case in the jury's hands confidently." He was impatient to testify and vindicate himself, he had asserted, and what he had to say would "startle Washington." And now he was to say nothing![28]

Ralph Potter, Crim's associated Chicago lawyer, ran with this point in the closing arguments: "Where is the man who speaks for Forbes?" Easby-Smith countered with: "Forbes did not have to prove his reputation." The judge gave a simple "no" and Potter agreed, "No, he does not." But the damage was done. The jurors would naturally be curious, even suspicious, when the defendants declined to testify. Judge Carpenter put the problem nicely after the trial: "I think such a statement [refusal to testify] would have influenced the minds of the jury strongly, that these defendants sat here for forty-four full court days and then uttered no word in their own defense." But even without the evidence of Forbes and Thompson, the defense had done a good job in their efforts to shake Mortimer's evidence to the level of reasonable doubt.[29]

The trial galloped to conclusion. Ralph Potter began final arguments for the government on January 23, 1925, ignoring Mortimer, who (as Potter pointed out) was not on trial, and getting to the guts of the prosecution's case. This trial was "one of the most important in the last half century" because a senior government official had betrayed his trust. Potter shouted as he paced to and fro before the jury: "This man was second only in responsibility to the president of the United States." The case struck at the "tap roots of republican government," at the "foundation of the integrity of the nation." Citizens had the right to an uncorrupted government. The jury would help save democracy. Mortimer's motive may have been "primitive," Potter said, but his testimony had been corroborated "in every essential point."[30]

Laughlin, for Thompson's defense, noted discrepancies in Mortimer's testimony and called Mortimer a "perjurer." Laughlin shouted, too: "Forget Mortimer's testimony. To hell with him." Senator Lewis described Mortimer as "a poor, unhappy man, suffering from some form of a mental aberration." Easby-Smith noted that Mortimer had evaded the draft during the war, reminded the jurors of Mortimer's vow to get revenge even if his soul went to hell and his body to the penitentiary, and pointed to one of the Ten Commandments on the wall: "Thou shalt not bear false witness." Chicago lawyer Stransky called Mortimer a "double crosser, crook, fixer, liar, confidence man." The trial stemmed from the political situation of 1923, he said, not from the disinterested pursuit of justice. After the final plea for the defense by Forbes's Chicago lawyer Elwood Godman, during which he claimed that the Republican administration had prosecuted merely to "save its face," Forbes, Thompson, and their defense lawyers were smiling, expecting an early acquittal.[31]

However, John W. H. Crim was still to come, and this was Crim's crowning moment. He addressed the jury for four hours on January 29, 1925, assuming the full force and conscience of the Coolidge administration. He plugged into visceral political themes and appealed to the jury's common sense and moral duty as Americans: "It is time to call a halt to skullduggery and rascality in Washington. It is for you to say." The explanation from the documentary evidence was the only possible one, Crim announced. Forbes and Thompson were "clever contractors and business men." Why, if Mortimer was as bad as blackened, was he the "buddy" and "pal" of these men? The two defendants deceived President Harding's sister, Mrs. Votaw, a "fine woman . . . of whom there is no question." In Crim's view, Forbes always had Mortimer in his sights for contracts and deliberately misled Harding. Everything wrong in the Veterans Bureau was Forbes's fault: "By this devilish intrigue a great department of the Government was placed in a position where it could not function." Crim's prose thundered toward conclusion: "Oh, the sins the friends of Warren Harding visited upon him. Oh, that they had stayed away from Washington. Oh, his untimely death; that he might have lived; that he might be living today to tell you how he was duped by his friends."[32]

Judge Carpenter's instructions to the jury followed on January 30, after he praised the jury and the lawyers: "We have had no wrangling. It has been, from my standpoint, an ideal trial." Jurors were not to accept what they might think the court's role was but make up their own minds. "The guilt of the defendants, if they are guilty, can be established only by evidence admitted at the trial." If after discussion they found the evidence to be as reasonably consistent with innocence as guilt, then they should return a verdict of not guilty. "You know what a doubt is and you have your idea as to what a doubt is that is reasonable." The law requires "absolute certainty," but, he pointed out, there is no such thing in human affairs. What is needed is "more than ordinary certainty of guilt"; not a "whimsical doubt" but an "honest and substantial misgiving, arising upon the evidence." You should be just as sure about this as you want to be about a "matter of the very highest importance to your business, to yourself or your family."[33]

Carpenter ran through the specifics of the case. Besides deciding whether there was a conspiracy, the indictment charged twenty-five or thirty overt acts. (Easby-Smith had argued that only three raised any real questions, and these were all innocent.) Carpenter emphasized: "One is enough." He addressed the question of fact: "You all know what direct evidence is. It is something that is produced before you. . . . On the other hand, people are sometimes charged with doing things, and the evidence is all around the circle; there is no direct evidence pointing to the fact that such a thing was done by the particular person, but circumstantial evidence is legal evidence, and it is to be regarded by the jury in all cases. . . . It should have its just and fair weight with the jury."

In the matter of the Northampton contract, if Forbes, "in good faith, believed that speed was necessary and desirable," then he had the right to award the contract to the Pontiac Construction Company. "You are the judges of the credibility of the witnesses in this case. You have seen them here on the witness stand. You have heard all about them." He addressed the key point of the defense: "As to the Witness Mortimer, who is a self-confessed accomplice, he had a right to testify . . . and if you believe that he told the truth, his testimony must be considered by you in reaching your verdict in this case." That was the bottom line: If you believe Mortimer, act on this belief. It followed that if jurors doubted him, there would be little or no evidence for conviction.[34]

At this point, Forbes tipped back his chair and winked at his lawyers. The defense was blinded by an undue sense of satisfaction. Yet to members of the press the substance of the defense seemed thin. The prosecution's view of "an insatiable greed among the conspirators" was a more likely tale and was certainly more newsworthy.[35]

Jury members retired at 11:30 a.m., debated for an hour and a half without a verdict, and were then escorted to lunch. At 3:45 p.m., they came out to ask for more information in response to a question posed by insurance man C. Dana Richardson: If the jury found there was a conspiracy, did this have to be connected with one or more acts in Chicago? Carpenter clarified that they must find "either that the conspiracy was engaged in here, inspired here or one or more overt acts had taken place here. That is a matter of my jurisdiction." A little later there was a false alarm that a not guilty verdict was forthcoming. Forbes exclaimed, "I hope it is true and I can go on my way rejoicing." Twelve ballots were taken by the jury. The first vote was 9–3 for conviction. The minority was eventually converted to the majority view. The vote moved to 10–2 and was then made unanimous. Jurors returned at about 5 p.m. to say they were ready. Judge Carpenter was called, and the foreman, Frank W. Hadlock, read the verdict at about 5:30 p.m.: "Guilty." The defense asked for a jury poll. Each juror voted guilty. Front-page news.

The defense group had been smiling and chatting. According to the United Press syndicate, in passing sentence the judge "bitterly denounced" both men, aiming mostly at Forbes, who "shook with emotion." Carpenter replied to a plea to remember Forbes's heroic war efforts: "The better the mind the more malignant the heart." A "mere shadow of the ponderous man" he had been in the Harding administration, Forbes gasped as sentence was pronounced, and would have fallen to the floor if "the strong arm of Randolph Laughlin" had not caught him. His face blanched from ruddiness to a sick pallor. Thompson groaned when he heard the verdict but retained his calm, and the defense attorneys were speechless. As Thompson slumped in his chair, his wife, accompanied by a group of women relatives and friends from St. Louis, appeared devastated: "The lips of the women were moving as if in prayer." There were murmurs that the verdict was unjust. Forbes seemed to have no other supporters at hand. Easby-Smith took his right hand and led him toward the door. "It is not over yet," Forbes said. He and Thompson remained free for the duration, continuing under their existing $10,000 bail bonds.[36]

The verdict was the second victory for the federal government on January 30. In the morning, flamboyant liar and former agent Gaston Means and shady lawyer Thomas Felder were convicted in New York for accepting money in a conspiracy to bribe former Attorney General Harry M. Daugherty. Means was sentenced to prison for two years, and Felder was fined. Daugherty seized the opportunity to gain some credit. Speaking from Columbus, Ohio, he claimed he had directed both the Means and Forbes cases and warned the public about officials who said they had "pull" or claimed they had been framed.[37]

On February 4, the court overruled a defense motion for a new trial. Among other points, Judge Carpenter dismissed Laughlin's claim that Mortimer made statements at the trial that conflicted with what he said at the Senate hearings. That issue was dead. Sentencing took place the same day. Carpenter spoke out: "What are we coming to when men in high places betray their trusts?" The two men had been proven guilty. "The jury has decided, and I can do nothing except mete out the punishment the law provides." He imposed the maximum sentence for conspiracy: two years imprisonment and a fine of $10,000 for each man. Forbes looked gray-faced and drawn. When the judge's comments suggested he was about to impose a strict sentence, Forbes "wiped his face with his handkerchief nervously." Both men appeared impassive as they listened.

Forbes's public statement followed: "I am clear in my conscience. I am innocent of the atrocious charge. I have been made the victim of circumstance." He said he would carry his case to the highest courts and "am confident that in the end I will be vindicated." Thompson reported that he was "drawn into the maelstrom of Mortimer's hate for Forbes." Public opinion was against both men. The journal the *Nation*, like the mainstream press, showed no surprise at the verdict: "So far as Colonel Forbes's guilt is concerned, there has been scant doubt of it since a congressional investigation unrolled a story of political debauchery which for sordid corruption has no rival in all our ugly pages of war scandal." There was "general satisfaction of the American people with the outcome."[38]

On February 10, 1925, Judge Carpenter took his wife to Europe for a few weeks. On March 6, Forbes's attorneys filed a seventy-five-page writ of error in federal court, which alleged, inter alia, a variance between the alleged conspiracy and evidence of a conspiracy, prejudicial, and irrelevant testimony by Mortimer and error in sending the jury home every night. As long as there were appeals, hope could be sustained.

PART

V

AFTERMATH

For Charles R. Forbes and John W. Thompson, the appeals that followed were dismal and convoluted—page after page of legalese, with Thompson footing the bill. An appeal to the US Circuit Court of Appeals for the Seventh Circuit, filed on July 10, 1925, covered thousands of printed pages and cited ninety-five errors in the proceedings and findings of the trial court. Appeal proceedings began on November 11, with Chicago lawyer Elwood Godman representing Forbes. "There was not a single thing in Mortimer's testimony that pointed to commission of a crime," he said. Judge A. B. Anderson was dismissive: "Well, the jury believed him. . . . What can we do about it?" The plaintiffs might as well have stopped right there. On January 2, 1926, the three-judge panel upheld the verdict and sentence on both men: Mortimer's story was "shockingly repulsive" but not disputed, neither defendant had testified, and the assignment of errors was "for the most part hardly worthy of consideration." On January 28, a rehearing by the Appeals Court was denied; on February 1, plans were announced to take the case to the Supreme Court of the United States; and on March 15, the Supreme Court declined to review the petition. End of the road.[1]

By mid-March 1926, Forbes and those close to him had been on tenterhooks for months. He had left his position as director of the US Veterans Bureau at the end of February 1923 and turned to his fledgling export-import business. President Harding died in August of that year. In October, sick and in the process of divorce, Forbes was surprised by news that the Senate hearings to investigate the bureau were set to demolish his character and reputation. In October and November, he had first been excluded from participating in the Senate hearings and then roundly "debunked" by a master interrogator (John F. O'Ryan)—backed up by an investigative team that had been gathering materials for months, and after damaging evidence had been given by two of Forbes's major foes (Elias Mortimer and Charles Sawyer). In February 1924, he had been indicted as a criminal in Chicago and in April in Baltimore. The need for a second grand jury had delayed the trial in Chicago until November 1924. He was found guilty in January 1925, sentenced in February, and then more than a year had passed on appeals.

In two areas, though, there was promise for the future. The first was his relationship with Katherine Mortimer. They married before he went to prison. The second was his resilience. Despite serious bouts of illness during the three years since he left the Veterans Bureau, he had not died, as Prosecutor Crim had once expected. He had retained a modicum of pride. Colonel Forbes would not be escorted to prison like a common felon. He would make the best of it.

On March 18, 1926, having got as far as Kansas City, Forbes telephoned Warden W. I. Biddle at the Federal Penitentiary at Leavenworth, Kansas, telling him he wanted to begin his sentence—thereby generating a flurry of communications across the wires between the warden's office, the Department of Justice in Washington, DC, and the Court of Appeals and the US District Court in Chicago, in an unsuccessful effort to get his commitment papers to the penitentiary before he arrived on its doorstep. Forbes appeared the same day, limping, and accompanied by an unidentified newspaperman. Warden Biddle greeted them as visitors and showed them around the plant. "Forbes Visits His Home-to-Be at Leavenworth" read a Chicago newspaper headline. As he left the penitentiary to return to the comfort of the Hotel Muehlebach, he said, "I wish I could start my term right now, for the sooner I start the sooner I shall be freed. Every day I am out counts one more day at the other end."[2]

His codefendant, John W. Thompson, had been admitted to a hospital in St. Louis on March 2. After a third operation for a hernia in two years, he became critically ill, and further endangered by a heart condition. On April 6, two government doctors rated him too ill to go to prison. On May 3, he died of heart disease at home, at the age of sixty-four. That left Charles R. Forbes as the lone survivor of the four coconspirators named by Elias Mortimer: Thompson, Black, Cramer, and Forbes.

Charles R. Forbes, Intake File No. 25021, was admitted on March 20, 1926, for a two-year sentence. Under normal rules, with maximum time off for good behavior, he would be eligible for release on October 27, 1927, but could be considered for parole before then. He went through the usual intake process: height 5 feet 8 ¾ inches, weight 160 pounds, hair mix of gray, eyes "gray pigment orange," complexion "florid," no facial hair. He was photographed and fingerprinted, relinquished his possessions, accepted blue denims and a leather-visored cap, and answered standard questions: civil engineer; Protestant; smoked but did not chew tobacco; drank but did not use opium or morphine; in case of sickness or death notify his mother, Christina Forbes of Plymouth, Massachusetts. He maintained secrecy about his marital status, wife's name, "K. Forbes," address "unknown at present." His tattoos were duly cataloged. The inmate clerk had problems describing the tattoos: shoulder, five-point star superimposed by other stars; left upper arm, a full-rigged ship "American Flags 1875 Sept. 13"; right upper arm, crescent in blue and red; below left elbow on front, a "hand holding a dagger piercing flesh red and blue" and an eagle and shield in red and blue; below and behind left elbow, an anchor and star-shaped flower; right outer forearm "bust sailor 2 American flags sailing ship red blue"; front of right forearm "eagle surmounting shield and flags forming breastplate"; chest, "8 point star superimposed by same"; right shoulder, "copy of a tattoo on his left forearm." Forbes had only to bare his arms at Leavenworth to show he was not a softy but a regular guy with experiences worth listening to.[3]

His first assignment was as a patient in the prison hospital. According to Leavenworth Penitentiary physician Dr. C. A. Bennett, Forbes was a "physical wreck." Medical observations: some paralysis on his left side, walked with a limp, knee brace on left leg. Admitting diagnoses: angina pectoris, arteriosclerosis, and partial paralysis. The prison hospital saved him. Though he had a life-threatening episode of illness in January–February 1927, when his hopes for a presidential pardon or release on parole were dashed, he left prison much healthier than when he went in. The hospital was surprisingly well run, given that the overworked penitentiary physician faced a wide variety of patients and had relatively little professional help. Though there were more than thirty physician inmates at Leavenworth, many were there on drug-related charges or for other reasons that made them unsuitable to care for patients. Among the patients: long-term inmates with problems of aging, effects of widespread drug addiction, accidents, and trauma. A large percentage of prisoners, by virtue of their former occupations, had acquired foreign materials such as bullets or operation plates in various portions of their bodies.[4]

In Washington, DC, the US Veterans Bureau steamed along under the direction of General Frank T. Hines. By mid-1925, all of the hospital construction planned by Forbes and funded under the second Langley Act was completed. The once-controversial project at Northampton, Massachusetts, was finished on May 14, 1925: a 462-bed neuropsychiatric hospital on spacious grounds, with multiple buildings, constructed from belowground up. Among others, new neuropsychiatric facilities had been built at Chillicothe, Ohio; Camp Custer, Michigan; and American Lake, Washington (the latter constructed by Charles B. Hurley, Forbes's old boss). Three new tuberculosis hospitals opened: at Tupper Lake, New York; Aspinwall, Pennsylvania; and the much-maligned, smaller hospital at Livermore, California (on the only site that was purchased). Altogether, the second Langley Act appropriation provided more than 4,000 new beds across the country in the space of three years, from funding to completion. Not a bad legacy. Of long-term relevance, the Forbes program affirmed a policy that continues in the twenty-first century: namely, that America's war veterans should be treated in separate, federally operated hospitals rather than in hospitals that serve the general civilian population.[5]

Forbes had served as bureau director for eighteen months. His successor, Frank Hines was beginning his fourth year. Hines had established three new divisions at the national level for investigation, evaluation, and standardization, respectively, cut back the number of subdistrict offices, set up a medical council, brought the Federal Board of Hospitalization into the bureau's orbit, and reorganized services at the local level.

Then, as later, the Veterans Bureau was by no means trouble-free. In May 1925, after renewed complaints heard in Washington about slowness in service and charges that the bureau was run by the same "clique" that ran it under Forbes, Hines had threatened to resign, by warning his supporters that he wished to take early retirement. President Coolidge got the message, rallied forces and praised Hines for "loyalty, efficiency and intelligence" and for saving taxpayers' money. The bureau was inevitably "political." Under pressure from veterans' groups, veterans' coverage was expanded when

Congress authorized the hospitalization of veterans of all wars, not just World War I, wherever appropriate space was available. Joined with the 1924 extension of hospital benefits to non-service-connected disabilities, veterans hospital facilities continued to expand. In 1923, there were fewer than 24,000 occupied beds in veterans hospitals; in 1930, more than 30,000; and 58,000 in 1941. Hines was to shepherd the bureau through its expansion into the US Veterans Administration in 1930. He stayed on the job until 1945, when the veterans system was transformed again for the young veterans of World War II.[6]

The months leading up to Forbes's imprisonment were filled with changes for others affected by his downfall. In January 1925, Katherine Mortimer's brother, Dr. Edward Tullidge, who believed (against reason) that he was deliberately kept out of the way in Leavenworth while Forbes's fate was decided (and who had not been permitted to work at the prison hospital, as he had expected) was released on parole on medical grounds (supposedly life-endangering tuberculosis). Otherwise, he would still have been there when Forbes went in. Undaunted, thirty-five-year-old Edward had rushed off, after his release, to Forbes's sickbed in Boston, purportedly as a specialist in tropical diseases summoned from Philadelphia to consult on Forbes's case.

Dr. George Tullidge, who had testified as a defense witness at Forbes's trial, died of apoplexy in March 1925, aged sixty-five. Katherine Mortimer was at her father's bedside when he died. Obituaries listed his many hospital affiliations and public service, noted his friendship with Warren G. Harding, and pointed to the testimony he had given against his son-in-law, Elias H. Mortimer. His widow, Katherine O'Donnell Tullidge, left Philadelphia for Milford, Connecticut, to establish a new life for herself. As national organizer of the National American War Mothers Association, she began to organize chapters of the association throughout Connecticut, with New England next on her agenda. Edward Tullidge opened a successful medical practice in Milford, to the gratification of his parole board, and completed his parole requirements, but, as earlier in Mexico, he was unable to keep a sufficiently low profile. In June 1926, Milford's police superintendent wrote the warden at Leavenworth for Tullidge's records and inquired, ominously, where he could obtain the full record of his court-martial proceedings. Dr. Edward Tullidge moved to Florida, where he passed the examination for the state medical board, was briefly married, but left that state when inquiries about him and his medical practice were being made by law enforcement officers, medical groups, and the US Narcotic Service. He lived a vagabond life after this, appearing briefly in different records as a crew member on the Holland American shipping line and as a doctor in Ohio, Arkansas, and Louisiana before going back to Mexico.[7]

Katherine Tullidge Mortimer finally freed herself of her husband, Elias H. Mortimer. Her divorce in the Court of Common Pleas, Philadelphia County, became absolute in June 1925, on the grounds of "cruel and barbarous treatment," and "indignities to the person." The latter was commonly used in Pennsylvania to signify a pattern of "indignities" that made life intolerable and burdensome to the party concerned. Cruel and barbarous treatment was physical abuse. The court had established that Elias Mortimer was violent and that Katherine had suffered, or was in danger of, serious injury. In the wake of her father's death, she was free to marry Charles R. Forbes.[8]

The two were very careful about how and where this would be achieved, if only to avoid potential headlines such as "Star Witness Wife Weds Crook." Deep secrecy was maintained even for family members. For years, Forbes's ex-wife, Kate, was under the impression that the marriage took place after Forbes was discharged from Leavenworth. But no. On December 31, 1925, in the village of Brewster, Putnam County, in New York's Hudson Valley, Charles Forbes (no middle initial) married Katherine Buckley (a misspelling of her noticeable middle name, Bulkeley) Mortimer. He was in his late forties. She had just had her thirtieth birthday. No reporters or gossips were in sight on New Year's Eve. Justice of the Peace James K. Smith married them. John E. Pugsley, the town clerk, was the witness. The groom was in poor health but was warm, unthreatening, straightforward, and reassuring. The bride was protective of him. It was her mission to make him happy and keep him alive and well, and this she did, waiting for him while he was incarcerated. Their marriage was to last until Bob's death, that is, for twenty-six years.[9]

Among others affected by Forbes's case was Katherine's younger brother George Tullidge, the alleged driver of a milk truck whom Forbes was accused of hiring at a large salary for doing nothing. George had expected to work in the Forbes import-export business in San Francisco. Instead he settled down with his wife in Staunton, Virginia, where his father-in-law, Thomas

Hogshead, owned a well-equipped drugstore with a magnificent soda fountain. He took a pharmacy course at the Medical College of Virginia and later entered the insurance business, on his way to becoming an esteemed Staunton resident. Tullidge Hall, now part of Mary Baldwin College, is named after him. Merle Sweet, who had committed himself to the overseas part of Forbes's business, had to start over when he returned to the United States. In 1930, he was the treasurer of an exterminating company in Chicago. His 1942 registration card for World War II shows him back in the federal government in the procurement division of the Treasury Department. With their lives upended, the two wives (Anne) Archer Tullidge and Marguerite Sweet, had reason to shudder at Forbes's shocking fall from grace.[10]

On the West Coast on Vashon Island, Bob's second wife, Kate, and their daughter, Marcia, suffered news of the trial and appeals long distance. "Awa" (Marcia) had her fourteenth birthday in 1926. At school, she was vulnerable to taunts from schoolmates about her wicked dad. In later life, she was not able to talk about him without bursting into tears. For both mother and daughter, the memory of family life in Hawaii grew more golden with the years. Kate coped well with her independent life. She was energetic, brimming with ideas, and kept up an active correspondence, even after an accident late in 1925 put her permanently on crutches. During Forbes's incarceration Kate claimed she was still his wife and sent sweet letters to the warden, explaining among other things that he was an expert drummer who might perform during recreation periods. She sent packages for Forbes, as did others. However, no parcels or packages were allowed because of pervasive drug-smuggling to inmates.[11]

For the government team that prosecuted Forbes the job was done. Other "Harding scandals" were quiescent in 1926. Harry Daugherty had gone back to private life. President Coolidge had appointed special counsel to review the oil scandals as a whole. As a political issue, the Teapot Dome case was quiet well into 1927, when corruption returned as a rallying cry for Democrats in the run-up to the 1928 elections.

Prosecutor John Crim had left the Forbes trial on the noon train to Washington in January 1925, while the jury was deliberating, to go home because his wife was ill. He received the news of the verdict on the train as he traveled east. Crim had come through for the Department of Justice and was ready to move into private practice. Attorney General Stone congratulated him on his "splendid handling of the case. . . . It was a tremendous task and I know the result is due to your untiring and intelligent labors." Crim moved out of the limelight of publicity. He is remembered at his alma mater, William and Mary College, not as a fiery crusader of justice but as a man who loved the college. A peaceful, romantic spot on the campus is named for him: the green and lovely Crim Dell.

Attorney General Harlan Fiske Stone, too, was in transition. In March 1925, he became an associate justice of the Supreme Court of the United States (becoming Chief Justice in 1941). Significantly for the future of the FBI, before Stone left the Department of Justice he appointed J. Edgar Hoover permanent director of the Bureau of Investigation, and gave that bureau a more central presence in the department by having its chief report directly to the attorney general rather than through an assistant attorney general. This gave young Hoover considerable authority in the job he held for almost five decades and made his professional life easier as he built standardized procedures and systems for his agents—and amassed extensive files on individuals of interest, as well as well-known criminals, on his way to enormous personal influence.[12]

J. Edgar Hoover and Assistant to the Attorney General William "Wild Bill" Donovan were of one mind about getting rid of Elias Harvey Mortimer, who had been put on the payroll under old-guard detective William J. Burns, and reported to Donovan. "I would like to know how much longer his services will be needed," Hoover wrote Donovan in February 1925. Donovan waited until he had received Mortimer's expense vouchers for February. In March, Donovan told the FBI that Mortimer might now be dropped. However, in April, a staff member was still trying to make sense of Mortimer's expense claims, and Crim was backing Mortimer on grounds that he had no money and was "dependent on the Government for income on which to live." For Donovan, working at the Justice Department was a temporary stopping place in a diverse career marked by the two world wars. In World War II, he became chief of the Office of Strategic Services (the intelligence/spy service known as OSS), which became the Central Intelligence Agency (CIA).

Elias Mortimer had been carried away by his government role. He hung on to his affiliation with the Department of Justice until March 1925, when Hoover wrote him his letter of termination. Dropped as being of no further use to the government, Mortimer went downhill fast—from stardom in a major trial to minor crimes and shoddy scams. The last known communication from Mortimer is a letter he wrote to Assistant Attorney General Willebrandt in March 1926: "I am very desirous of obtaining all of my papers that I gave to the department in the 'Langley case' and also the 'Forbes Thompson case.'" The letter was written on his letterhead, 489 Fifth Avenue, New York, with three phone lines listed, the trappings of a successful man, but Mortimer was always excellent at trappings. Willebrandt wrote a negative letter back: the Langley papers were part of the evidence on that case, and the Forbes-Thompson case was not yet finished.[13]

In June 1925, J. Edgar Hoover sent Colonel Donovan a report from a special agent that described Mortimer as "continually running to Washington and Chicago, always on the verge of getting some big contracts." His old ways no longer worked. For example, the charge of graft Mortimer tried to make in New York against Stephen O'Connor, son of the director of the Shipping Board, reads simply like a boozing binge (in which Mortimer participated). An excerpt from a report by a federal agent, citing Mortimer, gives the gist: "Every Saturday afternoon O'Connor frequented a bar-room known as 'Hogan's' on Greenwich Street. His regular hang-out was the 'The Steam Club' on the same street. O'Connor made almost daily visits to a bar in an office at 29 Broadway, and also daily visited an office on the 18th floor at 30 Broad St., which led to an adjoining room in which liquor was kept in a large safe. Mortimer further stated that O'Connor always drank whiskey with a beer 'chaser.'"[14]

Unexpectedly, but such is fate, within three years Elias Harvey Mortimer died of a brain tumor (a malignant glioma). Mortimer went home to his widowed mother in Minneapolis, was ill for about a year, and died at the age of forty-four in August 1928 in the house he grew up in, 2104 Glenwood Avenue. He was buried in the family plot in Lakewood Cemetery. In death he received an obituary description he would have appreciated: former agent of the Department of Justice, and major witness in the trial against Colonel Charles R. Forbes.[15]

In 1926, Charles R. Forbes, the only major figure in the Harding scandals yet convicted, adjusted to life behind bars, while Albert B. Fall was waiting for the next shoe to drop in terms of his legal status, crooked or clean. The US Penitentiary at Leavenworth was a sixteen-acre city within walls, containing 3,000 crowded men sentenced there from a year (white collar crimes) to life (murder). A great dome, still under construction, soared above the columns of the Rotunda Building, joining two stentorian flanking blocks that faced down the outside world. Beyond the walls, hundreds of acres of federal land served the prison's needs. Inmate assignments included work on the penitentiary's two large farms, in its sawmill to process the penitentiary's lumber, its shoe factory, substantial construction program, well-stocked library, printing press, and penitentiary newspaper, and in multiple office and menial jobs. Selected inmates worked at the prison hospital.

Assistant Attorney General Mabel Walker Willebrandt, tough as ever, had had Warden Sartain of the federal penitentiary in Atlanta dismissed on charges of mismanagement, favoritism, and bribery, with the help of undercover agents infiltrated into the institution, and was now gunning for reform at Leavenworth. Drug use, smuggling, and trafficking were rife in both penitentiaries. Morphine, cocaine, and heroin circulated widely in American society in the late 1920s. In December 1927, a Mrs. Elaine Battier was caught trying to sell dope to federal agents in Chicago and sentenced to two years for helping supply narcotics to an "inside" syndicate at Leavenworth run by her incarcerated husband. Forbes later estimated that one-third of the Leavenworth inmates were on drugs. Willebrandt could have inserted her own agents into Leavenworth without telling Warden Biddle, whom she considered "crooked" and "incompetent." She was trying to fire him in the spring of 1926. President Coolidge blocked this. Biddle resigned in November. As Veterans Bureau chief, Forbes had made a special visit to investigate the drug problem at the Atlanta penitentiary (in 1923), thereby enraging the Justice Department for trespassing on its turf. (Forbes remembered Daugherty telling him it was none of his "damn business.") His interest in drug control would have commended him to Biddle, and in the Justice Department they also had a common foe. Biddle welcomed Forbes as a positive presence in the institution. In turn, Forbes's experience there was more tolerable and productive than anyone might expect.

The next warden, Thomas B. White, also looked on Forbes with favor and supported him (unsuccessfully) for early release. In a recommendation for clemency for Forbes in September 1927, White wrote, "I can say, without reservation, that he has rendered as much service as a great many of our employees." Meanwhile, Willebrandt continued as a force to be reckoned with, exercising continuing vigilance against prohibition scofflaws wherever possible (though there was no overt sign of her agents at Leavenworth). Mabel Walker Willebrandt left government in 1929 amid scores of letters thanking her for her contributions, returned to private practice with offices in Los Angeles and Washington, and established a successful career that included advising and lobbying for two up-and-coming corporate conglomerates: the Hollywood movie business and the burgeoning aircraft industry.[16]

Less than a month after arriving, Forbes was well enough to work in the office of the superintendent of construction, one of the best assignments in the place, and was soon reported to be "getting along very well." He drew up plans, made drawings, and estimated building costs. His usefulness grew when he became an outside Trusty in March 1927, able to work beyond the walls. Colonel Charles R. Forbes designed, built, and installed a septic tank at the flying field at Fort Leavenworth, the neighboring military base. "It was a good piece of work," the fort's quartermaster wrote to Warden White, and saved the War Department money. Forbes had assisted the construction office "materially" in various projects, including the Administration Building, the warden wrote in September, and "has just today completed drawings of the contemplated remodeling of the stone shop so it may be used as a warehouse and a broom factory." Besides this work, he read widely while in prison, conducted a voluminous correspondence, and developed ideas for a post-prison career.[17]

He also began to write, thanks to a fortuitous meeting in the hospital with Dr. Frederick A. Cook, inmate 23118—the famous Arctic explorer, then in his sixties, who claimed he had beaten Admiral Robert E. Peary to the North Pole in expeditions of 1907–1909. (Peary was strongly favored, though debate still continues as to whether either of them reached the Pole.) Cook had been convicted, with others, of mail fraud in 1923 for using the mails to promote stock in the Petroleum Producers' Association while he was its president, promising returns on the shares that could not be realized. Cook pleaded not guilty. His sentence: fourteen years, nine months in a federal penitentiary plus a fine of $12,000 and a lecture from Federal Judge John M. Killits: "This is one of the times when your peculiar and hypnotic personality fails you, isn't it? You have at last got to the point when you can't bunco anybody." The inner strength for the rigors of Arctic exploration was in all likelihood a good preparation for prison. Cook entered Leavenworth in April 1925 with his enthusiasm for life intact and found ways to make prison as constructive an experience as he could. After six months at Leavenworth, he became night warden in charge of the hospital between 4 p.m. and 8 a.m. and moved to a comfortable well-lit single room so he could be on call. His intelligence, stoic qualities, romanticism, travel tales, writing skills, and work ethic appealed to Forbes. Above these, he brought hope and friendship.

In 1926, in addition to his hospital responsibilities, Cook became editor of the penitentiary's well-regarded monthly newspaper, the *Leavenworth New Era*, assisted by a secretary, Joseph Weil, a former bank robber and swindler. Cook convinced Forbes to write for the paper on top of his construction duties. Volunteering for the newspaper was therapeutic. (Cook was released on parole in 1930 and pardoned by President Franklin D. Roosevelt in 1940.)[18]

The seriousness of inmate Forbes's interests as a prison journalist contrasted dramatically with his popular image outside the walls as a member of the Harding Gang, conspiratorial looter, and shallow partygoer. He published a series of front-page articles on Hawaii (seen through a soft, romantic lens) in the *New Era* in the spring and summer of 1926 and then turned to famous people he had met. One of them was Kaiser Wilhelm II, whom he had observed, he wrote, when he was traveling as a youth in Europe. (Forbes did not say that he was the marine fifer on board when the kaiser visited the USS *New York* at Kiel, Germany.) Another was Warren Harding: a man "steadfast in the faith of his friends . . . genuinely sincere, honest of purpose, and fearless in the discharge of duty."

By September 1926, almost six months in, Forbes was engaged in a "nine months course of intensive training," as he put it—his words for continuing education. Soon he was ready to discuss his theories of penology, based on the belief that prisoners could be rehabilitated through education. He drew up a plan for a "prison without walls"; recommended that the 20 percent of inmates in federal penitentiaries who were illiterate should be required to attend night school as a condition of their parole; called for drug addicts to be segregated from other inmates in the penitentiary so that certified nonaddicts could receive gifts from outside; published an analysis of the penitentiary's farms, with 900 acres under cultivation, drawing from a report he wrote for the warden in 1927; and recommended a formal training program for selected inmates in the business of agriculture so they could acquire a useful trade on their release. His prison without walls would replace the usual "high gruesome wall" with a waterless moat, thirty feet wide and thirty feet deep, with walls extending only three feet above grade, watchtowers at the corners, and drawbridges. Forbes liked his plan sufficiently well to send a set of his drawings to Washington. He wanted penitentiaries to become self-supporting and pay a decent wage to men for their work so that they could send money home to help support their families. He hoped to share his views on release.

Taking his own advice to use prison as a means of education, he researched (and supported) Frederick Cook's claim to have been the first to reach the North Pole. In April 1927, he reported, he had just finished reading Will Durant's *The Story of Philosophy: The Lives and Opinions of the Great Philosophers of the Western World* and was reading John Erskine's new novel *Galahad* and Emil Ludwig's recently translated biography of Napoleon, all published in 1926.[19]

Releasing inmate 25021 on parole was blocked from the beginning. Public opinion outside the walls ran viciously against Forbes, as well as against Fall and Daugherty. All were subject to public shaming, but at this point Forbes, the only major figure so far confined, carried the weight for the misdeeds of all three. To release him could prove politically disastrous for President Coolidge and the Republican Party. And on what grounds? He had been convicted of a serious crime in federal court and had had a full run of appeals. Members of the Coolidge cabinet who had served in the Harding administration fell into line, for they were fair game for criticism by Republican opponents: how could they not have known what was going on in all these scandals? "It would have seemed unnecessary to deny that such conspiracies were ever so communicated," was the way Commerce Secretary Herbert Hoover remembered it: "But the statements were so persistent that Secretary Hughes, my other colleagues and I found it necessary to denounce them." That is, denounce the conspirators, including Forbes, in the sharp division that was being made between the Coolidge and the Harding years.[20]

In June 1926, longtime Democratic Senator Henry Ashurst of Arizona announced in Congress that he had heard of a petition being circulated to release Forbes on parole and condemned any such action. The Department of Justice was solidly against, as was federal Superintendent of Prisons A. H. Conner, a presidential appointee. Forbes, Fall, and Daugherty had each become enmeshed in a tangled web of interweaving charges that made simple statements of guilt or innocence virtually irrelevant. In the public mind, each was corrupt; guilty by fiat. Harry Daugherty was prosecuted for conspiracy to defraud the US government, but acquitted in March 1927 by one jury vote. (Eleven members of the jury voted to convict; the holdout was a woman who worked as a hotel florist.) Albert Fall, caught up in multiple cases arising from the Teapot Dome scandal—the chief corruption question in the 1928 election—finally went to prison in New Mexico in 1931, during the administration of Herbert Hoover, who refused a petition to pardon him.[21]

Forbes was formally denied parole in January 1927, no reason given. He wired his sister Marie: "keep this from mother . . . am standing it as any good soldier should." When he fell sick, he deflected all visitors except his sister Marie, who sent a touching entreaty to the warden as she set off for Leavenworth: "Take care of my poor boy." With the approval of the Department of Justice, Forbes was sent to the university-connected Kansas City Hospital for consultation and treatment, arriving back at the end of February "made much improved" after a diagnosis of acute nephritis. His recuperative powers kicked in, and he was soon reengaged in prison work. He drafted a telegram to a friend that he strongly believed the denial of parole was "prearranged" in the same way he was "convicted before [he] went to trial" (but the warden's office censored this), and to another friend (in a wire that did go through) that although his was one of many petitions turned down, it was a "heartbreaker especially in view of all the promises." There is no way to know whether there were promises, and if so, what those promises were or from whom, but if there were, Forbes was ill-advised to count on them. During his illness, friends lobbied the White House for executive clemency for reasons of illness. In principle, Coolidge was not averse to granting clemency. During his administration, he approved 1,545 clemency actions, including pardons, which ranked him number two in the presidential clemency stakes to that point, with Woodrow Wilson in the lead. But not for Forbes. The theme of no clemency joined that of no parole.[22]

On the outside, times were good in 1926 and 1927. The Coolidge administration had settled down; the stock market pointed up. The ideal statesman, according to the editors of *Barron's*, the business periodical, "never rocked the Ship of State and gave business the go-ahead signal." Coolidge's image of New England probity, reticence, and common sense balanced the enchantment of the marketplace. Stores bulged with consumer goods and catchy tunes were everywhere, old and new: "I Want to Be Happy," "Look for the Silver Lining," "I'll See You in My Dreams," "Bye Bye Blackbird," "Blue Skies." Theatrical productions and movies flourished. The play *Chicago* opened a successful run on Broadway in December 1926, with Forbes's former acquaintance Francine Larrimore playing the lead as Roxie Hart. Popular newspapers, chasing dollars from advertising, served up emotional fare. The press provided "a thrill, an opiate," wrote Silas Bent, a contemporary critic of modern communications: "Its product sells, but so does hooch. The man who drinks does not register approval of the bootlegger's decoction by purchasing it; he buys it because he can get nothing else."

Melodrama infused political observations and was relished. Barb-jabber pundit William Allen White denounced the late Warren G. Harding as incapable: "child in heart and head, set down to fight the dragon," a "henchman of the Republican machine," uneducated, unprepared, overwhelmed, and ruled by the Ohio Gang, which was "collecting money in blackmail wherever it could"—a man for whom death was his "best friend." White also wrote, "Probably no other American President had to run the gauntlet of cruel malice and public odium as Harding ran it during the first four years that followed his death." Those years were late 1923 through late 1927, critical years for Charles R. Forbes.[23]

Into this mix Samuel Hopkins Adams—former muckraker, author of the racy novel *Flaming Youth*, Hollywood screenwriter, Will Irwin's friend—dropped a biting, entertaining novel, *Revelry*, in November 1926, a hard-hitting parody of the Harding administration based on then-current stereotypes that became a smash hit, in its tenth printing in February 1927, with sales eventually topping 100,000 copies. *Revelry* burst into view after the midterm national elections. The jury was being selected for the Teapot Dome trial of Albert Fall and California oilman Edward Doheny. Prospective jurors were asked whether they had read the book because if they had, they might be biased against the defendants. Forbes read a copy in Leavenworth soon after it was published—the prison library was excellent. There, in the book, was Harding as "Willis Markham" from Michigan; Daugherty as "Dan Lurcock"; Mortimer as "Henry Forrest," longtime bootlegger to the Senate and cabinet; and not least, among a string of others, Forbes as "Charles M. (Charley or Cholly) Madrigal," a charmer, sensual, self-indulgent, vain, a "great and confident talker" who carried himself with "jaunty resiliency." The whole gang was there, engaged in a ridiculously complicated plot. In one scene, involving drinking and playing cards in the White House, a heavily drunk Forrest enters and accuses Madrigal: "You stole my wife, you bastard." Forrest has a gun, shoots, misses. Madrigal faints. Secret Service agents rush in. Forrest threatens to expose the whole group and is locked in a room to sleep it off but dies suspiciously of a gunshot wound during the night. In a subplot, Madrigal is offered up as a fall guy to save the others from impending disgrace and agrees to be a "sport and take my medicine," assuming he will have a short sentence and be rescued by executive pardon. Instead, he is killed by guards following an altercation. He has left behind him incriminating evidence about the oil scandal (another part of the plot). President Markham dies of self-inflicted poison and becomes a martyr.[24]

"I read myself into the story as Madrigal," Forbes said on his release from Leavenworth. He wrote an unsigned, negative review that appeared in the January 1927 issue of the *New Era*. He disliked the book intensely—"If you like 'dirt for dirt's sake,' you will like 'Revelry'"—and expressed the hope that someday the full truth might be told. Later in 1927, sparked off by the negative, "murky" tone of this book, Forbes started work on his own views of the Harding administration, preparing a manuscript to be published in the press after his release.

Revelry provoked unease in high places. Its character drawings were too near the bone. A reviewer in Appleton, Wisconsin, summarized the problem: "The reader cannot get rid of the bothersome knowledge that he has of the actual events of the administration that is described." For a Progressive editor in Iowa, on the other hand, it was "the most toothsome morsel ever rolled under a Washington tongue; men outside administration circles shook with laughter, while those on the inside turned ashy white." The author, Adams, observed that "congressional investigations live and flourish, not on fact and evidence, but mainly on the sensational interest of the scandal-hungry public." He included caricatures of betraying presidential friends. A character called Senator Thorne, "tall, white, charming, scholarly, corrupt, and influential," delivers the novel's terrific final sentence: "Friendship in politics undermines more principles than fraud, and gratitude is a worse poison than graft."[25]

The novel and the subsequent play, which opened (for a short run) in the fall of 1927, made it difficult for anyone to separate fact and fiction. This was further illustrated when the jury was picked for the second conspiracy trial of former Attorney General Harry M. Daugherty and former Alien Property Custodian Thomas W. Miller early in 1927, in relation to the transfer of $7 million assets of the American Metal Company, which had been seized as an alien foreign asset during World War I. (The first trial ended in a mistrial.) Again, *Revelry* appeared as a material factor in jury selection, this time because it might have biased jurors against "certain types of politicians," such as political fund-raisers, fund disbursers, managers and organizers. Daugherty was one of said politicians. His lawyer reminded the court that the book was "just fiction." Nonetheless, the judge excused several jury candidates who admitted they had read the book. Daugherty later called *Revelry* a "coarse, filthy screed" and "scurrilous," but he too had read it, as had President Coolidge, who reportedly discussed the book with indignation at a cabinet function and was "annoyed" at being put down in the persona of the fictional vice president. Adams certainly got publicity.[26]

Returned to vigor and looking forward to life on the outside, inmate Forbes regained a sense of purpose, expressed in his work on an ingenious prefabricated house-construction system, which he hoped would form the base of a thriving post-prison business: "no studding, no siding, no shingle, no paper, no sheathing, no window frames, no casings either inside or out, no mouldings of any kind, no finished floors, no plastering or lathing and absolutely tight and free from dampness and cold and the structure when erected in its frame it is finished inside and outside and ready to occupy." He was back thinking big; "several million" could be made, he announced. He got in touch with several of his friends to scout out sites, sent blueprints and a model of the patent to his lawyer, James Easby-Smith (who promised to send the materials to a first-class patent lawyer), and made efforts to involve members of his first family in the venture: his son, Russell Markham Forbes, and son-in-law, Carlos (Carl) Sands. Forbes-as-Dad assumed they would be as enthusiastic as he was over his new project. He sent Russell copies of the design for HOME-O-BLOCK, and asked him for his opinion. Russell, who worked for a construction firm, was noticeably unresponsive. The proposal was ill timed, the gesture had come far too late, and the proposed CEO was an incarcerated convict without funds. After a while, nothing more was heard of this venture. Prospective riches vanished.[27]

Near the time of his expected release in October 1927, Forbes was hounded by the Department of Justice for payment of his $10,000 fine, which was in addition to his prison sentence. The punitive intent of Judge Carpenter, the sentencing judge in Illinois, was clear: "stand committed until said fine is paid." Forbes must remain in Leavenworth after his release date for as long as it took, until the fine was paid. In theory, that could be years.

In an extraordinary gesture, Warden White stepped in to help his trusty inmate nullify the ruling by assisting Forbes and his attorneys with having Forbes declared a pauper. The Certificate of Discharge of Poor Convict for prisoner number 25021 was issued through the Federal Court, Kansas Division, First District, under section 1042 of the Revised Statutes of the United States, on Friday, November 25, 1927, the day after Thanksgiving. According to the paperwork, Forbes had served thirty days solely for the nonpayment of his fine of $10,000 and costs imposed by the court. Queries and rumblings from Chicago were ignored.[28]

As an essential part of the process, Forbes produced a signed statement of his debts. As of July 14, 1927, he owed $104,500 (more than $1.4 million in twenty-first-century terms) to nine parties, the largest being the Bernie Thompson estate c/o Randolph Laughlin, Bank of Commerce Building, St. Louis, Missouri ($90,000)—in short, Forbes had borrowed heavily from his codefendant, J. W. Thompson, and his heirs, presumably to pay for legal fees. Laughlin was Thompson's trial lawyer. Among other debts, Forbes owed $1,000 to his lawyer James S. Easby-Smith; $4,000 to his ex-wife, Kate Marcia Forbes; and $3,500 on his mother's mortgage. His debt to Kate most likely included unpaid payments for child support. Borrowing on the mortgage on his mother's house was a statement that Forbes had indeed come to the end of his financial resources, for she was the last person he would wish to hurt. Forbes was now a designated pauper relieved of debt and could be released. He had served more time in Leavenworth, more than twenty months, than he had spent as director of the US Veterans Bureau.

He left Leavenworth immediately after midnight on the morning of November 26, 1927, with $20 for transportation to his mother's home in Plymouth, Massachusetts, the $2.31 in cash he went in with, plus his civilian clothes, a watch, some buttons, and some stamps. (Kate Forbes had sent the warden some socks for Forbes to wear on his release, which he apparently did not receive.) Warden White had gone to bed. "Hello, boys—you don't know how good it feels to be out," Forbes said to reporters who greeted him, holding a pet raccoon in his arms named Susie. Frederick Cook accompanied Forbes to the exit, trying to hold back tears. Cook wrote a farewell to Forbes in the *New Era*, describing him as "physically ten years younger than when he arrived . . . keen and active." Leavenworth, he wrote tongue-in-cheek, had proved a "splendid health resort."

Forbes produced a prepared statement on his wish to spend time in the future to improve prison conditions: "The present day penitentiary is nothing more than a combination prison and insane asylum; a school for post-graduate work in crime, specializing in moral perversity." The addict "is not primarily a criminal, but is a sick person, more of a subject for the modern psychiatrists and the practical implementation of psychology." And more. The reporters were not much interested in this stuff. Forbes changed gears to a more newsworthy topic. His ability to stimulate an audience had not diminished: "I'm going to heave bombs among the persons responsible for my imprisonment, regardless of where they light. I don't want to besmirch characters of anyone but I will clear myself." He said he had data (never publicly produced) to clear the name of Warren G. Harding: "I shall have some startling facts to reveal, facts that will put to shame a lot of sycophants and calumniators, whose chief purpose seems to be the destruction of the good character of one of the noblest men it has been my privilege to know." The task of vindicating Harding was the "most important mission of my life."

After these exchanges and Forbes's assertion, in tribute to his friend, that Cook had reached the North Pole before Peary, a journalist from St. Louis drove him away in an automobile. The announced plan was to go first to St. Louis to meet with attorney Randolph Laughlin, and then on to visit his mother in Plymouth, Massachusetts. The *New York Times*, taking a folksy line appropriate for family reading, reported Christina's first words as she greeted him at her home: "God bless you, my son."[29]

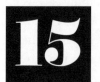

CHARLIE AND BOB, MASKS AND MIRRORS

Charles R. "Bob" Forbes and his wife, Katherine Tullidge Forbes, achieved a life of normalcy after his release from Leavenworth. It was as if they had turned off a switch marked Fame-Thrill-Infamy and dimmed themselves out of public view for the next quarter-century. Meanwhile "Charlie" Forbes, his distorted mirror image, continued in press accounts, histories, and popular literature into the twenty-first century. The Harding scandals remained as moral tales, transportable to other times and political situations. Forbes published a long article soon after he left prison. But after that, as we'll see, there was virtually no input into the continuing narrative of the Harding years from the man at the center of the Veterans Bureau scandal.

After his release from Leavenworth, Forbes testified on the problem of narcotics addiction in the Leavenworth penitentiary as a follow-up to charges he had made that drugs could be had by any prisoner who had the money to buy them. The US Department of Justice ordered a federal grand jury to be called in Kansas City, Kansas, in December 1927. Leavenworth Warden T. B. White and the regional federal narcotic agent also testified. This experience was, however, a footnote to his prison experience, not the start of a new career. Instead, Forbes spoke to reporters about his plans for a future flight to the South Pole with Dr. Frederick Cook, once Cook was released from Leavenworth. They expected to ship the plane as far south as possible and then take off for the pole, he said; two experienced pilots had already been identified. Reporters wrote down this tall tale. If only for a twinkling minute, Forbes was back in his old form.[1]

While Forbes was still in Leavenworth, two newspapers, the *St. Louis Post-Dispatch* and the *New York World*, had commissioned him to write a feature story about the Harding administration to be syndicated by Pulitzer and the Press Publishing Company. He had pounded out his script on the typewriter he used when writing for the prison newspaper. Limits were drawn in the resulting article. There was nothing in it about the Veterans Bureau. He focused instead on descriptions of Warren Harding and his administration as he reportedly remembered them. Bob Forbes, an extrovert who had gone out of his way to blur his own past, assumed an eerie distance from his topic, as if he were a journalist who happened to have had access to the Harding White House. The article appeared on the front-page of major newspapers on Sunday, December 4, 1927, little more than a week after he left the penitentiary.[2]

The result was peculiar. Forbes's messages were not the ones he said he had hoped to convey; notably, restoring Harding's reputation. Rather, he drew on then-popular themes, such as those in the widely read novel *Revelry* by Samuel Hopkins Adams. The *New York World* made the connection explicit by telling readers in an editorial insert that Daugherty's associate Jess Smith, whom Forbes mentioned, was "Jeff Sims" in *Revelry*, and reminding them that Sims was murdered (in the novel) because he "knew too much." Forbes described a Harding who was betrayed by his friends without naming himself as one of the friends who was accused. Harding's good qualities were weaknesses in public life, Forbes wrote, and would have destroyed him if he had lived. Forbes's vivid, fluently written, frequently negative reminiscences of the Harding administration shored up existing concepts of the Harding administration as a gang of hard drinkers. By then, he may have been angry or simply not have cared. And he needed money. His fee was not revealed.[3]

The Veterans Bureau was an independent federal organization. Forbes seemed genuinely ignorant of other aspects of the administration and of what Harding did as president outside of social gatherings. His anecdotes about Harding, plucked as if from a pack of cards, were of a man who was depressed and easily fooled, a poker player offering alcoholic drinks, and, in one case, an accessory to an overtly illegal activity. That was Harding's attendance, with other officials, at a party given by newspaper owner Ned McLean when a smuggled-in film was shown of the famous fight between heavyweights Jack Dempsey and Georges Carpentier (in July 1921). Dempsey won. It was illegal to transport a boxing film across state lines. Another vignette was of Christmas Day 1921, when Carolyn Votaw phoned Forbes to "come on over" to the White House because "Wernie wants to talk to you." (Carolyn used her nickname for her brother.) Forbes found Harding alone in his office: "This is a hell of a Christmas," Harding said, as he chewed tobacco and Forbes smoked a cigarette. Forbes asked what the matter was. Harding: "Everything is the matter." Later in the day Forbes met Sawyer, who told him that Warren and Florence Harding had "a hell of a row this morning." On another occasion Harding wept as the two men sat on a bench in the gardens of the White House: "he told me how unhappy he was and how empty his life had been."

Forbes did not say in this telling, or anywhere else, what his own feelings were toward life, or examine his own doubts and failings. His reminiscences gleam mysteriously through a series of prisms: what actually happened; what Forbes remembered happening; and what he wrote when recalling the incident. He did not mention the role of Florence Kling Harding in her dedicated work for veterans or her generosity in inviting the newly arrived Kate Marcia Forbes to write about her and the White House and gave no hint as to why relations between Forbes and the First Lady apparently soured (at about the time Dr. Sawyer was attempting to stop the sale of government supplies at Perryville), or whether Forbes viewed the rift in their relationship with regret. The First Lady was Harding's "strong-minded and ambitious wife," who had propelled her husband to the presidency.

According to the article, Secretary Fall tricked Harding in the transfer of the oil leases, and Secretary Daugherty, the "evil genius" of the Harding administration, knew all about it. Daugherty came in for special opprobrium: he corrupted Jess Smith, used cronyism to select judges, decided pardons (many of which were for bootleggers) on the basis of the influence and pocketbooks of their friends; tampered with the office of the Alien Property Custodian, Thomas W. Miller; and put money in his own pocket. Describing himself as a "drinking man," Forbes said his best liquor came from Daugherty's supply, delivered under the protection of the Department of Justice to a house on H Street owned by Ned McLean. There was drinking in the private quarters of the White House, which while not illegal was not an ideal example for the populace. Mrs. Harding instructed the president's valet: "Brooks, mix the Colonel a cocktail." Harding kept whiskey at his home in Marion, Ohio, in the bottom section of the sideboard in the Harding dining room, with a backup supply stored at Sawyer's White Oak Sanitarium and at the Marion Club. Forbes described a poker party on a steaming-hot day in the White House library with Harding, the host, at one end of a rectangular table, and Will Hays (the postmaster general) at the other, accompanied by Albert Lasker (chair of the Shipping Board), Harry Daugherty, Mr. and Mrs. McLean, and Colonel Forbes, while Mrs. Harding, a nonplayer, sat with them. Lasker took off his coat, revealing wide red suspenders. Hays and Forbes won the game and pocketed their winnings.

And what of the late General (Dr.) Charles E. Sawyer, Harding's White House physician and health and welfare policy adviser? Here is Sawyer pressuring Forbes to provide a well-paying job at Perryville for the husband of Sawyer's lady friend, who then became Sawyer's spymaster, and Sawyer enlisting an unnamed assistant director (most likely Dr. Hugh Scott) to frame Forbes by placing several bottles of whiskey from the Perryville depot in a closet at his home, which Forbes found and sent back. Sawyer wreaked havoc in government departments. He was a "vain, strutting little creature" who "fancied that he had a great attraction for women," and visited Harding every morning to "feel the President's pulse and to advise a new brand of pills."

Forbes did not explain why others believed he was one of Harding's betrayers, but he did offer a response to criticism he said he had received for failing to testify at his trial. The answer was that his testimony would lead to unhappiness in the lives of others who were "victims of Elias H. Mortimer's villainy" and that his innocence had been fully proved. He said nothing about his relationship with Mortimer and how he got into such a mess, though he could plainly see what happened to others who tangled with Mortimer and his ilk. Hence his statement that his good-natured friend Tom Miller, who was prosecuted with Daugherty, had been imposed on by "shrewd men who knew what they wanted and who wove about him a net of companionship for ulterior purposes." The effect at times was to taunt readers to disbelieve him: in claiming, for example, that he could produce a witness who was still in government service, who overheard his conversation with President Harding on the occasion when, rumor had it, Harding allegedly grabbed him by the throat, and could attest that the conversation was "extremely friendly"; yet he offered no clue as to who this witness might be. Similarly, he said he had lunched at the White House after he left the Veterans Bureau and had advised Harding on this occasion not to go to Alaska on what would be his final trip. A date (even an approximate date) would have made this statement much more plausible, as Forbes must have known. He was writing as the journalist he had become in prison, tailoring his prose to his audience. And in this, he was successful.

Forbes's article had a wide circulation. Newspapers that did not carry the full text referred to it, pulling out generic points: "Harding Duped by 'Ohio Gang' Says Forbes. White House Poker Party Described" (*Chicago Tribune*); "President 'Betrayed by His Friends,' Says Convicted Man's 'Memoirs'" (*Los Angeles Times*). These messages sold newspapers and were not an unfair summary of what Forbes said. The *New York World* reported that the article caused considerable comment in official and social circles in Washington, with particular interest in Forbes's comments about Sawyer, who was appointed brigadier general by President Harding in the face of resistance from regular army officers and became a "sort of a bull in a china shop." Clerks in more than one department in which Sawyer was "meddling" had reportedly hissed at him as he walked the corridors. Several senators seconded Forbes's description of Harding as a man caught up in the self-interested agendas of others. According to Senator Lee Slater Overman, Democrat of North Carolina, who described himself as Harding's friend: "The Forbes story is remarkable in that it tallies with the reports we used to hear around the Capitol and in hotel lobbies while those various escapades of prominent men and women of that Administration were taking place." Quite so. Harry Daugherty remarked, "I have not personally seen the article and of course have nothing to say."[4]

Because this was the most Forbes ever said in print about Harding and the social milieu of the White House, his article was to be widely used as a source for historians. With its publication, Forbes's participation in public life was done, except for a few sightings over the years, as we'll see. He had arrived in Washington in 1921. He retired from view as 1928 was about to begin.

As a topic, however, the Harding scandals remained in the public eye. The oil lease (Teapot Dome) hearings resumed in the Senate in January 1928, with Albert B. Fall as mouse on a treadmill. (He was convicted in October 1929 for accepting a $100,000 bribe from oilman Edward L. Doheny for leasing naval oil reserves at Elk City, California, to a Doheny corporation.) After President Coolidge announced that he would not seek the presidential nomination in 1928, old stories gained force and new ones rippled to the surface. In one, Harding signed the transfer of the oil reserves when he was drunk. The former (maladroit) Governor of Puerto Rico, E. Mont Reily, appointed by Harding, suggested that Forbes had effectively killed him: he "broke the president's heart and thus brought him to an untimely death." Later, loud-mouthed detective Gaston Means, after a stint in the Atlanta Penitentiary, accused Mrs. Harding of poisoning her husband. She was a "bitter, calculating, determined woman," Means wrote, who confessed and said "I have no regrets." A book by a young woman from Marion, Ohio, Nan Britton, added to the flames by describing her affair with Harding and the birth of their daughter Elizabeth Ann. Britton reported that "six burly New York policemen" and the agent for the Society for the Suppression of Vice, brandishing a warrant, had seized the plates and printed sheets at the press, but these had been returned to complete the process after a magistrate's decree. As Harding's reputation went, so did those of his discredited cronies. Images of devious fraudsters and corrupt administrations merged with those of dangerous crooks. Gangster Al Capone, one of the principals of a crime syndicate that supposedly generated $75 million a year (in 1920s dollars), left Chicago for a recuperative stint in St. Petersburg, Florida, with the message, "I've been spending the best years of my life as a public benefactor. ... I've given people the light pleasures, shown them a good time.... Say, the coppers won't have to lay in the gang murders on me now."[5]

Oil was a "new devil god," wrote observer William Allen White: an industrial force that raised fortunes and encouraged speculation, powered factories and machines, and fed the urge for new, faster automobiles. In February 1928, the Senate arrested the chairman of the board of Standard Oil of Indiana for refusing to answer its questions, which he considered irrelevant. Senator Gerald P. Nye, Republican-Independent, of North Dakota warned a Boston audience that the oil scandal was the "most flagrant example" of the use of money to control the American government. Recriminations flew. Democratic Senator James A. Reed of Missouri (no relation of Senator David A. Reed, who chaired the Veterans Bureau hearings) charged President Coolidge with malfeasance in office, for protecting the "arch criminal" Harry Daugherty, acting at the "bidding of selfish interests," and sitting "mum as an oyster," while Fall, Denby and other senior officials ran roughshod over government.[6]

No one wanted to be associated with members of the Harding Gang. In March 1928, Secretary of War Dwight F. Davis released a list of certificates his department had sent everyone who had been awarded army decorations since the time of the Civil War. Forbes's name was listed for his Distinguished Service Medal. One immediate conclusion was that he had been given the medal while in prison; others maintained that he should receive a "medal of dishonor" or the government should go to the "last extreme" to wrest the medal away. Secretary Davis parried with a political excuse: Forbes's medal was awarded during the last Democratic administration. The now-convicted Tom Miller was working his way through the appeals courts. Though part of his argument was that he could not be convicted of conspiracy when his alleged coconspirator Harry Daugherty had been acquitted, Miller's conviction was upheld unanimously by the US Circuit Court of Appeals in New York.[7]

Having scored a resounding victory for the Republican Party in the 1928 election, Herbert C. Hoover was sworn in as president on March 4, 1929, a rainy day. Calvin Coolidge had left the country in apparently good order. "There was a remarkable simplicity about Coolidge that is still attractive," historian Robert Ferrell has remarked about his presidency, "and it helped him in his moves upward politically." But Coolidge did not understand the market speculation that was evident to those who looked for it. The New York stock market crashed in October 1929. A cascade of actions swept the economy toward collapse: rapidly rising unemployment, plunging stock values, loans called in and businesses retrenched or closed, and banks stressed to failure as individuals panicked and pulled out cash. If the business of America was business, as the famous Coolidge quote would have it, the nation was rapidly headed toward failure. Fears of insurgency, class warfare, communism, and revolution joined prospects of economic chaos. Senator David A. Reed (of the Veterans Bureau hearings) was heard to remark, in the fearful climate of the early 1930s, "If this country ever needed a Mussolini, it needs one now."[8]

Forbes had moved with his third wife, Katherine Tullidge Forbes, to California, where he became involved in oil politics at the local level. His birth family remained remarkably cohesive; in 1929, all three of his surviving siblings plus himself and his widowed mother lived within the sprawl of Los Angeles County. In Pasadena, automobiles packed bustling streets and used-car lots were full. Forbes was a proprietor of a gas station, Raymond Service, at 193–95 North Raymond Avenue. His brother-in-law, Harry Judkins, was manager of an auto accessories business. California was overproducing gasoline, and the big companies, such as Sinclair, were forcing down retail prices at the pump. In March 1929, Forbes unveiled his plan to the press to consolidate seventy independent gas stations in Pasadena—the first such merger in the United States, he said—as the first step in forming a national organization with a common code of ethics, designed to develop mass purchasing power. Forbes was president—and back to thinking big. The *Los Angeles Times* reported that the organization had already received its first shipments of oil and gas and that the goal was to prevent a price-cutting war in the future. No connection was made between businessman Forbes and Colonel Forbes from Washington, DC, at least immediately. But that is all that is known. Press coverage disappeared, and so did Forbes. When his mother died in 1931, Colonel and Mrs. Forbes moved back east.[9]

Albert B. Fall, the prime target of the national oil scandal, published his version of the Harding scandals in 1931, and Harry M. Daugherty published his version in 1932. Fall's fifteen-part newspaper series on the Harding administration, coauthored with Magner White of the *San Diego Sun*, appeared in daily installments from mid- to late July 1931. Fall's version of Warren Harding was of a sentimental man who tended to follow "instinctive intuitions" and nearly always overestimated the abilities of his closest friends. Fall said that he had declined Harding's wish to make him secretary of state, that Navy Secretary Denby had initiated the oil lease transfers, and that he, Fall, had been ignorant of the scale of the oil deal, "astonishingly innocent." Then "the whole thing flamed." Yes, Fall had accepted a loan of $100,000 from Edward Doheny, plus other help from Harry Sinclair, and stupidly wrote a "false letter" about the loans when he had a high fever and was on narcotics. Doheny lent him money because he was grateful for his support of American oil production in Mexico when Fall was chair of the Senate Foreign Relations Committee. The Carranza government had confiscated American properties in Mexico in 1917; Fall "went to bat" for American firms as a "matter of high American principle" and saved their investments; and Doheny, a very old friend, had been the largest of the oil investors. In short, the $100,000 had nothing to do with the naval oil reserves.[10]

Harry Daugherty jumped into the fray with collaborator Thomas Dixon with a book that was so misleading and self-serving that it was, and has continued to be, widely discounted. A contemporary reviewer summed it up nicely: "From its pages there emerge two men [Harding and Daugherty] viciously and wrongfully attacked by their political enemies, uncomplainingly sacrificing themselves for the good of their country." Daugherty's Forbes was "handsome, genial, plausible and very popular," particularly with the ladies, not dishonest, but "not big enough for the job," and not to be trusted. Forbes's article was a "vicious tirade against me." Of all experiences in the White House, Daugherty wrote, the one with Forbes was "the only one that cut Harding deeply." However, the alleged incident on which this was based happened in January–February 1923, when Daugherty was incapacitated, on the verge of a nervous breakdown, and in danger of a stroke, and he was still unable to work in March and April. At least some of his memories were false.[11]

On the basis of what each of the three memoirists claimed, there was no common cause or camaraderie among them such as might be expected from imputed members of a "gang." Fall saw Daugherty as his enemy, as did Forbes. Each plowed his own administrative domain: Forbes with regard to veterans' services when organization was fractured and demand was at its peak; Fall wrapped up with conservation disputes and the contentious question of oil leases; Daugherty struggling, for better or worse, with questions of law, order, prosecutions, and civil rights. Daugherty had the most concern about sanitizing his reputation, Fall took the loftiest stance, and Forbes seemed careless of how he was viewed.

Back in the eastern United States, Bob and Katherine Forbes established homes in Washington, DC, and Boynton Beach, Florida; exactly when and how is unknown. A reporter recognized Forbes in Washington in August 1933—the first year of the Democratic administration of Franklin D. Roosevelt, when new federal agencies were created in efforts to turn the economic tide. According to the press, Forbes denied rumors that he had received $17,500 from the garment trade for acting as their agent in negotiations with the National Recovery Administration (a short-lived effort to make cooperative agreements between government and major industries, ratified by negotiated trade codes). He said he had accompanied New York attorney Sidney Cohen, who represented the garment trades, to a meeting with NRA officials as "a friendly act to Cohen" and received no payment. Forbes was reportedly selling coffeepots to hotels and restaurants for a firm called Sensational Plans Company of New York. He volunteered the news that he had been gathering and organizing information for a book on his Harding days, which would be a sensation when published later in the year. Both of these stories deflected attention to New York—usefully so, if he was living in Washington. No book was ever seen.[12]

Katherine Tullidge Forbes reestablished connections with influential Democratic friends in Washington. She took and passed the federal civil service examinations, qualified to operate a Monroe calculating machine, and started as a statistical assistant at the newly formed Civil Works Administration (CWA) in December 1933. Apart from a brief gap after that agency was terminated in 1934, she worked for the federal government until she retired in 1957, mostly as a placement (personnel) officer at the General Accounting Office. No stranger would have recognized the retired army officer known as Colonel C. Robert "Bob" Forbes, an active member of the Chamber of Commerce in Boynton Beach, Florida (while also living in Washington), and Katherine T. Forbes, hard-working, well-connected, gracious civil servant, as the Forbes and Mrs. Mortimer portrayed in the Harding scandals. And so their lives continued, marked by work and play (sailing in Forbes's case), visits with family and friends, joy and sadness, like the rest of us, through the 1930s and World War II.[13]

Charles Robert Forbes died in Walter Reed Hospital at the age of seventy-five on April 10, 1952, after a long course of cancer. Katherine Forbes organized a magnificent military funeral for the man who had put his career on the line and saved her from Mortimer's mental and physical abuse. The funeral four days later began with a well-attended memorial service at the eighteenth-century-style Old Post Chapel at Fort Myer, next to Arlington National Cemetery. (Fort Myer was the base from which Forbes had deserted from the US Army more than half a century earlier. Since then, he had risen, fallen, and then risen again. He was home.) After the service, his coffin was carried to a horse-drawn caisson and driven in slow procession with other vehicles to ceremonials at the gravesite on a peaceful hill. Colonel Forbes was buried with full military honors, with escort and riderless horse, keening bagpipes, a resonant bugle sounding taps, and the finality of three volley shots firing a salute. Almost sixty years later his grandson Richard F. Barry recalled the funeral in detail, with, at the end, the removal of the Stars and Stripes from the coffin, its folding, and presentation to the widow, who then presented it to young Richard, telling him his grandpa would want him to have it. At least one influential Washingtonian, Leslie "Les" Biffle, secretary of the US Senate, known as the president's "helpful pal and backstage fixer" in the Truman years (1945–1953), was noted at the reception following the ceremonies. Bob Forbes's farewell was managed by Democrats.[14]

But "Charlie" lived on in print—a characterization that developed during the life of Bob, and then moved on beyond him. Historians and other serious analysts in the 1920s, 1930s, and 1940s accepted the betrayed president theme without question, with Daugherty and Fall as supportive stock characters: an ambitious lawyer entangled in politics and graft, from Ohio (where the phrase "Ohio Gang" embraced that state's long-established Republican Party machine), and an arrogant westerner with frontier morals. Forbes's image was more difficult to pin down but had the advantage of flexibility; he could be a dolt or an intelligent rogue, vain or slovenly, rough-necked or handsome, playboy or hick. He could be fixer Mortimer's back-slapping crony, investigator O'Ryan's crooked fool, debunker Will Irwin's adventurer, *Revelry*'s high-living jester. A political scientist, writing in otherwise measured academic prose about federal health administration, burst forth with a colorful description when he got to Charles R. Forbes: "this drummer-boy-Signal Corps deserter-colonial public works executive-contractor-war hero," also a "political-industrial adventurer" (1928). A historian referred to the novel *Revelry* as a "bitter but largely truthful depiction of the Harding regime under a thin veil of fiction" and stated that Forbes and his fellow conspirators looted the Veterans Bureau (1930). Frederick Lewis Allen, in what he called an "informal history" of the 1920s (1931), associated Forbes with scandals that were "juicier and more reeking" than the oil scandals. This "buccaneer of fortune" went on a "notorious junket across the country" to select hospital sites that had already been selected, while $200 million "went astray in graft and flagrant waste." Morris Werner, in a valuable analysis of the Senate hearings on the major Harding scandals (1935), described Forbes as a "difficult, disorderly witness," who "made every effort to blacken Mortimer's character." Allen quoted William Allen White's comment that Harding was "almost unbelievingly ill-informed," moved on to explain that Harding could not "distinguish between honesty and rascality" and was "ready to follow the lead of Daugherty or Fall or Forbes," and referred to him as a martyred president, who may have committed suicide. White restated his views about Harding and Forbes in his biography of Calvin Coolidge (1938); namely, Harding's "chief worry was his friends," and he had denounced Forbes and expelled him from office. One account ratified or improved on a previous version, like elders recounting tales around a fire.[15]

President Hoover gave such accounts a sheen of respectability in his speech at the dedication of the Harding Memorial in Marion, Ohio, in June 1931. Honor demanded that he say something complimentary about the man he had served as secretary of commerce, but from whom he had distanced himself in the Coolidge administration; indeed, he had praised Coolidge for taking vigorous action against corruption and indicting the major malefactors. The best he could do was damn Harding with faint praise: "Here was a man whose soul was being seared by a great disillusionment. Warren Harding had a dim realization that he had been betrayed by a few of the men whom he had trusted." He did not need to name the Judas-like friends, merely to declaim against the disloyalty and crime of betraying the public trust. Hoover had been near to Harding in his final weeks of life; thus, his assertion was taken as an accurate historical statement.[16]

Viewed from the economic deprivations of the 1930s, the Harding scandals belonged to a distinctly different, unreal period: the Roaring Twenties, prosperous, boozy, risqué, glamorous, corrupt, and dangerous. Repeal of national prohibition in December 1933 through the passage of the Twenty-First Amendment to the US Constitution pushed the allegedly booze-stoked Harding stories further into myth. Charles Forbes, Albert Fall, and to some extent Harry Daugherty lived on in public memory as folk villains surrounding a weak chief. Forbes was listed as an item in a historical "Mile Post" of notable events from the past. "Ten years ago today," the *Washington Post* announced on March 1, 1934, "Charles R. Forbes was indicted on a bribery charge by a Chicago Grand Jury." That was the entire message about him. He appeared in the company of two twenty-year-old items: armed Texas Rangers invading Mexico to reclaim the mutilated body of a Texas rancher, and the sixth arrest of "militant suffragette" Sylvia Pankhurst, in London, both in 1914. This squib about Forbes was an item that needed no explanation.[17]

The most-balanced interpreter of the Harding period in the 1930s was Washington political journalist Mark Sullivan. In June 1935, Sullivan looked for Forbes and other living participants in Harding's twenty-nine-month administration, asking them to check facts and make suggestions on one of fifty sets of page proofs available for the sixth volume in his historical series *Our Times,* this one titled *The Twenties.* Forbes had done a vanishing act. Officials at the Veterans Administration (as the bureau was then called) told Sullivan they had no knowledge of his whereabouts. Official ignorance of where he was continued though the 1940s. After a Forbes seeker was turned away from the VA in May 1945, looking for Forbes's heirs to settle an ownership question, someone in the office added an exasperated handwritten inscription on the file copy: "Col Forbes is not deceased! His Wash DC address is 2700 Conn Ave."[18]

History belongs to the victors, it is said, but it also belongs to others who contribute to the records as history is being written, and those who keep their records for posterity. Charles R. Forbes, shucking off his past, consistently absented himself from the creation of his own public history. Mortimer had served as his chronicler at the hearings and at the trial, and Will Irwin had served those roles in between those two events. Harry Daugherty was to be a major interpreter of the Harding administration for Sullivan in the 1930s. Daugherty spent days with Sullivan and sent detailed letters, which remain in Sullivan's archives at the Hoover Institution.

Forbes's silence extended to the absence of his own records. Harding's correspondence file with Forbes had reportedly been taken from the White House by Mrs. Harding and destroyed before the Forbes trial. Forbes took his personal files with him when he left the Veterans Bureau—a stack of papers five or six inches thick—and he must have had other documents. It is still possible some of these may emerge (scholarly detectives are always optimistic), but they were most likely discarded as he moved on with his life or thrown away after his and Katherine's deaths. Katherine Forbes died in California in 1967 after having been disabled for several years. Her nephew Thomas H. Tullidge remembered accompanying his father, the George Tullidge who was once connected with Forbes's failed import-export business, to clean out the Forbes storage unit in Washington, and objecting—to no avail—as his father tossed out files without examining what was in them. Sufferers are unlikely to keep reminders of unpleasant periods. Mark Sullivan summarized initial reactions to rumors about the Harding scandals: "Some cynically believed all. Others, their sensibilities wounded, hating to believe but unable to deny, refused to talk about them or listen to them."[19]

Sullivan did the best he could with available sources. The former chair of the Senate committee on the Veterans Bureau, Senator David A. Reed, wrote forcefully to him along familiar lines: "Mr. Harding was a very poor judge of men and his blind loyalty to those whom he considered to be his friends was a horrible handicap to him." And again: "I was with Mr. Harding when Dr. Sawyer brought back from Perryville conclusive evidence that Forbes was grafting in the crudest possible manner. Harding was in tears. He had completely forgotten that he had ever been warned about Forbes and the shock of his disclosure had nearly broken his heart." Another respondent, Charles G. Dawes, supported his old friend, the late Dr. Sawyer, and praised his "initiative and consequent discovery of Forbes's dishonesty." Taking various views into account, Sullivan came up with a Forbes who was a breezy, glib go-getter, compounded of "animal energy and a shrewd workaday knowledge of applied psychology, which a decade later came to be known as 'muscling in.'" Forbes was a superb "muscler-in," Sullivan wrote. "To his skill in that art he owed his lone-handed capture of one of the best jobs Harding had to bestow."[20]

This was a valiant attempt to acknowledge that the real Forbes must have been smart and in many ways effective, but in retrospect it, too, is unsatisfying. If Forbes had had a shrewd knowledge of applied psychology, he could have avoided the mess he ended up in. The problem was that he did *not* have the psychological insight to understand the motives of others, including those of Mortimer and Sawyer, whose motives were practically worn on their sleeves. If Forbes had muscled-in successfully for the job he wanted, he would not have served at the War Risk Bureau but on the Shipping Board or somewhere else more to his taste. Harding shoehorned him into the job. If the War Risk Bureau and the Veterans Bureau were such great jobs, where were the better-qualified candidates clamoring to take them?

Why did Harding have to fall back on someone with Forbes's limited experience, after failing to inspire a General Leonard Wood or a General Charles G. Dawes? Forbes did not see the job as a plum.

Other descriptions followed. Samuel Hopkins Adams, author of *Revelry*, came back to put a final gloss on how the Harding scandals were presented in the 1930s and beyond, in a history of the life and times of President Harding entitled *Incredible Era* (1939) and marketed as "the story of our Great Speakeasy Age and its rococo leader." To provide some gravitas, he used the notes and help of a graduate student at Syracuse University, Harold F. Alderfer, who had chosen Warren Harding as his thesis topic. The assessments of the two men were close. For Alderfer, Harding was "no leader"; he "played personal politics all his life," and although he tried to change he could not bring himself to "oust his former friends," and Daugherty and Forbes were friends, linked together in the game of spoils. Adams cautioned the reader that he relied on hearsay as well as facts, but having said that, he was free to roam. Forbes was a "fine flower of Capital night-life," who in Hawaii "cannily laid the foundations of a friendship that was to close in catastrophe." Mrs. Harding was a dupe, who "fell for his camaraderie, his boisterous, high-pitched familiarity, his flattering hand on her arm and his jovial 'Hello, Duchess. What about a little drink for a thirsty hombre?'" Charlie was known for "entertaining royally." There was "glorious whoopee" on the western trip, including a swimming party in full evening dress. Harding's disillusion because of Forbes's betrayal drove him to make his final trip to Alaska. Harding "died in time," relieved of his burdens.[21]

On December 7, 1941, Japanese planes bombed the active American base at Pearl Harbor, Forbes's old workplace, precipitating American entry into World War II. With the upheavals and tragedies of a new war, it would be reasonable to expect stories of the Harding scandals to die a natural death, but they did not. They lived on as examples of corruption, greed, and dangers to the body politic, ready as a touchstone for subsequent scandals, elections, and presidential administrations. In 1948, a popular history defined the Harding scandals as warnings of new dangers of right-wing extremism, conspiratorial relationships among America's leaders, and ever-present threats from gangs of crooks: Secretary Fall and the "boys from Ohio" were "as unsavory a gang of psychopaths and thieves as ever invaded a national capital this side of the Balkans." Among them, "drunken Charley Forbes." In 1952, a journalist questioned whether corruption was as bad under Harding as it was then and concluded that the 1950s were much worse because in the Harding scandals there was no "covering up," no "tucking it under the bed," but vigilance in federal affairs, with malefactors punished—and seen to be punished. And so the stories continued.[22]

Even when revisionist histories of Harding appeared in the later twentieth century and early decades of the twenty-first century, including those by Robert K. Murray and John W. Dean, the secondary characters were taken as given, except for the role of Albert Fall, who received attention through historical interest in the oil politics of Teapot Dome. An Internet search in 2015 repeated the old stories of Charlie Forbes as a "dashing playboy" who embezzled approximately $200 million selling hospital supplies, took kickbacks from contractors, and accepted a $5,000 bribe in the Drake Hotel, Chicago, and that Harding allowed him to leave the country to escape prosecution.[23]

President Hoover took credit for an "entire revolution" in veterans' affairs, including the transformation of the Veterans Bureau into the Veterans Administration in 1930 by incorporating the separate National Homes for disabled volunteer soldiers and the Pensions Bureau into the new VA, with each keeping its special status—though this was a relatively simple piece of government reorganization compared with what Forbes had to do. Hines's title changed to administrator instead of director. By the end of the Hoover administration in March 1933, 853,000 disabled, sick, and destitute veterans or their dependents were receiving federal benefits compared with 376,000 at the beginning of his administration.[24]

Like his two Republican predecessors, President Hoover resisted continuing pleas for full cash payment of the soldiers' bonus, though laws had been relaxed to allow borrowing on the value of what was effectively a life insurance policy, payable on death or in 1945. In a now familiar story, in the early summer of 1932, a "Bonus Army" estimated at 40,000 veterans and their families arrived in Washington, DC, via truck and train, settling on the flats across the Anacostia River as they waited in vain for Congress to give them their full cash benefits. Settlers were forcibly removed by armed cavalry, tanks, and infantry of the US Army, led by General MacArthur and his aide Major Dwight Eisenhower—soldiers against former soldiers, soldiers against civilians, in a totally overmatched, small-scale civil war. "I can see the soldiers now, rushing here and there with torches," a journalist remembered in horror: "The fire crackled and the flames rose and the smoke billowed upward." Veterans finally received the $1,000 bonus (or what was left of it after borrowing against the certificate) in 1936. President Harding had chosen to build veterans' services, including hospitals, as an alternative to the bonus. In the end, the veterans got both. The bonus issue was finally settled, while the veterans' health system grew.[25]

After World War II, the Veterans Administration reorganized its hospitals, creating major affiliations between VA hospitals and medical schools that emphasized scientific research and education. In theory, by bringing veterans hospitals into the medical and technological mainstream, services to all veterans would be enhanced by providing them with the "best." That was the creed of Colonel Forbes for services to veterans of World War I, when the most urgent long-term needs were hospitals for psychiatry and tuberculosis.

In the second decade of the twenty-first century, the US Department of Veterans Affairs operated more than 150 hospitals, 120 nursing home units, and 800 community-based clinics for military veterans, provided specialty training opportunities for a majority of US physicians and conducted major biomedical and health care research programs, plus other programs, in facilities located across the American subcontinent. That remarkable set of developments can be seen in the long-ago hopes, actions, and accomplishments of Colonel Forbes.[26]

In many ways, the early 1920s would seem weird, outmoded, and hard to understand if we were suddenly plunged back there: segmented by race, ethnicity, gender, occupation, profession, education, and immigrant status; shadowed and excited by the effects of prohibition; enlivened by unfamiliar slang; threatened by sickness and lack of effective medications; and fearful, shrill, and snobbish, as individuals hustled for advantage and social status. Nevertheless, the political milieu of that time has some basic similarities to our own. Modern democracy came with hustling groups of politicians, rival political parties that were further split by sectional and ideological interests, a stomping herd of lobbyists, deal-makers and publicists, and journalists after the next big story or juiciest scandal, preferably both at once. Social media in the twenty-first century merely extend the opportunities for shaming, and, as we are well aware, despite ethics panels and legal probes, there are still high-status government officials who play beyond the rules. Reputation in the 1920s, as now, was a prized possession, something to be nourished, groomed, polished, and suitably displayed. Gentlemen in high positions were expected to know how to avoid trouble and how to succeed —smoothly and with restraint.

Charles R. Forbes was a man with a mission who had a poor understanding of the official environment of Washington and the nuances of professional and bureaucratic etiquette, including the value of keeping a low profile, achieving more than one promises (rather than less), and not offending people unnecessarily. He successfully brought the bureau into being and established the veterans hospital system, handing these over to a more polished and experienced successor. Forbes's problems at the Veterans Bureau may be attributed to an education unsuited to his government role; his expansive, ornery personality; his unusual, mysterious life history (colored by the abandonment of a marriage and a military desertion, and the creation of fabulous stories); his unexpected elevation to a highly visible, politically important government position in 1921; his misunderstanding of what "independent" meant for the Veterans Bureau as an independent federal organization; to hubris; to the sheer difficulty of his mission; or to a mix of some or all of these, or more. It is impossible to know; that's just the way he was. General Drain, in reviewing the decisions made in the rushed sale of surplus property at Perryville, concluded that the Perryville sale was the result of stupidity rather than cupidity. The evidence bears out that observation for other incidents as well. Like Harry M. Daugherty and Albert B. Fall, Forbes made decisions that a polished, upper-crust bureaucrat of the time would not have made: organizing an injunction against striking railroad workers (Daugherty); planning to transfer oil leases from one department to another without proper consultation (Fall); ignoring warnings about a conniving contract-seeking friend, and selling the contents of a military-surplus supplies depot in such a rushed way that it seemed suspicious on the face of it (Forbes).

Was Forbes guilty of criminal behavior? And, if so, what was he guilty of? The answer that has come down through history is the simplest: He was found guilty in a federal court of conspiracy to commit fraud against the federal government; appeals, properly filed, sustained the verdict. Ergo, he was guilty. Though he was convicted on the evidence of Elias H. Mortimer, the jury believed Mortimer, as an appellate judge remarked at the time, and that was that. And, yet, Mortimer was a compelling liar with a destructive personal agenda. Take him out, and the case fails. It would have done in any case, if any of the three jurors who initially voted for acquittal had held firm.

A central question, then, is why Mortimer was believed. Why was his testimony, an indigestible accumulation of suppositions, facts, and lies, taken at face value by the prosecution, the judge, and the jury when skepticism about Mortimer was apparent at the time? As shown, the defense included reputable witnesses who testified they would not trust what he said under oath. A leading Chicago journalist described Mortimer at the trial as having a mind "seeped in scandal and dirt"; having a relentless attitude and speaking to the court through "snarling lips"; and as a "torrent unleashed," giving a performance at the top of the "witness class" of dubious figures of the time, including the notorious liar Gaston Means. Clearly he was not a pattern card of an American gentleman. His deficits were ignored. Mortimer, though a proclaimed coconspirator, got a free ride. He spoke for the government. He embraced a popular agenda. He said what people wanted to hear.[1]

Most of us are lucky enough to go through life without getting entangled with a sociopath; but charmers such as Mortimer are still with us. He displayed antisocial characteristics that have been medically defined in the twenty-first century: lack of remorse, no guilt, no compunction about lies and cheating; a narcissist who demands special attention, charming, glib, and grandiose; able to manipulate and exploit; treating his family and significant others with indifference and needing to punish loved ones; yet with an attractive exterior in terms of looks and manners. This person seeks powerful people and sometimes seems to be playing a game; deceit is a way of life. He constructs a "line" (a story). An outer display of social approval is important to him. He is smooth—able to present an image of himself as he would like to appear. He has the ability to con and builds conspiratorial situations by co-opting people. And Mortimer himself? He was a manipulator of others who became, for a brief time, a government tool. The role of General Charles E. Sawyer was also important, if only as a second string, for Sawyer's accusations against Forbes gave credence to the more dubious stories of Mortimer.[2]

The outcome of the Forbes-Thompson trial was widely praised. Ferreting out scandal had become a social movement in which an accusation became a certainty, a skewed stereotype of an individual became a justification for punishment, and the will to convict outpaced evidence. The evidence against Forbes was suggestive but thin. Forbes may have borrowed sums of money from Mortimer, as others did, but there was no evidentiary proof, such as a cash receipt or checkbook record. Forbes had no reason to enter a conspiracy. There were no kickbacks from selling hospital sites (he bought no sites); there was no ready money in the management of contracts (which were handled by the army and navy); he signed a construction contract for the Northampton hospital, which resulted in the contractor missing the completion date and favored government rather than Forbes. Forbes had no reason to rely on Mortimer in any business way. His weaknesses were that he valued Mortimer as a friend, relied too much on his own judgment, and did not listen to warnings.

Charles R. Forbes was found guilty of conspiracy to commit fraud against the federal government. And conspiracy is a charged word in this great nation. Conspiracy to destroy the government is one of America's most chilling fears, especially when corruption comes from within. Vigilance is an essential message in a democracy, but fear is liable to take processes too far—now as then. Conspiracy charges can whip up a destructive culture of contempt that extends to legislators, senior officials, prosecutors, and judges. The Veterans Bureau scandal offers a salutary warning. Forbes and building contractors John W. Thompson and James W. Black, and their families, down to the second and third generations in Forbes's case, were victims of a vicious movement. When all aspects of the case are considered, it is reasonable to conclude from the evidence that Forbes was found guilty of a crime he did not commit.

However, Forbes was not without guilt, when guilt is defined in terms of social inadequacies, managerial failures, and behavioral sins. He was not an out-and-out villain but he was by no means a perfect human being. Far from it. His gaffes and prevarications made him an ideal scandal victim. So-called cultivated American gentlemen, such as Haven Emerson, the eminent public health physician whom he fired, and John F. O'Ryan, his interrogator at the hearings, found him despicable. In the Washington world of the 1920s, appearances mattered. They do today. The Harding scandals exposed the need for accepted standards of behavior (ethics and etiquette) for government officials—and for those officials to stick with them. The business of government is not the same as the government of business. The problem is defining which is which.

As a social movement, the Harding scandals had a momentum of their own. For the public, they were sociopolitical morality plays. Besides gripping stories, they offered a touchstone for behavior, a sense of common purpose in a diverse population, and a goad for needed policy reforms. Like gladiator matches at the Roman Coliseum centuries earlier, they were public entertainments. Scandal plays a similar role today. The hearings and trials that were at the core of all the Harding scandals offered the nation a spectacle of the look-on-and-shiver kind: bad things were happening. Bad people were threatening the fabric of the nation—but they were being brought to justice. "Star witnesses" became sensations as they made one extraordinary accusation after another. It is as folklore rather than history that such stories continue to engage us.

A cascade of events made the 1920s ripe for scandal. Among them: suspicions of illegal business deals in World War I and in the postwar economy; political hysteria about subversive foreign agents, undesirable immigrants, and fears of corruption in government in those areas; and, by no means least, the effect of prohibition as a hotbed of crime, including collusion with public officials. Modern communications were in play, via a corps of journalists well-versed in the art of muckraking and witticisms, newspapers looking for melodramatic stories, and a population that was attuned to sensation. As writer Clinton Gilbert remarked: "We like to see the masks pulled off our actors. . . . We like to see our strutters strut in a little fear of us."[3]

The most obvious value of the Harding scandals was as a multipurpose political tool in the Coolidge years: useful, that is, for each political party, for creating mass opinion, and for government reform under the banner of efficiency. And reform was achieved. The Interior Department, the Veterans Bureau, and the Department of Justice were modernized under the successors of Fall, Forbes, and Daugherty, respectively. Criticism of a previous president is fair game during the administration of the next incumbent; and criticism of Harding in the Coolidge years was in some ways an extreme version of this process. Multiparty buy-in added to the process. Blaming the Harding administration served Democrats as a rival party but also served Republicans by clearly disassociating the reforming "cool" of Republican Coolidge from the scurrilous "heat" imputed to Republican Harding and his associates. Congressional investigations, running in parallel, promised to bring those responsible to justice. For a while, under Coolidge, each element of government could claim to be functioning for the common good.

There was no direct connection across the administrative domains of Forbes, Fall, and Daugherty nor strong personal connections among the three. This was no national Mafia. The connections were ones imposed by convenience. Harding had appointed each of them; and each case was brought into prominence at about the same time. But there were at least three common themes. The first was the push to redefine and modernize government in the Harding, postwar years, the second the need to establish clear limits of executive authority for each major government agency. Third, as demonstrated to the full in Forbes's behavior as a charismatic leader, acceptable manners, etiquette, and deportment are essential in carrying out a long term set of policies—from making a good impression to projecting a personal code of ethics.

Identification of the Harding administration with scandal masked, or overshadowed, subsequent investigation of underlying challenges to American government in the years 1921–1923—years of lagging postwar reconstruction, readjustments between Congress and the White House, and attempts to make government institutions more effective. The equivocal role of General Sawyer as a White House adviser without portfolio, who hampered Forbes in his role as director of an independent federal agency (and vice versa), points up broader problems in the history of relationships between White House staff and executive agencies. Sawyer was a one-man representative of an otherwise absent White House advisory team. Forbes never felt secure about Sawyer's role. Secretary Fall's apparent assumption that he had authority over government oil and forests raises questions not only about the authority granted to cabinet members at different times but also about how well the president is briefed in each domain (and by whom), and whether and in what ways the Harding period was unique. Government reorganization was a major theme of the Harding administration, as we've seen; but how the "business" of government is defined is still an open question.

Forbes's experience in forming one organization out of three mutually skeptical government cultures deserves comparative analysis with other, larger attempts at government reform since then. If Forbes's Washington story had stopped when he resigned in February 1923, and not been overwhelmingly defined as a scandal, it could have served as an illuminating case study of the risks that exist for anyone who takes on the thankless task of consolidating diverse, established pieces of government into a single agency, a phenomenon that is by no means unique. Two other examples are the creation of the Defense Department after World War II and of Homeland Security in the early 2000s, each of which instances exhausted able leaders. Each of them, in turn, illustrates the challenges Forbes faced in 1921. There is a big gap between efficiency on paper and cooperation in the field. Forbes's challenge was smaller than either of these but just as contentious, and his reforms should be acknowledged.[4]

In the world of realpolitik, identifying Forbes as a crook was of considerable value to the subsequent development of the US Veterans Bureau. The bureau's second director, General Frank Hines, was boosted by the twofold characterization of Forbes as failed director, and then as corrupt conspirator. Veterans' services expanded in parallel to the growing crop of stories about the Harding scandals. By 1931–1932, the total expenditure on World War I veterans in the United States was reportedly greater than the combined totals of expenditures for comparable veterans in France, Germany, and the United Kingdom, each of which had fought four years of bloody war. The US Veterans Bureau phased out its vocational rehabilitation program in the late 1920s, but the extension of hospital and medical benefits to non-service-connected disabilities in 1924 gave US veterans an expanded status as American civilians: access to a free health service and related benefits.

Forbes's story thus provokes a mixed set of observations. The Harding scandals were not as scandalous as portrayed. Charles R. Forbes was found guilty of a crime (conspiracy to commit fraud) he almost certainly did not commit. His role in the Harding administration was to take the hit for the disruptions that were necessary in establishing the Veterans Bureau, a massive job, which he did. The first stage ended with dissatisfaction and conflict, ready for the second stage of management by way of readjustments and routine. Forbes fought successfully for modern health care for World War I veterans and can be seen as the founder of the extensive veterans hospital and health care system that exists today. The history of what is now the US Department of Veterans Affairs needs revision.

The ongoing history of Warren G. Harding and his presidency deserves more attention to the set of scandals as a phenomenon—scandals that were imputed to his presidency but did not become full-blown until the Coolidge administration. Despite convincing revisionist accounts of Harding and his presidency, Warren G. Harding is still considered one of America's corrupt presidents, if only by association with his "cronies"—a labeling that assumes the culpability of the central characters in the Harding scandals. Take the supposed gang members out of a "gang" and absolve them from looting the federal government (indeed it is difficult to see how any of them could pry large amounts of money out of the bureaucracy at the time, though they could take bribes), then what becomes of the powerful concept that Harding was betrayed by his friends?

Because it has been assumed that Forbes was the character played by the irresponsible "Charlie" in the historical literature, and that he was guilty as charged, no detailed reassessment has been made of his case until this one. Added to research by others on the Teapot Dome scandal (which focuses on the culpability of Albert Fall) and inconclusive findings on the Justice Department scandal (in which Harry Daugherty was not convicted), *A Time of Scandal* helps tip the scale of history for the Harding scandals as a whole.

Policies are designed and carried out by human beings, such as we are. The characters we have met here—our ancestors in many cases—are very much as we are now: complicated and flawed, filled with emotions, struggling to make life as good as possible, overly credulous or fearful at times, and not always rational in behavior. Things happen that are unplanned, tragic, or absurd. In Forbes's life: a collapsed gangplank, an unanticipated pregnancy, a chance meeting with a future president, and a prison sentence that restored his health. Warren Harding embarked on an ill-fated cross-country mission to take his presidential agenda to the voters, as had President Wilson before him. Wilson suffered a stroke during his trip; Harding died before he got home, and Wilson outlived him. Charles G. Dawes, chair of the Dawes committee, made an editorial decision he had not fully thought through, which established the Veterans Bureau as an independent federal entity. Elias Mortimer, the noted wheeler-dealer, had his life cut short by a brain tumor—an ending that in fiction would surely seem contrived. The shooting of the Mortimer character in the White House in the novel *Revelry* (1926), is much more satisfying as a story. Families matter. Private lives and public actions merge more than they should. Woe betide anyone caught in Washington's predatory coils. We are both a hopeful and an imperfect species.

Acknowledgments

My first set of thanks is to all who have contributed to the rich, variegated literature that now exists on the 1920s, without which this book could not have been written. Names are cited in the text and referenced in the notes. Additional thanks go to present-day scholars of the early twentieth century for help, lively views, and excellent advice, not all of which I have taken: Jessica Adler, Larry Brown, Carol Byerly, Jennifer Gunn, Susan Lindee, Beth Linker, Ron Numbers, Wendy Oliver, Stephen Ortiz, David Rosner, and Megan Wolff.

When I first became interested in Forbes in the 1980s, I did an initial search for documents and read the Senate hearings on the Veterans Bureau, plus materials in the National Library of Medicine, which also drew largely on the hearings. David Babbitt, a graduate student in history at the University of Chicago, worked with me on this, but it soon became obvious that the search for further resources would be difficult, and other parts of life intervened. I returned to the project after moving from Philadelphia to New York in 2005. Not having a research assistant, I benefited from the wonderful research team at History Associates Inc., located in greater Washington, DC. Their staff chased up materials; located and copied materials for me in Washington, Chicago, and elsewhere; organized a Freedom of Information Act request; and became enthusiastic about the Forbes project. All appreciated. My thanks to them all, but particularly to government historian Jamie Rife, with whom I speculated about the meaning of various findings, and to Laura Moore and others who did archival work on my behalf.

The National Archives are a treasure, and their archivists are a joy to work with. This book draws from National Archives in Washington, DC; College Park, Maryland; Chicago (for the trial); St. Louis (for personnel records); and Kansas (Leavenworth Penitentiary). In Chicago, I had a fruitful discussion with Judge Rebecca R. Pallmeyer, US District Court, Northern

District of Illinois, the court in which Forbes was tried. In New York, Tom Harvey, a former senior official at the Veterans Administration, reminded me of the links that exist between past and present.

My thanks to Jack Gumbrecht at the Historical Society of Pennsylvania and librarians at the Urban Archives at Temple University (both for materials about the Tullidge family); Shelly Bronk (Phillips Exeter Academy), Carol Salomon (Cooper Union), and Jocelyn Wilk (Columbia) who checked reports on Forbes's education (he was not visible at any of these educational institutions); Charles Brodine (Naval History Center), Robert Aquilina (US Marine Corps History Division), and Mike Ressler (chief librarian, US Marine Band) for Forbes's early military experiences; Ev Chasen and Darlene Richardson (Veterans Health Administration); Jack Metzler (Arlington National Cemetery); and others referenced in the text and notes. The papers of Warren G. Harding (on microfilm) were available in New York at the Mina Rees Library, CUNY Graduate Center. My thanks to the helpful librarians there.

The Internet has made materials not previously reachable available with a few clicks. Without it, I would never have found Julie Degenhardt, who is researching the McGogy family with Sherry McGogy (Kate Marcia Forbes's family), or Cathryn Vannice, a professional genealogist who did invaluable work on the project on the West Coast and was a great, if far-off, colleague.

Especially important were members of the Forbes family and their spouses, who welcomed my husband, Jack, and me into their homes and gave us access to family papers. Thank you, Dick and Eileen Forbes, Joan and Arnold Marsh, Richard and Judy Barry, Robert and Rachel Barry, and Barry and Karyn Marsh. Their materials included some letters from Harding, letters between Charles and Kate Forbes, other letters, menus and lists, old newspaper clippings, wartime maps, and memorabilia. Barry Marsh, Forbes's great-grandson, generously shared the research he had done on Forbes's army career and gave me three spare brass buttons from Forbes's World War I military jacket. Richard Forbes graciously shared memories of his family (from Forbes's first marriage) and produced copies of documents he had rescued that had been disintegrating in a barn. Judge Thomas Hogshead Tullidge kindly opened boxes of records and photos of the Tullidge family at his home. We had an enjoyable time looking through all of these materials. Since these meetings, Dick Forbes and Tom Tullidge have died. The generations roll on through time.

Dr. Richard Harding, Warren Harding's great-nephew, talked with me about his relative. Members of the Richardson history seminar at Weill Cornell Medical College gave valuable feedback. Special help came from Katherine Dalsimer and Ted Shapiro. Members of my own extended family joined in. William Wallace offered trenchant but kindly brotherly criticism from London, much needed at the time he gave it. Marcia Wiss pursued the career of Forbes's lawyer, James Easby-Smith, at Georgetown University. Janine Barchas, professor of English, critiqued my prose. Isaac Barchas read part of the manuscript. Judy Cohen gave me her professional opinion on the psychology of Elias Mortimer. Gene Cohen shared his newspaper database on Spokane, Washington, where Charles and Kate Forbes once lived. Larry Lieberman gave us a fascinating and informed tour of areas relevant to Forbes in Hawaii. Mark Barchas read parts of the book and approved, which meant a lot. Friends requested oral updates on the Forbes story. Thank you, Don Haynie and Tom Hamlin, and Bill and Paula Frosch, for your continuing enthusiasm.

At Weill Cornell Medical College, Pamela Trester has been a marvel in tracking down appropriate images for the book (we avoided stiffly posed portraits as far as possible) and followed through on obtaining permission to use them. Richard and Judy Barry moved heavy boxes to find the photo that graces the cover (which in the original includes General John J. Pershing as well). Carl Sferrazza Anthony, the biographer of Florence Harding, found the best possible photo for her in the company of Forbes.

The New York Community Trust and its DeWitt Wallace Program at New York Presbyterian Hospital and Weill Cornell Medical College provided partial support for the research.

The detective work on research was fun. Getting the book into shape for publication requires a different form of energy, and grounding in the present. I am very fortunate to have Peter W. Bernstein for my agent in New York and Jacqueline Wehmueller as editor at Johns Hopkins University Press.

Appreciation above all goes to my husband, Jack Barchas, who read every version of every chapter as it came through and became a de facto part of the project. Thank you, Jack, for being a tower of strength and the most splendid man there could be.

Time Line for Significant Characters, 1914–1929

....

1914: World War I begins in Europe . . . *Charles R. Forbes* becomes superintendent of Public Works in Hawaii . . . *Warren G. Harding* is elected US senator.

1915: Harding meets Forbes in Hawaii.

1916: President *Woodrow Wilson* elected to a second term.

1917: United States enters World War I . . . Forbes deploys to France as a divisional signal officer . . . *Elias H. Mortimer* of Minneapolis joins a crowd of deal-makers and fixers in Washington.

1918: Republicans gain control of both Houses of Congress . . . Crippling influenza epidemic in the spring, second outbreak in the fall . . . Armistice ends hostilities November 11.

1919: Prohibition ratified . . . Volstead Act establishes guidelines for national prohibition of manufacture, transportation, and sale of intoxicating liquor nationwide, effective August 1920 . . . Mortimer marries (and enters the family of) *Katherine Bulkeley Tullidge* . . . Third wave of pandemic influenza in the spring . . . "Red Scare" against suspected communist cells in the United States . . . *J. Edgar Hoover* manages antiradical program at the Department of Justice . . . Forbes works for Harding in Republican primary campaign.

1920: Ex-soldiers demand compensation for high civilian wages lost during the war and campaign for a "soldiers bonus" . . . The American Legion (established 1919) gains strength as a lobby for war veterans

... Women have the vote for the first time ... In November, Harding elected president by a landslide.

1921: Harding's inauguration in March ... Outgoing President Wilson signs the first Langley Act for constructing hospital beds for World War I veterans, named for Rep. *John W. Langley* of Kentucky ... Committee run by *Charles G. Dawes* recommends consolidating scattered federal services for World War I veterans into one organization ... Harding makes White House physician *Charles E. Sawyer* his aide on health and welfare policy ... Forbes becomes director of the Bureau of War Risk Insurance ... Creation of the Bureau of the Budget and the Office of Comptroller General with Dawes as first director of the budget ... Establishment of the US Veterans Bureau with Forbes as its first director ... *Carolyn Harding Votaw* part of Forbes's team ... Establishment of Federal Board of Hospitalization, with Sawyer as chief coordinator ... Second Langley bill introduced for additional hospital construction ... At instigation of Interior Secretary *Albert B. Fall*, Harding signs executive order transferring oil reserves from the navy to the Interior Department, which later sets off the Teapot Dome scandal.

1922: Coal strike begins ... Attorney General *Harry M. Daugherty* under fire ... Forbes meets Mortimer ... *Kate Marcia Forbes* leaves for Europe and stays away fifteen months ... Forbes makes major trip west ... Railroad shop workers' strike ... Daugherty arranges injunction to stop strike ... Forbes and staff decide on a quick sale of army surplus goods at Veterans Bureau depot in Perryville, MD ... Harding vetoes Bonus Bill in the cause of a balanced budget ... Forbes breaks with Mortimer ... November elections: Republicans lose congressional seats ... Harding halts the Perryville sale ... Charges of impeachment against Daugherty ... At Harding's second annual message to Congress, Republicans greet him with cheers ... Albert Fall leases oil reserve no. 1 to oilman *Edward L. Doheny*.

1923: Interior Secretary Fall resigns ... Backlash against "military influence" at the Veterans Bureau ... Forbes departs for Europe ...

Harding announces Forbes's resignation ... *Frank T. Hines* becomes
bureau director ... Senate authorizes investigation of the Veterans
Bureau, conducted by Senators *David A. Reed* (chair), *David I. Walsh*,
and *Tasker Oddie*; with *John F. O'Ryan* as counsel ... Veterans
Bureau lawyer *Charles F. Cramer* commits suicide ... *Jesse "Jess" W.
Smith* commits suicide ... Harding leaves Washington with a large
party on trip to Alaska ... Forbes goes to West Coast to establish
a business ... Harding dies ... *Calvin Coolidge* becomes president
... Kate Forbes returns to United States, files for divorce ... Senate
investigative hearings on the Veterans Bureau and Senate hearings
on oil leases begin, both in late October ... Senate investigation of
the Veterans Bureau ends in December ... *James S. Easby-Smith* rep-
resents Forbes.

1924: Drama at the oil hearings in January ... Critical reports on the Veterans Bureau investigation published ... Senate passes joint resolution
calling on Coolidge to appoint a special committee to investigate oil
scandals ... Grand jury investigation summoned for Veterans Bureau
case in Chicago, with *John W. H. Crim* as government prosecutor and
Mortimer as chief witness ... Resignation of Naval Secretary *Edwin
L. Denby* ... Articles by *Will Irwin* depict Forbes as one of Harding's
betraying friends ... Grand jury indicts Forbes and businessman *John
W. Thompson* ... Mortimer works for Assistant Attorney General
Mabel Walker Willebrandt as informer on prohibition cases ... Senate investigation of Daugherty opens ... Mortimer testifies against
two congressmen on liquor charges ... Langley indicted, convicted,
and goes to prison ... Bonus Bill passes after Congress overrides
Coolidge's veto ... Daugherty resigns ... Baltimore grand jury indicts
Forbes and a Boston businessman over the sale of surplus goods
at Perryville ... Political party conventions highlight the Harding
scandals, singling out Fall and Forbes ... Sawyer dies ... Coolidge/
Dawes presidential ticket wins in November ... Trial of Forbes and
Thompson begins under federal judge *George A. Carpenter.*

1925: Guilty verdict for Forbes and Thompson ... Civil suit to cancel Teapot Dome lease to *Harry F. Sinclair* begins in Wyoming ... Albert

Fall indicted for conspiring with Doheny . . . Appeals by Forbes and Thompson unsuccessful.

1926: Forbes begins prison term, Thompson dies . . . *Samuel Hopkins Adams* publishes influential satire of the Harding administration . . . Fall-Doheny oil trial testimony ends . . . Daugherty and *Thomas W. Miller* tried in New York on illegal sale of alien property, Miller convicted.

1927: Supreme Court invalidates Teapot Dome lease . . . Trial of Fall and Sinclair fails, jury discharged, and new trial set . . . Forbes released from Leavenworth in November . . . Publishes his account of the Harding years.

1928: Senate hearings on the oil leases resume, end in May . . . Fall continues under legal scrutiny . . . Mortimer dies . . . *Herbert Hoover* elected president.

1929: Sinclair enters Washington jail in May, leaves in November . . . Fall found guilty of accepting a bribe from Doheny, sentenced to one year. (After appeals fail, Fall enters prison in Santa Fe in July 1931, released May 1932.) . . . New York stock market crashes . . . Forbes resumes private life . . . Forbes dies in 1952.

Abbreviations

AdeCP: Andre de Coppet Papers: Manuscripts Division, Princeton University Library, Andre de Coppet Collection, C0063.

ARVB: Annual Report of the Director, United States Veterans Bureau.

BDG: Boston Daily Globe.

BWRI: Bureau of War Risk Insurance.

CDT: Chicago Daily Tribune.

CES: Charles E. Sawyer.

Consultants on Hospitalization: NARA-CP, RG 121, Records of the Public Buildings Service, Records of Collaborating Boards and Committees, Board of Consultants on Hospitalization. General Correspondence and related records, 1921–1923, Entry 164.

CPR: Civilian Personnel Records, NARA, National Personnel Records Center, St. Louis, MO. (Personnel files for federal civilian employees, some richer than others.) CPR-CRF refers to Forbes's file, CPR-MWW to the file of Mabel Walker Willebrandt, and so on.

CRF: Charles R. Forbes.

Dawes Papers: Charles G. Dawes Papers, Charles Dearing McCormick Library of Special Collections, Northwestern University Library.

Digest of Testimony: NARA-CP, RG 60, US Department of Justice, DOJ Central Files, Straight Numerical Files Enclosures, 225367–225387, Box 1199: Digest of Official Testimony, April 23, 1925, 225387, Typescript, 191 pages.

DOJ Central Files: NARA-CP, RG 60, US Department of Justice, Central Files for 225387.

DOJ Director File: US Department of Justice, Federal Bureau of Investigation, FOI-PA No. 109495-000 (under the Freedom of Information Act), Subject: Charles R. Forbes, FBI Headquarters File 62-3552.

EHM: Elias H. Mortimer.

EKT: Edward Kilbourne Tullidge.

FBH: Federal Board of Hospitalization, NARA, RG 51, BB series 21.5, Records of the Federal Board of Hospitalization.

FBI: The bureau was called the Bureau of Investigation (without "Federal" at the beginning) in the 1920s. For the sake of clarity, instead of "BOI," I also employ the familiar, if anachronistic, "FBI," which has been used since 1935.

HP: Harding Papers, Warren G. Harding Papers, Ohio Historical Society (microfilm edition). The papers of Charles E. Sawyer form a separate part of this collection.

JWHC: John W. H. Crim.

KMF: Kate Marcia Forbes.

LAT: Los Angeles Times.

LF: Leavenworth File: NARA, RG 129, Records of the Bureau of Prisons, Kansas City, 1895–1931, Inmate Case Files. Here for Forbes (CRF) and Edward Tullidge (EKT).

LOC: Library of Congress: Papers for Theodore Roosevelt, Jr., and Joel T. Boone.

MWW: Mabel Walker Willebrandt.

NARA: National Archives and Records Administration. NARA-CP means NARA collections at College Park, MD.

NYT: New York Times.

NYW: New York World.

SH: Senate Hearings, US Senate, Committee on Investigation of the Veterans Bureau, 67th Cong., 4th Session, pursuant to S. Res. 466. Hearings, October 22 to November 7, 1923. Printed in two volumes, Washington, DC: Government Printing Office.

Sullivan Papers: Hoover Institution Archives, Stanford, California. Mark Sullivan Papers, 1883–1952.

Trialdoc: United States Circuit Court of Appeals for the Seventh Circuit, October Term AD 1924, No. 3615, Charles R. Forbes v. United States of America, Transcript of Record, and No. 3616, John W. Thompson v. United States of America, Transcript of Record Vols. 1 and 2. Filed July 3, 1925.

USVB Director's Files: NARA DC, RG 15, Records of the Veterans Administration, NM 60/2A. Director's Files, 1927–ca. 1935.

WGH: Warren G. Harding.

WP: Washington Post.

Notes

CHAPTER 1. Hidden Stories, Fateful Meetings

1. US passport applications from the National Archives are accessible online via ancestry.com.

2. Information on the Harding visit: *Honolulu Star-Bulletin*, January 28, February 2, 3, 13, 1915. The May visit included ten US senators and twenty-seven members of the House, plus families, for a stay of eighteen days, designed to show "what the actual facts concerning the Islands are." *A Souvenir of the Trip of the Congressional Party to Hawaii in 1915* (Honolulu, HI: Advertiser Press, 1915), courtesy Joan Barry Marsh.

3. Forbes's work: Territory of Hawaii, Superintendent of Public Works, "Report of the Governor for the Year Ended June 30, 1915," Honolulu, 1915; "looking down . . .": CRF, *NYW*, December 4, 1927; Kate Marcia Forbes, "The Volcano Kilauea," *Honolulu Star-Bulletin Press*, 1915; Jack London to Kate Forbes, January 18, 1916, courtesy Richard F. Barry.

4. Kate Marcia Forbes described the dinner party later: *WP*, December 18, 1921, 8; "every few days . . .": WGH to CRF, July 30, 1915, courtesy Joan Barry Marsh.

5. Square-rigger story: Charles R. Forbes, Director of the Veterans Bureau, undated typescript, courtesy Forbes's great-grandson Barry Marsh, who received the document on April 13, 1990, from the National Photo Collection, LOC, related to a photo of Forbes. The story also appears in *Outlook*, August 4, 1921, 632.

6. Sources include British National Archives, Kew; Alan Ramsay Skelley, *The Victorian Army at Home: The Recruitment and Terms and Conditions of the British Regular, 1859–1899* (London: Croom Helm, 1977). Database of birth, marriage, and death certificates; census data (Scotland and United States); and ships' manifests available online at ancestry.com.

7. NARA Northeastern Region–New York, Court of Common Pleas, New York City, Naturalization Records, Charles Forbes, Bundle 577, Record No. 1, and index card F 612; enlistment: NARA DC, RG 127 U.S.M.C. Box No. 288, "Case Files, Enlisted Men F–G, 1893"; envelope: "Forbes, Charles R., Dec. 5, 93"; D. Michael Ressler, "Historical Perspective on the President's Own U.S. Marine Band": U.S. Marine

Band, ca. 2006; first voyage: *Dictionary of American Fighting Ships*, vol. 5 (Washington, DC: US Navy Department, Office of the Chief of Naval Operations, Naval History Division, 1970), 70.

8. *NYT,* June 20–30, 1895; quotes: *NYT,* July 26, 1895, 1.

9. Medical condition as reported later in LF-CRF; Surgeon General, US Navy to Commissioner on Pensions, November 2, 1897, Navy Disability Records, 1897–1900, Charles R. Forbes; medical discharge report: NARA DC, RG 127 U.S.M.C. Box No. 288, "Case Files, Enlisted Men F–G, 1893"; Charles R. Forbes, Bugler, Declaration for Navy Invalid Pensions, received by the Navy September 4, 1897; US Government, Navy Disability Records, 1897–1900, Charles R. Forbes, No. 42655.

10. Surgeon's Certificate in Case of CRF, No. 42,655, May 18, 1898, Massachusetts; CRF to Commissioner of Pensions, August 20, 1898, Certificate No. 27,748, Navy Invalid, CRF, Fifer, US Marine Corps, issued February 24, 1899, Navy Disability Records.

11. 1900 US Census, June 1. Forbes Sr. also mentions golf instruction in the Somerville, Massachusetts, Directory 1899. In 1900, Forbes's sister Marie was a private-duty visiting nurse; George, an "electric light trimmer"; and Christine's husband, Edgar Newcomb, a train dispatcher. In the 1910 Census, Sarah (no longer Sadie) Markham described herself as a widow. She and the children still lived with her parents. Times became difficult after her father died in 1911.

12. Hay's remark is often quoted. Here it is from Walter Karp, *The Politics of War: The Story of Two Wars Which Altered Forever the Political Life of the American Republic* (1979; repr. New York: Franklin Square Press, 2003), 3. The Hudson scene was described by Charles G. Dawes in Bascom N. Timmons, *Portrait of an American: Charles G. Dawes* (New York: Henry Holt, 1952), 76–77; NARA-DC RG 94, Entry 53, "Regular Army Muster Rolls"—Signal Corps, Box 2107, Company B, February 29, 1904, to April 30, 1904; enlistment papers United States Army: NARA, RG 94, Entry 91 (Second series), Box 438; stopping the pension: Navy Disability Records, Charles R. Forbes, No. 42655; on divorce proceedings: Will Irwin, February 11, 1924, 2.

13. Forbes was hospitalized from November 23 through December 24, 1906. NARA, RG 94, Entry 52, "Regular Army Muster Rolls"—Signal Corps, Box 2107. The identification as typhoid fever comes from LF-CRF. On the work of the Corps: Harry Meyer Davis and F. G. Fassett, Jr., *What You Should Know about the Signal Corps* (New York: W. W. Norton, 1943), 62–65.

14. Herbert Hunt, "Charles B. Hurley," in *Tacoma, Its History and Its Builders; a Half Century of Activity* (Chicago: S. J. Clarke, 1916), 2:312–14; 1911 Polk Tacoma City Directory, 337; Vashon Island home: Joan Barry Marsh, personal communication; Forbes's "water-boy" quote: Will Irwin, *Atlanta Constitution*, February 11, 1924, 2.

15. Paolo E. Coletta and K. Jack Bauer, *United States Navy and Marine Corps Bases, Domestic* (Westport, CT: Greenwood Press, 1985); postcard: "Kittie and Bob" to Mr. and Mrs. H. D. Spielman, June 18, 1912, courtesy Richard F. Barry.

16. On descriptions of Hawaii, see *Hawaiian Almanac and Annual for 1913*, esp. 100, 180–83; on the "duck pond district": *Honolulu Star-Bulletin*, clipping no date [January 1915], courtesy Richard F. Barry; quote on politics: Robert M. C. Littler, *The Governance of Hawaii: A Study of Territorial Administration* (Stanford, CA: Stanford University Press, 1929), 89.

17. The "best politics": Leonard Schlup, "The Available Man in Hawaii," *International Review of History and Political Science* 25, no. 3 (1988): 15; also H. Brett Melendy, "The Controversial Appointment of Lucius Eugene Pinkham," *Hawaiian Journal of History*, 17 (1983): 185–208.

18. CRF, *Dad's Den*, childhood magazine, Honolulu, May 1915, 283, courtesy of Robert A. Barry; Pinkham to KMF, June 30, 1921, courtesy Richard F. Barry.

19. August 1914 issues of the *Pacific Commercial Advertiser*. Forbes sent Senator J. M. Wadsworth a pamphlet, *The Duty of Japan towards Asia*, in 1916, which Wadsworth found "intensely interesting": Wadsworth to CRF, November 11, 1916, courtesy of Joan Barry Marsh; Territory of Hawaii, Superintendent of Public Works, "Report of the Governor for the Year Ended June 30, 1915," printed by the *Honolulu Star-Bulletin*, 1915.

20. "dynamo of industry" and related quotes: Editorial, *Honolulu Star-Bulletin*, September 16, 1915, 4; "Memorandum for Mr. Pedigo," War Department, Adjutant General's Office, August 28, 1916, signed by H. P. M. Cain, Adjutant General, NARA-CP, RG 60, DOJ Central Files for 225387, Enclosures, Box 1203.

21. "Charles R. Forbes," NARA-CP, RG 60, DOJ Central Files for 225387, Enclosures, Box 1205, F: Exhibit 76. See also Bureau of Investigation, Department of Justice, Director File: 62-3552-79 and 62-3552-80.

22. "Experts Denounce Forbes and His Plans for Piers," *Pacific Commercial Advertiser*, March 17, 1917, clipping, courtesy Barry Marsh.

23. WGH to CRF, July 30, 1915, courtesy Joan Barry Marsh. Forbes was in Washington from mid-December 1915 through mid-January 1916, testifying to committees of the House of Representatives on at least eight separate occasions. The Forbes/Silva headline is from [*Pacific Advertiser*], March 13, 1917, clipping, courtesy Joan Barry Marsh.

24. WGH to CRF in Hawaii, June 20, 1917, courtesy Richard F. Barry.

25. Major General Hunter Liggett, *A.E.F., Ten Years Ago in France* (New York: Dodd Mead, 1927), 1.

26. Reporter's quote: Thomas L. Stokes, *Chip Off My Shoulder* (Princeton, NJ: Princeton University Press, 1940), 60; 2,400 agencies: National Archives, *Handbook of World War Agencies and Their Records, 1917–1921* (Washington, DC: Government Printing Office, 1943), vii.

27. For background: J. Leonard Bates, *The Origins of Teapot Dome: Progressives, Parties, and Petroleum, 1909–1921* (Urbana: University of Illinois Press, 1963).

28. Colleague: James Kelly to Chief Signal Officer in Frederic Louis Huidekoper, *The History of the 33rd Division A.E.F.* (Springfield: Illinois State Historical Library, 1921), 2:554–55; W. K. Naylor to Adjutant General AEF, December 22, 1918: Reproduced in the transcript record for Forbes's appeal; George Bell, Jr., Major General, USA, Headquarters 33rd Division, AEF, APO 750, Luxemburg, February 2, 1919, ibid.; CRF to Marcia Forbes Barry, November 11, 1936, courtesy Robert A. Barry.

29. Mary Roberts Rinehart, *My Story* (New York: Farrar & Rinehart, 1932), 329. The mayor was Ole Hanson, *Americanism versus Bolshevism* (Garden City, NY: Doubleday, Page, 1919). The Centralia massacre is well known.

30. Spencer Ervin, *Henry Ford vs. Truman H. Newberry: The Famous Senate Election Contest; a Study in American Politics, Legislation, and Justice* (New York: R. R. Smith, 1935).

31. WGH to CRF, December 19, 1919; CRF to WGH, December 19, 1919; CRF to HMD, December 19, 1919; WGH to CRF, January 5, 1920; CRF to WGH, February 17, 1920; CRF to WGH, February 25, 1920; WGH to CRF, March 16, 1920; WGH to CRF, April 1, 1920: HP Roll 29, Boxes 87–89.

32. John W. Dean, *Warren G. Harding* (New York: Times Books, 2004), 43–44; telegram: WGH to CRF, November 13, 1920: AdeCP.

CHAPTER 2. Washington, DC, March–April 1921

1. There is a rich literature on Wilson, Harding, and Coolidge and on their administrations. I have limited my footnotes to quotations and information that may not be familiar or easily accessible. Specific details of the parade and the inauguration are drawn from contemporary newspapers: *NYT, WP, CDT,* and *LAT,* March 4 and 5, 1921.

2. "finely cut . . .": John Maynard Keynes, *Essays in Biography*, 2nd ed. (1933; repr. London: Mercury Books, 1961), 20. Economist John Maynard Keynes, part of the British delegation to the Paris Peace Conference, was markedly unimpressed by Wilson's diplomatic skills. For background, see Robert H. Ferrell, *Woodrow Wilson and World War I, 1917–1921* (New York: Harper & Row, 1985).

3. See Randolph C. Downes, *The Rise of Warren Gamaliel Harding, 1865–1920* (Columbus: Ohio State University Press, 1970), 470–71; and Carl Sferrazza Anthony, *Florence Harding: The First Lady, the Jazz Age, and the Death of America's Most Scandalous President* (New York: W. Morrow, 1998), 219–20.

4. On Harding's family and personal background: John W. Dean, *Warren G. Harding* (New York: Times Books, 2004). Also Nan Britton, *The President's Daughter* (New York: Elizabeth Ann Guild, 1927).

5. Quotes from Robert K. Murray, *The Harding Era: Warren G. Harding and His*

Administration (Minneapolis: University of Minnesota Press, 1969), 168; Evalyn Walsh McLean, with Boyden Sparkes, *Father Struck It Rich* (Boston: Little, Brown, 1936), 217–18.

6. David Cannadine, *Mellon: An American Life* (2006; repr. New York: Vintage Books, 2008), 267–68, 278, 280; Herbert Hoover, *The Memoirs of Herbert Hoover, 1920–1933: The Cabinet and the Presidency* (New York: Macmillan, 1952), 47–48.

7. Albert D. Lasker, *The Lasker Story, as He Told It* (Chicago: Advertising Publications, 1963), 58; "you are the only . . .": quoted by Jeffrey L. Cruikshank and Arthur W. Schultz, *The Man Who Sold America: The Amazing (but True) Story of Albert D. Lasker and the Creation of the Advertising Century* (Boston: Harvard Business Review Press, 2010), 370; "deliberate, when time . . .": Charles G. Dawes, *The First Year of the Budget of the United States* (Harper & Brothers, 1923), 2; WGH, "First Annual Message to Congress," December 6, 1921.

8. Mark Sullivan Diaries, 1922–1927, Box 1, Folder June 18–December 13, 1922; entries for July 13, 1922 ("gift for telling stories . . ."), and July 14, 1922 ("cool capacity"): Hoover Institution Archives; "fretful sullenness" and "cock-eyed world . . .": Mark Sullivan, *Our Times, 1900–1925*, vol. 6, *The Twenties* (C. Scribner's Sons, 1935), 115 and 2, respectively.

9. "a disturbingly dull mind": reported by Secretary of Agriculture (later Secretary of the Treasury) David F. Houston, *Eight Years in Wilson's Cabinet 1913 to 1920: With a Personal Estimate of the President* (Garden City, NY: Doubleday, Page, 1926), 2:17; and see A. Scott Berg, *Wilson* (New York: G. P. Putnam's Sons, 2013), 618; for "mediocre mind . . .": Houston, *Eight Years*, 2:93; "the faith in which I was bred . . .": quoted by Ray Stannard Baker, *American Chronicle: The Autobiography of Ray Stannard Baker* (New York: C. Scribner's Sons, 1945), 485; "old Solomon": WGH, *Our Common Country: Mutual Good Will in America* (Indianapolis, IN: Bobbs-Merrill, 1921), 15.

10. "tired of men . . . more or less afflicted . . .": William Allen White, *Masks in a Pageant* (New York: Macmillan, 1928), 410; "region of fictions . . .": Clinton W. Gilbert, *Behind the Mirrors: The Psychology of Disintegration at Washington* (New York: G. P. Putnam's Sons, 1922), 159, 202; "an escape, a thrill . . .": Silas Bent, *Ballyhoo: The Voice of the Press* (New York: Boni and Liveright, 1927), 197–98.

11. Walter Lippmann, *Public Opinion* (New York: Harcourt, Brace, 1922), 125; Bruce Bliven, "Charlie, Warren and Ned," *New Republic*, May 28, 1924, 9 (fourth installment in the story of the "Ohio Gang").

12. "modern type . . .": Anonymous [Clinton W. Gilbert], *The Mirrors of Washington* (New York: G. P. Putnam's Sons, 1921), 4; F. Scott Fitzgerald, *The Vegetable: Or, from President to Postman* (1923; repr. New York: Macmillan, 1976), "bloviate" was a favorite Harding word; Gilbert, *Behind the Mirrors*, 140.

13. *LAT*, March 4, 1921, 13.

14. "A stranger . . .": *LAT*, March 4, 1921, 11. See also *WP*, March 6, 1917, 6; *NYT*, March 6, 1917, 1.

15. Movies listed in *WP*, March 6, 1921, 53; federal arrests in *NYT*, February 25, 1921, 6.

16. *WP*, November 9, 1920, 1; *NYT*, November 15, 1920, 2; *NYT*, November 26, 1920, 12; December 1, 1920, 3; *WP*, December 5, 1920, 1.

17. "give the best . . .": *LAT*, December 7, 1920, 11; see also *WP*, December 7, 1920, 1; "the best minds . . .": Harding quoted, *WP*, January 23, 1921, 1; "the greatest job dispenser . . .": *NYT*, December 5, 1920, 104.

18. Gilbert, *Behind the Mirrors*, 138; Harding's cabinet in 1921 was as follows: Charles Evans Hughes, Secretary of State; Andrew W. Mellon, Secretary of the Treasury; John W. Weeks, Secretary of War; Edwin Denby, Secretary of the Navy; Albert B. Fall, Secretary of Interior; Henry C. Wallace, Secretary of Agriculture; Herbert C. Hoover, Secretary of Commerce; James J. Davis, Secretary of Labor; Harry M. Daugherty, Attorney General; William H. Hays, Postmaster General.

19. David H. Stratton, "Behind Teapot Dome: Some Personal Insights," *Business History Review* 31, no. 4 (Winter 1957): 388, 389. The five Hoover said "stood above the others" were Hughes, Mellon, Weeks, Denby, and Hays. Another commentator would of course have included Hoover. Hoover, *Memoirs*, 40.

20. The four men served without pay as a committee of consultants on hospitalization to plan for hospital provision for veterans and to distribute the available funds, backed up by government officials, with direct report to Secretary Mellon. See Rosemary Stevens, "Can the Government Govern? Lessons from the Formation of the Veterans Administration," *Journal of Health Politics, Policy and Law* 16, no. 2 (Summer 1991): 281–305; William P. Dillingham, *Federal Aid to Veterans, 1917–1941* (Gainesville: University of Florida Press, 1952); and Jessica L. Adler, *Burdens of War: Politics, Necessity, and the Birth of the Veterans Hospital System* (Baltimore: Johns Hopkins University Press, forthcoming).

21. See *CDT*, March 5, 1921, 1; *NYT*, March 5, 1921, 1.

22. For the reaction in Los Angeles: *LAT*, March 5, 1921, 1.

23. Forbes's appearance in the social news: *WP*, April 14, 1921, 7.

24. *CDT*, March 15, 1921, 1; WGH to CRF, December 14, 1920, courtesy Robert A. Barry; US Shipping Board, File 40, Folder 53, "Charles R. Forbes": HP, Roll 152, 1921–1923. Hoover memo to WGH, April 2, 1921; ibid., about the successful candidate for the Shipping Board, Meyer Lissner. Same HP reference for other letters cited. On London: *Tacoma Daily Ledger*, April 22, 1921, courtesy Robert A. Barry.

25. WGH to CRF, April 7, 1921, AdeCP. CRF, *NYW*, December 4, 1927, 1.

CHAPTER 3. The Dream of Efficiency in Government

1. The best contemporary account of the work of BWRI is by Forbes's predecessor Richard G. Cholmeley-Jones, *Scientific Monthly* 12 (March 1921): 228–35. His quote is from this source. For Forbes: *NYW,* December 4, 1927, 2.

2. Quote and Women's Day: Randolph C. Downes, *The Rise of Warren Gamaliel Harding, 1865–1920* (Columbus: Ohio State University Press, 1970), 510–13.

3. Statement of Brigadier General Charles E. Sawyer: US Senate and US House of Representatives, Committees on Education, *Hearings on S. 1607 and H.R. 5837, Bills to Establish a Department of Public Welfare and for Other Purposes,* 67th Cong., May 11, 12, 13, 18, and 20, 1921, quotes at pp. 4, 5.

4. For the 97 percent figure: Howard W. Odum, "Public Welfare Activities," in [Herbert Hoover] President's Research Committee on Social Trends, *Recent Social Trends in the United States,* chapter 24, 1261, table 6. On federal policy up to the 1920s, see Theda Skocpol, *Protecting Soldiers and Mothers: The Political Origins of Social Policy in the United States* (Cambridge, MA: Belknap Press of Harvard University Press, 1992).

5. CRF: *NYW,* December 4, 1927, 2.

6. US House of Representatives, Committee on Interstate and Foreign Commerce, Subcommittee on Consolidation of Government Agencies for the Benefit of Disabled Ex-Service Men, *Hearings on Consolidation of Government Agencies for the Benefit of Disabled Ex-Service Men, H.R. 3, Part 1, April 29, 1921,* 67th Cong., 17.

7. Ellis W. Hawley, *The Great War and the Search for a Modern Order: A History of the American People and Their Institutions, 1917–1933* (New York: St. Martin's Press, 1979), 19; Robert K. Murray, *The Politics of Normalcy: Governmental Theory and Practice in the Harding-Coolidge Era* (New York: Norton, 1973), 34–35.

8. "shilly-shallying" and "mind made up": Marcus E. Ravage, *The Story of Teapot Dome* (New York: Republic, 1924), 25–27; Murray, *Politics of Normalcy,* 34–35; on Denby: Herbert Hoover, *The Memoirs of Herbert Hoover: The Cabinet and the Presidency, 1920–1933* (New York: Macmillan, 1952), 40.

9. Daugherty and Burns: *NYT,* April 1, 1921; Murray, *The Harding Era: Warren G. Harding and His Administration* (Minneapolis: University of Minnesota Press, 1969), 414–15; *Fingerprint and Identification Magazine* 4, no. 1 (1921): 4.

10. Dawes's committee report, included as Exhibit 1 in US House of Representatives, Committee on Interstate and Foreign Commerce, Subcommittee on Consolidation of Government Agencies for the Benefit of Disabled Ex-Service Men, *Hearings on H.R. 3, Part 1, April 29, 1921,* 67th Cong., 41–44; quote is at p. 43. Sawyer, too, wanted someone in authority who would "get all of the forces headed in the proper direction." Ibid., 51; quote is at p. 49.

11. Charles G. Dawes to Milton J. Foreman; Dawes to F. W. Galbraith, Jr.; Dawes to Sawyer, all on April 26, 1921. HP, Roll 196, Folder 312-1.

12. Statistics are from *Historical Statistics of the United States: Colonial Times to 1957*, Table Y, "Select Characteristics of the Armed Forces, by War," 735; shipment of coffins: *NYT*, May 23, 1921; August 2, 1922, HP, Roll 175, File 95; Veterans' Affairs, Folder 5.

13. US Congress, H.R., Committee on Interstate and Foreign Commerce. Bureau of Veteran Reestablishment, *Hearing . . . on H.R. 14961, January 7, 1921*, 71; US Congress, Senate Committee on Finance, Subcommittee, Establishment of a Veterans' Bureau. *Hearings on H. R. 6611 [Sweet bill]*, 67th Cong., July 5 and 7, 1921, 63.

14. American Legion membership dropped off between 1920 and 1925 and then picked up, soaring to more than a million members in 1931, in the hope that the "soldiers' bonus" would finally be achieved. William Pencak, *For God and Country: The American Legion, 1919–1941* (Boston: Northeastern University Press, 1989), 82–83. For the New York parade, see Stephen R. Ortiz, *Beyond the Bonus March and GI Bill: How Veteran Politics Shaped the New Deal Era* (New York: New York University Press, 2010), 25–26.

15. Regarding Cholmeley-Jones, see Robinson E. Adkins, *Medical Care of Veterans* (Washington, DC: Department of Veterans Affairs, 2009), 107–9; and see Richard Seelye Jones, *History of the American Legion* (New York: Bobbs-Merrill, 1946), 128. Forbes's comments: SH, 913.

16. Sawyer to Dawes, May 7 and 14, 1921. Dawes Papers, Northwestern University, Box 93, Folder 33. Mark Sullivan, *Our Times, 1990–1925*, vol. 6, *The Twenties* (C. Scribner's Sons, 1935), 237–38.

17. Forbes to Dawes, May 28, 1921: Dawes, Box 94, Folder 24; for the "meat ax," see Dawes committee proceedings, included as Exhibit 2 in US House of Representatives, Committee on Interstate and Foreign Commerce, Subcommittee on Consolidation of Government Agencies for the Benefit of Disabled Ex-Service Men, *Hearings . . . on H.R. 3, Part 1, April 29, 1921*, 67th Cong., 44–130; quote is on p. 49; Dawes to CRF, June 1, 1921, Andre de Coppet Papers: Manuscripts Division, Princeton University Library, C0063 (hereafter AdeCP).

18. ARVB, 1922, 26. On general aspects of hospital provision: William P. Dillingham, *Federal Aid to Veterans, 1917–1941* (Gainesville: University of Florida Press, 1952); and for an in-depth study of politics and policy making for veterans hospitals, Jessica L. Adler, "A Solemn Obligation: Soldiers, Veterans, and Health Policy in the United States, 1917–1924" (PhD diss., Columbia University, 2012).

19. Sawyer to Charles G. Dawes, April 11, May 15, and May 26, 1921, and Sawyer to J. E. Bute, April 21, and related correspondence: Dawes Papers, Box 93, Folders 33 and 26. Minutes of proceedings of the meeting called and chaired by President

Harding in the auditorium of the Interior Department, June 29, 1921, Typescript, HP, Roll 262. Charles E. Sawyer Papers, 1914–1926.

20. US Congress, Senate Committee on Finance, Subcommittee, Establishment of a Veterans' Bureau, *Hearings on H.R. 6611 [Sweet bill]*, 67th Cong., July 5 and 7, 1921, 10–11, and passim.

21. Jones, *American Legion*, 47. Jones knew Taylor, ibid., 362; SH on the Sweet bill, p. 11.

22. SH on the Sweet bill, 15, 16.

23. Ibid., 40, 44, 54, 60–62; WGH to CRF, July 28, 1921, AdeCP.

24. The four naysayers were Hamilton Fish (NY), Rosenblum (WV), Lineberger (CA), and Blanton (TX); *CDT*, August 2, 1921, 3; August 3, 1921, 1; August 5, 1921, 5.

25. *NYT*, August 10, 1921, 5.

26. Charles G. Dawes, *The First Year of the Budget of the United States* (New York: Harper & Brothers, 1923), 52, 57, 64, 69, respectively; *WP*, July 17, 1921, 3. According to historian Carl Sferrazza Anthony, Sawyer was "planting spies" in BWRI in the summer of 1921, motivated at least in part by jealousy of Mrs. Harding's "blind admiration" of Forbes and her close relationship with him. Anthony, *Florence Harding: The First Lady, the Jazz Age, and the Death of America's Most Scandalous President* (New York: W. Morrow, 1998), 334.

27. "Why Harding Takes the Helm," *Literary Digest*, August 6, 1921, 11–13; *WP*, August 11, 1921, 3; *CDT*, August 14, 1921, 7.

28. Mr. and Mrs. Walter Brown were also present; *WP*, August 14, 1921, 30. Kate Marcia Forbes, "What Happened When I Was a Guest at the White House," *WP*, December 25, 1921, 25.

29. Andrew W. Mellon to CRF, August 15, 1921, AdeCP.

30. Hoover, *Memoirs of Herbert Hoover*, 4.

CHAPTER 4. Harding's Flagship Program

1. For vocational education, see W. Stull Holt, *The Federal Board for Vocational Education: Its History, Activities and Organization* (New York: D. Appleton, 1922), 11. Figures are for August 15, 1921.

2. ARVB 1922, 17–26, 55. Further extension of services was made in legislation of April 19, 1922, when veterans of the Spanish-American War, Philippine Insurrection, and the Boxer Rebellion who suffered from neuropsychiatric illnesses or tuberculosis were covered for hospital and medical services, whether or not the condition was service related.

3. *WP*, August 28, 1921.

4. NARA-CP, RG 60, DOJ Central Files, Box 1202, F: Sweet, Merle L., 1–2, 7; and SH, 1319–38: Sweet.

5. Forbes's quotes: *NYT*, August 11, 1921, 3.

6. On June 30, 1922, the Veterans Bureau reported 29,746 employees, of whom 4,758 were in central office, 14,247 in district offices, 10,416 working in Veterans Bureau hospitals, and 325 at the US vocational school at Chillicothe. ARVB, 1922, 562.

7. WP, August 21, 1921, 2; *CDT*, August 21, 1921, 15; for national training centers: *NYT*, August 20, 1921, 11.

8. Forbes's quotes: WP, October 6, 1921, 1; WP, October 18, 1921, 9; for the thirty-two schools "disallowed": WP, October 19, 1921, 2; Rose C. Feld, "The New War Cripples' School," *NYT*, March 19, 1922, 107.

9. ARVB, 1922, Table 95, 382–89; officers' quotes: ARVB, 1922, 317 and 287; Forbes quote: WP, October 19, 1921, 2.

10. The December conference was chaired by John H. Finley of New York. Participants included among others the secretary of labor (James J. Davis), the chair of the American Legion's major rehabilitation committee (A. A. Sprague), and the celebrated author Mary Roberts Rinehart, who was a committed advocate for veterans. *NYT*, December 30, 1921, 30; WP, December 30, 1921, 9; *CDT*, December 30, 1921, 4; Dean's and Forbes's parting shots: *NYT*, January 17, 1922, 13; and *New York Post*, n.d. [January 16, 1922], NARA-CP, RG 121. See Records of the Public Buildings . . . Board of Consultants on Hospitalization, General Correspondence and Related Records, 1921–23, Entry 164, Box 21, Binder, Press Notices.

11. Haven Emerson (1874–1957) was commissioner of health for the city of New York before World War I and then served as a colonel in the Army Medical Corps with a special interest in communicable diseases, including tuberculosis. He was an acknowledged expert on hospital organization. Obituary and Emerson quote: *American Journal of Public Health* 47, no. 8 (1957): 1009–11. Emerson was the man Dr. Sawyer had wanted Forbes to fire from the Bureau of War Risk Insurance, apparently because Emerson disdained Sawyer's medical field, homeopathy.

12. *Oakland Tribune*, September 1, 1921, 1.

13. *NYT*, January 17, 1922, 13; WP, September 14, 1921, 1 and 6; also *Modern Hospital* 27, no. 4 (October 1921): 282; *The Survey*, September 24, 1921, 719.

14. Emerson, *Outlook*, April 5, 1922, 545–46.

15. The Reminiscences of Haven Emerson (ca. 1952, exact date not given), No. 54, Columbia University Oral History Collection; Forbes's testimony at the Senate hearings: SH, 1096.

16. Sprague: Minutes of Meeting of Legion Representatives of First and Second Districts with the Director of the Veterans' Bureau and Managers of Districts 1 and 2, May 1922, NARA I, RG15, Records of the Veterans Administration, Director's Files, NM/2A 1917–1935, Box 115, quotes at 30, 34.

17. *The Survey* 46 (September 24, 1921): 698; Charles G. Dawes, *The First Year of the Budget of the United States* (New York: Harper & Brothers, 1923), 393; ARVB, 1922, 562; Leon Fraser to John J. Walsh, June 22, 1922; NARA DC, RG 15, NM60/2A, Box 114, Waddle to Wit. (Someone had fun here in dividing the Ws.)

18. Meetings of representatives: Fred E. Hamilton, Chief, Administrative Division, Veterans Bureau) to Major Leon Fraser, Executive Officer, Veterans Bureau, January 26, 1922, NARA DC, RG 15, NM60/2A, Box 123, 023-1. The first meeting was in Kansas City, the second in Indianapolis.

19. *WP*, December 28, 1921, 5; *WP*, December 30, 1921, 9.

20. ARVB, 1922, 48, and 44, respectively. In October, the task of vetting private dental bills was also decentralized to district offices, where oversight was easier to do (46).

21. ARVB, 1922, 27. *CDT*, August 31, 1921, 3; *NYT*, August 31, 1921, 16; on Sergeant Crossland: *The Crisis*, May 1918, 35.

22. Minutes of Meeting of Legion Representatives of First and Second Districts, May 18, 1922, NARA I, RG 15, Records of the Veterans Administration, Director's Files, NM/2A 1917–1935, Box 115, 32.

23. Details of Forbes's travel: CPR-CRF. The example here is for October 11–14, 1921.

24. Lila Cramer's role in Washington: *WP*, September 23, 1921, 7; December 5, 1921, 7; April 21, 1922, 7; June 22, 1921, 7. The 1919 trip: A letter from a certain E. Manifold Raeburn of the British Ministry of Shipping Office in New York, dated April 16, 1919, states that the purpose of Cramer's trip was to discuss "important matters in which the British Government are interested." Cramer, Passport Application file.

25. CRF to Secretary of the Treasury, June 7, 1921, NARA-CP, RG 60, Box 1207; Cramer to Johnson, June 6, 1918, Hiram W. Johnson Papers, 1895–1945, Part III, Bancroft Library, UC Berkeley.

26. Cramer's recommendation to Forbes: Report as of September 22, 1921, appended to Charles F. Cramer's report of November 29, 1921. For the Treasury reaction: A. W. Mellon to CRF, December 7, 1921, reported at SH, 955.

27. Dawes, *The First Year of the Budget of the United States*, 73, 79; James A. Tobey and New York Academy of Medicine, *The National Government and Public Health* (Baltimore: Johns Hopkins Press, 1926).

28. Dawes, *The First Year*, 98–101. Senator Borah: *CDT*, February 16, 1922, 4. A million dollars a day: *NYT*, August 11, 1921, 3. Most of the expenditure for the Veterans Bureau was accounted for by statutory monetary benefits.

29. *NYT*, March 25, 1922, 23.

30. LOC, Joel T. Boone Papers, Box 40, F: No Title (Typed Diary), unpaginated: entry for Wednesday, May 24, 1922; Salmon to Sprague, April 23, 1922, and Sprague to Salmon, April 18, 1921: NARA-CP, RG 60, DOJ Central Files for 225387, Box 1203, F: Sprague.

CHAPTER 5. High Stakes

1. CRF to "Kate and Awa," August 22, 1922, courtesy of Robert A. Barry.

2. On health policy in this chapter, I draw from my previous work: Rosemary Stevens, *In Sickness and in Wealth: American Hospitals in the Twentieth Century* (New York: Basic Books, 1989), updated with a new introduction (Baltimore: Johns Hopkins University Press, 1999); Stevens, "Can the Government Govern? Lessons from the Formation of the Veterans Administration," *Journal of Health Politics, Policy and Law* 16 (1991); Stevens, "The Invention, Stumbling and Reinvention of the Modern US Veterans Health Care System, 1918–1924," in *Veterans' Policies, Veterans' Politics: New Perspectives on Veterans in the Modern United States*, ed. Stephen R. Ortiz (Gainesville: University Press of Florida, 2012). In *A Time of Scandal*, I focus on the Veterans Bureau scandal. In parallel, wonderful work has been, and is being, done by others on medical aspects of the history of the US health system for veterans and its relationship to military medicine. I have specially benefited from the work, help, and colleagueship of Jessica Adler, Carol Byerly, Beth Linker, Sanders Marble, Stephen Ortiz, and Wendy Moffatt. On Carl Bronner: *NYT*, December 12, 1921, 14.

3. ARVB, 1923, table 6, 64.

4. *Hearings . . . on H.R. 8791, Report No. 14, Additional Hospital Facilities*, Committee on Public Buildings and Grounds, February 8, 1922, 7.

5. "It is absolutely senseless. . . ": CES to WGH, August 10, 1921, CESP, Roll 262, Collection 95; for the context of the budget: Thomas A. Rumer, *The American Legion: An Official History, 1919–1989* (New York: M. Evans, 1990), 145; for other Sawyer quotes: *WP*, August 21, 1921, 7.

6. US Treasury Department, *Report of the Consultants on Hospitalization, Appointed by the Secretary of the Treasury to Provide Additional Hospital Facilities under Public Act 384 (Approved March 4, 1921)* (Washington, DC: Government Printing Office, 1923), 58. The first Langley Act: Public Law 66-384.

7. FBH minutes, January 10, 1922, 1; *Hearings . . . on H.R. 8791*, 11, 14, 25; Treasury Department, *Report of the Consultants on Hospitalization.*

8. *Hearings . . . on H.R. 8791, Additional Hospital Facilities*, Committee on Public Buildings and Grounds, Report No. 10, January 14, 1922 (Washington, DC: Government Printing Office, 1922), 25.

9. On Fox Hills, see *NYT*, February 14, 1922, 14; March 5, 1922, 8; March 9, 1922, 7; March 18, 1922, 9; and CRF to WGH, March 17, 1922, HP, Roll 175, Folder 14, applications for Hospitals for Disabled Veterans.

10. Conference, Director's Office, April 18, 1922, typescript of proceedings, NARA DC, RG 15, Records of the Veterans' Administration, NM 60.2A; Director's Files, 1927–1935, Box 115, NM 60.02, State of New York, pp. 1, 7, 16. This was a meeting

between Veterans Bureau staff and members of the New York congressional delegation to try to resolve some of the problems. The meeting seems to have gone well.

11. Rogers: SH, 811. Salmon: *Hearings . . . on H.R. 8791*, 21.

12. *Hearings . . . on H.R. 8791*, 6 (Forbes), 15 (Fraser).

13. FBH minutes, February 10, 1922, 3; February 11, 2, 4.

14. The newspaper series, as published in the *Washington Post*: Kate Marcia Forbes, "Mrs. Harding's Favorite Portrait of Herself Hitherto Unpublished, and What Happened When I Was a Guest at the White House," *WP*, December 25, 1921, 2, also January 1, 8, and 15, 1922.

15. Biographer Stacy A. Cordery described Mrs. Longworth neatly as the "social doyenne in a town where socializing was state business": *Alice: Alice Roosevelt Longworth, from White House Princess to Washington Power Broker* (New York: Viking, 2007), viii; examples of the system: Mary Roberts Rinehart, *My Story* (New York, Farrar & Rinehart, 1931), 339, and George Wharton Pepper, *Philadelphia Lawyer: An Autobiography* (Philadelphia: Lippincott, 1944), 257–58; for Kate's listing: Louis S. Lyons, ed., *Who's Who among the Women of California* (San Francisco: Security, 1922), 155; for Mrs. Harding's teas: Carl Sferrazza Anthony, *The First Lady, the Jazz Age, and the Death of America's Most Scandalous President* (New York: W. Morrow, 1998), 593n16.

16. In the Forbes family tradition, Marie Judkins had no qualms in stating on an official form that she was forty-three years of age on her appointment to the Veterans Bureau, when actually she was fifty-one. Forms were to be manipulated—even, perhaps, a form of red tape (CPR-Judkins). Forbes laid out his expectations of a wife in letters to Kate that have survived; notably CRF to KMF, August 22, 1922, courtesy Robert A. Barry; on Kate's condition: CRF to Dr. L. Vernon Briggs in Boston, replying to his inquiry about Kate, February 17, 1922, NARA DC, RG 15, NM 60/2A, Box 117-02 004; on Forbes's only recorded visit to Johns Hopkins: Robert U. Patterson to George B. Christian, April 7, 1922. HP, Roll 147, April 7, 1922, File 21: 81.

17. About Dr. Cole: *NYT*, May 26, 1921; about Forbes meeting: Nan Britton, *The President's Daughter* (New York: Elizabeth Ann Guild, 1927), 178.

18. Typed copy of an originally handwritten letter, Votaw to CRF, February 10, 1922, NARA, RG 60, DOJ Central Files for 225387, Box 1205 F, Exhibit 76. Harding's younger siblings, including Carolyn, were raised as Seventh-day Adventists; see Bill Knott, "The Nearly Adventist President," *Adventist Review*, http://archives.adventistreview.org/article/307/archives/issue-2006-1503/the-nearly-adventist-president; CPR-Carolyn Votaw.

19. *WP*, February 14, 1922, 3; for the hearings: Rep. Martin Madden (IL), chair, Second deficiency appropriation hearings, House Committee on Appropriations, February 15, 1922, 106–10, and 97–99.

20. Second deficiency hearings, February 15, 1922, 28, 55.

21. Public Law 67–194. Richard Seelye Jones, *A History of the American Legion* (Indianapolis, IN: Bobbs-Merrill, 1946), 173–74; Langley to WGH, March 22, 1922, HP Presidential Case File, Roll 175, File 95, folder 15.

22. NARA-CP, RG 60, DOJ Central Files, Straight Numerical Enclosures, Box 1201, F: From Mr. Crim; and see FBH minutes, April 6, 1922.

23. NARA-CP, RG 60, DOJ Central Files, Straight Numerical Enclosures, Box 1201, F: From Mr. Crim; FBH minutes, May 10, 1922. Present were two heavyweights, Surgeon General Ireland of the US Army and Surgeon General Cumming of the US Public Health Service, plus Captain Pleadwell, representing Admiral Stitt of the US Navy; Dr. Noyes, representing Dr. William Alanson White, superintendent of the federal St. Elizabeths Hospital; and a Mr. Merritt, representing Commissioner Burke of the Bureau of Indian Affairs. The bare-bones specifics were as follows. For Northampton, Massachusetts, a new neuropsychiatric hospital in District 1. For District 2, a 250-bed hospital for tuberculosis to be located somewhere in Upstate New York. In District 5, the purchase of a fully equipped private general hospital in Memphis, at a cost of $4,000 a bed: "a going modern hospital, the best I have ever seen," Forbes said. In District 6, the bureau was trying to get land donated in Mississippi. The PHS hospital there was unsatisfactory. PHS Surgeon General Cumming remarked, "We had a lot of trouble about malaria." In District 7 (Ohio, Indiana, and Kentucky), the bureau was considering a 400-bed neuropsychiatric hospital at Chillicothe, Ohio. However, Forbes reported, President Harding preferred not to put more federal money into his home state. This was clarified at another meeting: Harding "did not want it to appear that he was fostering [federal] hospitals in Ohio." Instead Harding recommended adding more beds to the Soldiers' Home at Marion, Indiana, which had just completed a neuropsychiatric unit, and which Sawyer favored. District 8 (Illinois, Michigan, and Wisconsin) raised questions of interstate conflict. Forbes recommended a 900-bed hospital on navy land at Camp Ross, Great Lakes, Illinois, and the board approved. (To Forbes's embarrassment, Harding later overturned this decision in favor of the competing political claims of Michigan.) In District 9, a 400-bed neuropsychiatric hospital at Kansas City or Fort Dodge, ideally on donated land. In District 10 a possible 350-bed neuropsychiatric hospital at Fort Snelling, Minnesota. District 12 included the site at Livermore, California. Surgeon General Cumming of the PHS was not entirely happy with the purchase there (quite rightly), but in the end, he agreed to go with Colonel Patterson, who recommended it, recognizing that Livermore was a done deal and by then the land belonged to the government. For District 13, a 250-bed neuropsychiatric hospital at Camp Lewis, Washington, and in District 14 a 200-bed neuropsychiatric hospital in northern Texas, whose representatives had argued that Texas had given more men to military service than Oklahoma and Arkansas (the initially favored possibility).

24. CES to WGH, May 11, 1922: HP, Roll 262, 1914–1926, Charles E. Sawyer Papers (Collection 95).

25. The full list of approved hospitals was for hospitals at Northampton, Livermore, Camp Lewis (Washington State), two in New York State (one within fifty miles of New York City, one upstate), at Gulfport (MS), and one in the Tenth District (MT, ND, SD, MN), which must be on government land. *NYT,* May 17, 1922, 9; for Sawyer's letter: CES to WGH, May 18, 1922, Harding Papers, Roll 262: 1914–1926, Charles E. Sawyer Papers (Collection 95). Forbes had said that Marion, Indiana, would not accept insane patients.

26. Forbes's quote, "You can't put these old men . . .": FBH, minutes May 26, 1922, 13. Forbes's second and third quotes: SH, Forbes testimony, 923 and 1045, respectively. Sawyer's quote: SH, 767.

27. Forbes quotes: SH, 1046.

28. CES to WGH, June 20, 1922, Warren G. Harding Papers, Roll 262, 1914–1926, Charles E. Sawyer Papers (Collection 95).

29. Major L. Walter Treadway performed the land-sea consultation before 500 assembled guests: *NYT,* April 16, 1922, 23; Patterson's quote: FBH minutes, June 5, 1922, 4. The Federal Board discussed the matter and agreed that the hospital should be patient-ready in all respects except for "expendable supplies such as drugs, food, office supplies and surgical dressings." Forbes's quote: FBH minutes, August 9, 1922, 17.

30. FBH minutes, June 12, 1922, 2, 12. Telegram, A. A. Sprague to C. E. Sawyer, June 30, 1922, telegram from Sawyer, July 1, and telegram, Sprague to Sawyer, July 3, 1922. Dawes Papers, Box 118, Folder 25.

CHAPTER 6. Hype, Hooch, and the Art of the Con

1. See Charles Merz, *The Dry Decade* (Garden City, NY: Doubleday, Doran, 1930), 330 and 162–63. The key character in Sinclair Lewis's popular novel *Babbitt* (New York: Harcourt Brace Jovanovich, 1922) also declares that "most folks are so darned crooked themselves that they expect a fellow to do a little lying. . . ." Signet edition, 1950, see pp. 38, 41.

2. Edwin P. Hoyt, *Spectacular Rogue: Gaston B. Means* (Indianapolis, IN: Bobbs Merrill, 1963). Quote from Gaston Means, *The Strange Death of President Harding: From the Diaries of Gaston B. Means, as told to May Dixon Thacker* (New York: Guild, 1930), 22.

3. R. B. Pixley, *Minneapolis Tribune,* n.d. [1924], to E. R. Mahoney, City Editor Chicago American, copy attached to a telegram from "Shiber" in New York [unknown] to "Mahoney" dated February 14, 1924. DOJ Central Files, NARA-CP, RG 60, Box

1208, F: Mortimer-Personal, Philip Kinsley, *CDT,* December 30, 1924, 9. "I fired him": Digest of Testimony, Box 1199, 106–7.

4. Report by John C. Updegrove, October 7, 1925, NARA-CP, RG 60, DOJ Central Files for 225387, Box 3856 and Box 1206; Lannen to Wm. J. Donovan, October 1, 1925, Box 3855; Mortimer to Crim, December 23, 1924, Box 1208; "fiend" quote: Lannen to Donovan, Box 3855.

5. Langley's quotes: John Wesley Langley, *They Tried to Crucify Me; or, The Smoke-Screen of the Cumberlands* (Pikeville, KY: J. W. Langley, 1929); for Mortimer's "$7500 car": Trialdoc, 437; for the fried egg story: *Owingsville (KY) Outlook,* August 11, 1921, 3. The other congressman was John C. Pringey of Oklahoma. The question of Langley's guilt or innocence is on my future research list.

6. Handwritten statement by E. H. Mortimer, undated, NARA-CP, RG 60, DOJ central files for 225387, Box 1206, F: Bank Account E. H. Mortimer: Commercial Trust Co., and Merchants Bank and Trust Co.

7. Reported Statement by Elias H. Mortimer, no date [1923] in DOJ Central Files, F: Mortimer-personal, NARA-CP, RG 60, Box 1208.

8. The canceled checks to Margaret Williams were as follows: February 7, 1921, for $325 (on Riggs Bank); $135 June 20, 1921 (on Merchants); and October 25, 1921, $300 (on Merchants), NARA-CP, RG 60, DOJ Central Files for 225387, Box 1206, F: Bank Account E.H.Mortimer.

9. When held as a spy, Tullidge told British authorities about a "passport factory" for American passports in Copenhagen and claimed that the German consul in Rotterdam had a supply of these—news that provoked an outcry of indignation against Tullidge from Germans and German Americans in the United States: *Philadelphia Evening Bulletin,* Newspaper clipping collection, July 11, 1915; Temple University, Urban Archives, Philadelphia. Tullidge published seven articles in 1916 in US medical journals based on his European observations. His article, "Military Surgery and the Surgeon in the Present European War" was extensively discussed in the Sunday issue of the *New York Times* in September 1916 as an important contribution from an intelligent, informed observer at the front: *NYT,* September 17, 1916, Section X, 12; court-martial: NARA, Central Plains Region, Kansas City, Leavenworth File, Edward K. Tullidge, No. 19554: Navy Department, Court Martial Order No. 69-1917.

10. Pennsylvania Department of Health, Death Certificate for Mary Louisa Tullidge, No. 4108805, copy issued June 7, 2007. *Philadelphia Inquirer,* September 28, 1918, 16; undated clipping, *Philadelphia Evening Bulletin,* [Sept 28, 1918], courtesy of Thomas H. Tullidge.

11. *Philadelphia Inquirer,* May 1, 1919, 3.

12. On Campbell: John Wesley Langley, *They Tried to Crucify Me,* 27, 30. Dahlberg: US Circuit Court of Appeals for the Seventh Circuit, October 1925 term, Nos. 3615–

3616, Summary 120–22; Mortimer's abuse: Forbes's lawyer, James S. Easby-Smith, listed Katherine Mortimer and Lieutenant Guy Burlingame of the Washington, DC, police as witnesses at the Senate hearings in 1923, to testify to "assaults and other violent trouble" between the Mortimers that occurred early in 1921. (They were not called to testify.) Easby-Smith to Select Committee on Investigation of the Veterans Bureau, US Senate, November 20, 1923. NARA-CP, RG 60, Box 1207 misc. Record of splits and reconciliations: Werner, *Privileged Characters*, 212.

13. SH, 1002, 1210; Trialdoc 1, 437.

14. Trialdoc 1, 446. For Forbes's understanding of the relationship: SH, 1002. The photo was reproduced in *The Bridgeport (CT) Telegram*, February 16, 1924, 15.

15. Trial Summary Statement, 5–6. Thompson's obituary, *Atlanta Constitution*, May 4, 1926. James Black died before the trial took place. Mortimer's boast about Thompson: SH, 199.

16. For Mortimer's statements: Trialdoc 1, 390. SH, 1005, 1002, and see SH, 199.

17. Trialdoc 1, 448, 455–56.

18. Trial summary statement, 4, 6.

19. SH, 1356; Trialdoc 1, 447; Trialdoc 2, 1423.

20. Joel T. Boone Papers, LOC, box 45 FXVI B Med-XVII. USS *Mayflower*-President Harding: Memoirs.

21. Herbert Hoover, *The Memoirs of Herbert Hoover, 1920–1933: The Cabinet and the Presidency* (New York: Macmillan, 1952), 48; Wardman Park: Trialdoc 1, 437.

22. Trialdoc, 389, 451, 455–56; SH, 1009.

23. Trial Brief for Crim re Edward Stockdale, NARA-CP, RG 60, DOJ Central Files for 225387, Box 1201.

24. *NYT*, May 26, 1922; NARA-CP, RG 60, DOJ Central Files, Box 1201, F: From Mr. Crim; NARA DC, RG 15. Director's files, 1917-CA 1935. SH, 1215.

25. Francine and Stella Larrimore were nieces of Jacob Adler, who was famous for his productions in Yiddish theater in New York. Mortimer claimed that he had found "cables from Europe" from Ms. Larrimore to Forbes, mysteriously hidden in Mrs. Mortimer's hatbox, but he did not produce the cables: SH, 1215, 387. Rachel Crothers was the author of *Nice People*, described as "one of the first to introduce the flapper as a stage personality": *WP*, May 2, 1922, 9; on the hotel bill: SH, 1166, 1259.

26. SH, 1212. Forbes testimony.

27. *Literary Digest* 74:10, September 2, 1922, 10–12.

28. H. L. Mencken, "On Being an American," in *Prejudices*, Third Series (New York: Alfred A. Knopf, 1922).

CHAPTER 7. Taking a Friend on a Business Trip West

1. Excerpt from Testimony of Catherine [*sic*] T. Mortimer, before U.S. Grand Jury No. 1471, on February 8, 1924, DOJ Files for 225387, Box 1201, F: From Mr. Crim; Mortimer's pleas: SH, 1003-05.

2. Milliken quotes and views: SH, 74, 521; DOJ files for 225387, Box 1199; Digest of Testimony, 72–73; Hurley's reaction: DOJ Central Files for 225387, Box 1201, F: From Mr. Crim; and SH, 524.

3. The mystery story analogy was apt. Mary Roberts Rinehart, Dr. Rinehart's wife, was the author (with Avery Hopwood) of *The Bat*, a play that ran on Broadway, August 1920–September 1922. Milliken: DOJ Files for 225387, Box 1201, F: From Mr. Crim; Mortimer: SH, 230; Forbes on his health: SH, 913–14.

4. Telegram, CRF to WGH, July 14, 1922, Director's Files, Box 108, 1922, filed with 005-03; job prospect: SH, 1015.

5. *Oakland Tribune*, June 18, 1922; *NYT*, June 18, 1922.

6. Wilmeth: *LAT*, April 1, 1922, 11; *BDG*, April 1, 1922, 1. Harding and Newberry: Robert K. Murray, *The Harding Era: Warren G. Harding and His Administration* (Minneapolis: University of Minnesota Press, 1969), 206–8; Murray, *The Politics of Normalcy: Governmental Theory and Practice in the Harding-Coolidge Era* (New York: Norton, 1973), 83; *NYT*, January 11, 1922, 1; Sullivan Papers, Entries for July 13 and 14, 1922 in Folder June 18–December 13, 1922; Thomas L. Stokes, *Chip Off My Shoulder* (Princeton, NJ: Princeton University Press, 1940), 96, 107.

7. Oil leases: *NYT*, April 8, 1922, 19; on Fall's declining role: *NYT*, March 12, 1922, 107.

8. Daugherty quote: *NYT*, June 3, 1922, 4.

9. James N. Giglio, *H. M. Daugherty and the Politics of Expediency* (Kent, OH: Kent State University Press, 1978), 127; Willebrandt: *SF Chronicle*, October 9, 1921.

10. Testimony of Katherine Mortimer before U.S. Grand Jury No. 1471, on February 8, 1924: DOJ Central Files for 225387, Box 1201, F: From Mr. Crim. For "delighted to take it out on his wife": SH, 1032; other quotes: SH, 1128, 1170, 1171, 1212, 1213.

11. Forbes's quotes: SH, 929–30.

12. SH, 1320–21.

13. Colombia project: SH, 1159, 1160–62; Milliken's role: DOJ Central Files for 225387, Box 1201, F: From Mr. Crim and SH, 1161. Trial summary statement, 3615–3616, 8–9, 10.

14. CRF, Report to the President of the United States on Inspection Trip—June 18 to July 19, 1922, with accompanying letter, CRF to WGH, July 21, 1922, Director's files, Box 117, 2–3; ARVB 1922, 30–33; radio broadcast: *WP*, June 21, 1922, 21.

15. *Oakland (CA) Tribune*, June 29, 1922, 20; *Modesto (CA) Evening News*, June 28, 1922, 23.

16. The meeting with Graupner and Quinn was on June 28, 1922: SH, 1091–92.

17. SH, 1206–07 and 947, respectively.

18. SH, 1093. William Pencak, *For God and Country: The American Legion, 1991–1941* (Boston: Northeastern University Press, 1989), 184.

19. Camp Kearney: SH, 996. Forbes, American Legion actions: Pencak, *For God and Country*, 183; SH, 998–99, 1721–22; on Milliken: SH, 74, 521; CRF on Cramer: SH, 1169.

20. CRF, Report to the President, 22–24.

21. CRF quotes: SH, 1165 and 1163, respectively.

22. SH, 1020, 1021, 1149.

23. WGH to CRF, July 24, 1922: AdeCP.

24. SH, 931, 939–42, and 335, respectively.

25. Pontiac's cost was $27,000 higher than Northeastern, but Pontiac was sixty days shorter and then required a substantial penalty. If you multiply the daily penalty charge of $450 by 60, the answer is $27,000. SH, 932–33.

26. SH, 934 and 345, respectively.

27. LOC, Theodore Roosevelt, Jr., Manuscript Collection, Box 1, Diary 2, June 16, 1922, 313–314; July 1, 328; July 9, 332; August 27, 375; Lee Garnett Day, President Bennett Day Importing Co. Inc. to John W. H. Crim, October 2, 1924, DOJ Central Files for 225387, Box 1205, F: Exhibit 76.

28. Vaughan to Shepherd, May 27, 1922, and H. E. Stafford to Hanford MacNider, July 11, 1922, DOJ Central Files for 225387, Box 1203.

29. *Hartford Courant*, August 4, 1922, 2. The square-rigger story is referenced in chapter 1, note 5. Sweet: Digest of Testimony, 8. Forbes's grandson Robert Barry, a teacher of American literature of the 1920s, brought up the Gatsby comparison in one of our conversations.

30. Automobile: FOIA, FBI Director File, 62-3552-160; travel: CPR-CRF, Sawyer and Sprague, Dawes Papers, Box 118, Folder 25; and telegrams: Sawyer to Dawes, July 25 and 28, 1922; Harding to Sprague, July 31, 1922, HP Roll 176, Presidential Case File; Veterans Affairs, Folder 16; also *NYT*, July 26, 1922, 7; *CDT*, July 27, 10; *NYT*, July 27, 13; *NYT*, July 28, 9; *CDT*, July 29, 3; *NYT*, July 29, 13.

31. "despite the worries . . .": *Hartford Courant*, August 4, 1922; clipping in NARA DC, RG 15, NM-60/2A, Box 117-005.04; "head over heels": CRF to KMF, August 22, 1922, courtesy Robert A. Barry; Forbes's medications: SH, 1324. Sweet, "preferred my going . . .": CRF to KMF, October 2, 1922, courtesy of Robert A. Barry.

32. CRF to Frank A. Guernsey, Stockton, CA, August 11, 1922, Director's files, Box 105, GR-GZ. Sweet to KMF, August 31, 1922, courtesy of Joan Barry Marsh. Sweet: SH, 1326, 1023.

33. On the "real information": SH, 945, 947; for "every department in the government": SH, 1009.

34. Drawn from: SH, 1398, 732, 944, 947, respectively; and Digest of Testimony, 99–103.
35. Wedding: *NYT,* September 21, 1922, 14; SH, 1230.
36. SH, 1035, 1003, 1221, 1238–39.

CHAPTER 8. Harding Resurgent

1. For the Sawyer-Sprague exchange: Dawes Papers, Box 118, Folder 25, July 10, 12, and 20, 1922; for those published: *NYT,* July 26, 1922, 7, and July 27, 13; *CDT,* October 20, 1922, and July 27, 1922, 10; for DAV: *NYT,* July 28, 1922, 9.
2. Marquis James, *A History of the American Legion* (New York: W. Green, 1923), 278–80; "Razberry" quote: *NYT,* October 25, 1922, 1. The meeting was in New Orleans, October 16 to 20, 1922.
3. CRF to KMF, October 25, 1922, courtesy of Robert Barry; Deegan's charge about Forbes's presence: *NYT,* October 15, 1922, 5. Also *Atlanta Constitution,* October 19, 1922, 1.
4. James, *History of the American Legion,* 279; LOC, Joel T. Boone Papers, Box 45, FXVI B Med-XVII, USS *Mayflower;* Wallace R. Farrington to CRF, October 25, 1922, USVB Director's Files, Box 117-005-09; for "lemon" quote: FBH minutes, October 23, 1922, 5.
5. *WP,* November 5, 1922, 1; for comments and analysis: *NYT,* November 8, 1922, 11; Edward Ranson, *The American Mid-Term Elections of 1922: An Unexpected Shift in Political Power* (Lewiston, NY: Edwin Mellen Press, 2007), 238–66; Lindsay Rogers, "American Government and Politics, First and Second Sessions of the Sixty-Eighth Congress," *American Political Science Review* 19, no. 4 (November 1925), 761–72; Frederic L. Paxson, *Postwar Years: Normalcy, 1918–1923* (New York: Cooper Square, 1966), 311, 285. In the Sixty-Seventh Congress, there were 60 nominally Republican senators and 296 representatives. In the new Congress, the Sixty-Eighth, there would be 53 Republic senators and 226 representatives.
6. The passage of the restrictive Immigration Act in 1921, strengthened and made permanent in 1924 legislation, fed into antiforeign hysteria. Daugherty's quote: Max Lowenthal, *The Federal Bureau of Information* (New York: William Sloane Associates, 1950), 271.
7. CES to WGH, September 16 and September 14, 1922, respectively; HP, Roll 262, Sawyer Papers (Collection 95).
8. Two different dates are shown in the archives for the evening meetings: November 13 and 14, and November 14 and 15. I use the date here in the official transcript: Conferences on Hospitalization of Ex-Servicemen, Held at the White House, November 14 and 15 [1922], NARA-CP, RG 121. See also Board of Consultants on

Hospitalization, General Correspondence and Related Records, 1921–1923, Entry 164, Box 4, Folder Conferences, November 13 and 14, 1922.

9. Conferences on Hospitalization of Ex-Servicemen, 1–2.

10. Mellon on Forbes: John K. Barnes, *The World's Work*, March 1924, 550; Mellon's proposal: *Washington Star*, January 11, 1923; clipping: Board of Consultants on Hospitalization, Entry 164, Box 21, Binder "Press notices," "Report of the Consultants on Hospitalization . . . Under Public Act 384 (approved March 4, 1921)," Government Printing Office, 1923; comments by Sawyer and Ireland: FBH minutes, January 3, 1923, 1–2, 9–10.

11. Forbes's comments on the hospital complexes and "problems in mechanical installation": FBH minutes, January 15, 1923, 4; Tullidge's background: Notes prepared by Crim on Forbes's testimony, DOJ Files for 225387, Box 1201, F: From Mr. Crim. Sawyer's comments: FBH minutes, November 20, 1922, 11. Other materials are from the minutes of the November White House meetings.

12. FBH minutes, November 20, 1922, 1, 2, 12; for "gold-brickers . . .": FBH minutes, January 3, 1923, 3.

13. Marquis James, "What's Wrong in Washington," *American Legion Weekly*, March 9, 1923, 11, 18–20, 21; Scott: SH, 982–83, 989, also Digest of Testimony, 81.

14. Notes on an informal conference held in the director's office, September 19, 1922: USVB Director's Files, Box 116, F: Conference re lease and contracts section in Dir. Office 9/19/22. Black had allegedly "carried a tale" outside the bureau, but Forbes refused to tell Black what this tale was—"it might embarrass you." See also Robinson E. Adkins, *Medical Care of Veterans* (Washington, DC: Government Printing Office, 1967), 122–23.

15. CRF to KMF, October 25, 1922, courtesy of Robert A. Barry; CRF to KMF, November 3, 1922, courtesy of Richard F. Barry.

16. Address of Col. C. R. Forbes at District Managers' Conference, September 18, 1922, DOJ Central Files, Box 1203, F: Sprague. This address was printed and presented to Congress by Republican Senator John W. Harreld of Oklahoma with the title "Work of the Veterans' Bureau," 67th Cong., 2nd sess., Document No. 260, LexisNexis US Serial Set Digital Collection, ID 7988.

17. CRF letter to Veterans Bureau employees, no date [December 1922]; Consultants on Hospitalization, Entry 164, Box 18, Folder US Veterans' Bureau, ARVB 1922, iii; *NYT*, December 14, 1922, 27; "propagandist": *NYT*, December 31, 1922, 84.

18. Sparks: FBH minutes, December 4, 1922, 37.

19. *BDG*, January 5, 1923, 22; *NYT*, January 11, 1923, 8; *BDG*, January 7, 1923, 7; *BDG*, January 11, 1923, 8; Stella Marks to Laura Harlan, January 15, 1923, Florence Kling Harding, HP Roll 242, Box 853; see Carl Sferrazza Anthony, *Florence Harding: The First Lady, the Jazz Age, and the Death of America's Most Scandalous President* (New York: W. Morrow, 1998), 389, and Adkins, *Medical Care of Veterans*, 124–25.

20. "Now Colonel . . .": FBH minutes, November 6, 1922, 26; maintenance cost: FBH minutes, August 21, 1922, 14; "Damned if we will . . .": SH, 967–68, Forbes; see also testimony of Scott; plan to dispose: SH, 599–600, 967, Forbes; Black's quote: SH, 690, Black; Forbes's quip: FBH minutes, November 6, 1922.

21. Forbes gave O'Leary authority to dispose of this property, if necessary, in ways "other than as is provided by Property Regulation No. 1, dated August 19, 1922": C. R. Forbes, Memorandum to Commander O'Leary, November 1, 1922, FBI FOIA, DOJ Director File: 62-3552, Section 3. O'Leary had been a supply officer in the navy. For other materials: SH, 606, 612, 973–74, and SH, 602, 608, 684. Thompson was no relation of John W. Thompson, the building contractor.

22. Sawyer, written testimony: SH, 754–55; and Forbes: SH, 969, 975–76.

23. FBH minutes, December 4, 1922, 10–13.

24. SH, 717, 741–42; and LOC, Joel T. Boone Papers, Box 40, F: No Title (Typed Diary), Unpaginated, November 22, 1922.

25. SH, 977, 980, Forbes.

26. SH, 993–94 and 991–92, respectively, Forbes.

27. For Sawyer's complaint: CES to WGH, January 24, 1923. FKH Papers, Roll 242, Box 853; Smith's quote: SH, 662–63; on the special committee: William H. Burns to WGH, December 20, 1922, HP, Box 210, File 800, Hospital Veterans—misc. Folder 1.

28. LOC, Joel T. Boone Papers, Box 40, F: No Title (Typed Diary), unpaginated; and ibid., Box 45, F: XVI B.Med.-XVII USS *Mayflower*-President Harding, Memoirs. Quotes are at pp. xvii, 118–19. Forbes's resignation letter was published after it was activated in February: *NYT,* February 17, 1923, 12.

29. Walter F. Lineberger to WGH, January 20, 1923, HP, Box 210, File 800, Hospital Veterans–misc. Folder 2; LOC, Theodore Roosevelt Jr. Manuscript Collection, Box 1, Diary 3, 434.

30. *NYT,* January 15, 1923, 15; *WP,* January 16, 1923, 3.

31. CRF to WGH, January 12, 1923. The letter is included in the Senate Hearings, SH, 738–39. See also CRF to WGH, January 13, 1923, HP Presidential Case File, File 95. Veterans Affairs. Folder 19, Applications for hospitals for disabled veterans.

32. Adkins, *Medical Care of Veterans,* 124.

33. J. Edgar Hoover, Memorandum for Mr. Burns: Bureau of Investigation, February 3, 1923; DOJ Director File: 62-3552-77, recorded and indexed May 23, 1924; follow-up: 62-3552-216. Mrs. Cramer "has no use for the Mortimers or Forbes," an FBI memo noted on another occasion: DOJ Central Files for 225387, Enclosures, Box 1208, F: Mrs. Charles Cramer. Hoover did not identify Mrs. Cramer in his original notes, but she was named later. US passport applications up to 1925 are available online via ancestry.com.

34. Crim sent an urgent telegram to Assistant to the Attorney General William J. Donovan at the Department of Justice, who passed the matter on to J. Edgar Hoov-

er: "Send me details of this by special delivery tomorrow"; Crim to Donovan, December 30, 1924, Crim to Edward J. Brennan, December 30, 1924, Hoover to Crim, December 31, 1924, and Hoover to Brennan, January 25, 1925, DOJ Director File, 62-3552, 205 and 216. Crim's inquiry was odd but not entirely fantastic, because when Thompson and Forbes were tried in Chicago in 1924, the federal judge was George A. Carpenter. Carpenter was the judge who had presided over the well-publicized case of John Arthur "Jack" Johnson, the famous African American world-champion boxer, who had been convicted under the Mann Act of taking his white mistress across state lines. Johnson left the country, returned in 1919, was reconvicted by Judge Carpenter in 1920, went to the federal penitentiary at Leavenworth, and was released in 1921.

Crim's additional, last-ditch lead to show Forbes was an adulterer was that an Emmett McBroom of Spokane had charged Forbes as co-respondent in his suit for divorce. Local Special Agent E. A. Morgan immediately investigated and found there was no report of any such co-respondent, nor indeed of any filing for divorce. Mrs. McBroom had been seriously ill and at the Mayo Clinic in Rochester, Minnesota, for five weeks, and Mr. McBroom was in constant attendance. She had returned ten days before this inquiry, and again her husband was constantly with her. The story was "merely a rumor without foundation." Bureau of Investigation, DOJ Director File, 62-3552-235.

35. Friends' reports: *WP*, January 31, 1923, 1, and *NYT*, February 2, 1923, 18; Forbes's money belt: SH, 1333; Sweet: BOI report, Bureau of Investigation, Department of Justice, Director File, 62-3552-71.

CHAPTER 9. Transitions in 1923

1. Charles R. Forbes, *Washington Star*, February 4, 1923; editorial, "Veterans' Bureau Troubles," *NYT*, January 22, 1923, 14, and February 25, 1923, E4.

2. For rumors: "Press Notices" collected for the White Committee, Consultants on Hospitalization, Entry 164, Box 21. Burns: *Washington Herald*, February 1, 1923.

3. KMF to Hester McGogy, February 25, 1923, Postcard, courtesy of Richard F. Barry. Robert A. Barry, personal communication, February 2, 2011. Quote on Forbes's resignation: Robinson E. Adkins, *Medical Care of Veterans* (Washington, DC: Government Printing Office, 1967), 125. Also *NYT*, February 16, 1923, 4. Dog show description, courtesy of Barry D. Marsh. Marcia: Personal communication, Joan Barry Marsh.

4. Forbes: *NYT*, February 26, 1923, 6; *NYT*, February 25, 1923, XX3. Sparks: FBH Minutes, February 19, 1923, 10. For other comments: *Outlook*, February 28, 1923, 133, 9, and March 21, 1923, 518.

5. For ship subsidy: *NYT,* February 25, 1923, E4; for Sawyer's comments and report of Harding's attitude: FBH Minutes, February 5, 1923, 2 and 4.

6. On the backstory of Teapot Dome: J. Leonard Bates, Senator Walsh of Montana, 212; Fall's resignation: *Brooklyn Daily Eagle,* December 21, 1922, 1; Harding's support of Daugherty, and the nomination: Sullivan diaries, February 20, and March 4, 1923; for June view: *WSJ,* June 25, 1923, 8.

7. Harding's health: *WP,* February 27, 1923, 19; and Robert K. Murray, *The Harding Era: Warren G. Harding and His Administration* (Minneapolis: University of Minnesota Press, 1969), 423; "yellow rat story": Will Irwin, *Atlanta Constitution,* February 11, 1924, 2; Samuel Hopkins Adams, *Incredible Era: The Life and Times of Warren Gamaliel Harding* (Boston: Houghton Mifflin, 1939), 297; Robert H. Ferrell, *The Strange Deaths of President Harding* (Columbia: University of Missouri Press, 1996), 236–37. Books that do not include the story are as relevant as those that do; for example, Mark Sullivan, *Our Times,* vol. 6, *The Twenties* (New York: Scribner's 1935); Morris Werner, *Privileged Characters* (New York: Robert M. McBride, 1935); and Thomas Sugrue and Edmund W. Starling, *Starling of the White House: The Story of the Man Whose Secret Service Detail Guarded Five Presidents from Woodrow Wilson to Franklin D. Roosevelt* (New York: Simon and Schuster, 1946).

8. WGH to Pomorene, February 28, 1923, HP, Box 210, File 800, Hospital Veterans-misc, Folder 3.

9. Hines: see *NYT,* February 28, 1923, 7, and Adkins, *Medical Care of Veterans,* 130. Sawyer on Perryville: FBH minutes, March 5, 1923, 7, and on Livermore: FBH minutes, April 15, 1923, 10; Silas Bent, "Veterans' Problems Seen by Gen. Hines," *NYT,* March 11, 1923, XX2.

10. Forbes's comments: *WP,* February 28, 1923, 5.

11. Unidentified newspaper clipping, February 12, 1923; Bureau of Investigation, DOJ Director File; *WP,* February 14, 1923, 2. Mrs. Tullidge is again described as Mrs. Pillage. On the "shovel": John Wesley Langley, *They Tried to Crucify Me; or, The Smoke-Screen of the Cumberlands* (Pikeville, KY: J. W. Langley, 1929), 34.

12. Mortimer's FBI records cannot be found: J. Edgar Hoover, Memorandum for Mr. Burns, BOI, February 3, 1923, DOJ Director File: 62-3552-77, recorded and indexed May 23 1924, and 62-3552-205.

13. NARA-CP, RG 60, formerly classified sub.corr. class 23-Liquor violation, Box 1059, F: 23-51-55; Felder: Werner, *Privileged Characters,* 228; Willebrandt and Mortimer: Digest of Testimony, 4 (Elias Mortimer); Mortimer's usefulness to DOJ: Memorandum for Mr. Burns from Willebrandt, March 31, 1924, NARA-CP, RG 60, Case 225387, Box 3855; Dorothy M. Brown, *Mabel Walker Willebrandt: A Study of Power, Loyalty, and Law* (Knoxville: University of Tennessee Press, 1984), 58–62.

14. James Duryea to WGH, February 1, 1923, HP Box 210, File 800.

15. A letter from "Harry Roe," evidently written by the same correspondent, was

timed for the Senate hearings in the fall and addressed to a New York newspaper. This, too, pointed to Forbes's army desertion and his status as a "wife deserter." It also included a glowing description of Sadie Forbes: She "has had to work all these years not knowing where he was. She gave her children an education and brought them up so that they are a credit to her. Col. C. R. Forbes you will note has never been divorced." The third letter, from "Charles Roe," addressed to the chief investigator of the Senate investigation of the Veterans Bureau, explained that exposure of who he was would "get the writer in trouble, being one of the few who knows all the facts," and reported that Forbes was trying to get a divorce from his first wife on the sly, "so he cannot be prosecuted by you as a bigamist." The names of the lawyers concerned were "Warner" and "Lee," the former described as the liaison between the two parties and the latter as an ex-congressman or senator. This letter noted that by then Russell and Mildred had met their father at New York hotels and once at a hotel in Washington, DC. Harry Roe to the *New York World*, October 25, 1923, and Charles Roe to Gen. John F. O'Ryan, December 7, 1923, DOJ Central Files for 225387, Enclosures, Box 1205, F: Exhibit 76. Russell Forbes had risen to clerk by 1920. His mother worked in a shoe factory, his grandfather was dead. Mildred, Forbes's daughter, had married Carlos Sands, a draftsman in a building firm. US Census, 1920.

Description of Sadie Forbes: Will Irwin, *Atlanta Constitution*, February 11, 1924, 2; anonymous: "Presumption of Death and Honest Belief in the Death of Absent Spouse As Defense to Prosecution for Bigamy," Select Committee on VB Investigation, General O'Ryan's personal file, Box 26.

16. Elias to Katherine Mortimer, November 23, 1922, SH, 1236.

17. SH, 1224–46 and 1249, and notes taken from SH testimony for Attorney Crim at the trial. DOJ Central Files for 225387, Box 1201, F: From Mr. Crim: Stephen Davis Timberlake; EHM to Campbell Corporation, November 1, 1922, SH, 1237.

18. W. W. Larsen to Mr. Mortimer, February 23, 1923, DOJ Files for 225387, enclosures, Box 1204, file F; SH, 1408, Mortimer.

19. *Congressional Record*, Sixty-Sixth Congress, 64:62, Senate, February 12, 1923, 3537 (S. Res. 489).

20. NARA, RG 46, SEN 6A-F22. US Senate, 69th Congress, Select Committee on Investigation of the Veterans Bureau. S. Res. 253 (S. Res. 466, 67th Cong.), Memorandum of First Meeting of Committee for Investigation of the Veterans' Bureau, March 4, 1923; Entry: Sen 68A-F22, Box 2, 3, and O'Ryan undated notes, March 3–6, 1923.

21. Because Cramer's death was proclaimed a suicide, which it clearly was, there was no inquest or autopsy. DOJ Director's File, 62-3552-132, 134, 136, 137; also Sullivan, *Our Times*, 6:241; Grafton Wilcox, *NYT*, March 15, 1923, 6; SH, 1356: Otto Koegel; also DOJ Files for 225387, Enclosures, Box 1208, F: Mrs. Charles Cramer.

22. Forbes on Cramer's death: SH, 1170, 1208; auction: Thomas Lunsford Stokes, *Chip Off My Shoulder* (Princeton, NJ: Princeton University Press, 1940), 147.

23. *NYT*, March 15, 1923, 6 and 1, respectively; *LAT*, March 15, 1923, 11.

24. *San Antonio Express*, April 3, 1923, 14; *Port Arthur News*, April 7, 1923, 1; Warden to Heber Votaw, August 16, 1923, LP-EKT.

25. *NYT*, April 27, 1923, 36; on Harry Daugherty's son, Draper: *CDT*, June 18, 923, 2; *NYT*, July 20, 1923.

26. John Corbin, *NYT*, April 15, 1923, XX3.

27. *LAT*, June 22 and 23, 1923, both on p. 12. Robert K. Murray gives an excellent account of the trip, *Harding Era*, 439–50.

28. CRF to Russell M. Forbes, n.d. [1923], courtesy of Richard Forbes.

29. On visiting Cuba: Irwin, *Atlanta Constitution*, February 17, 1924, 9; Sweet to Hurley, August 2, 1923, DOJ Central Files for 225387, Box 1202, F: Sweet, Merle L.

30. CPR-Marie Forbes Judkins: this file includes the report of the investigation of Chief Nurse Judkins from Fred E. Hamilton to the Director [Hines], June 4, 1923. Other information in this paragraph is also from the personnel file.

31. DOJ Central Files from 225387, Box 1202, F: Sweet, Merle L.; Statement by Mrs. Merle L. Sweet, February 18, 1924, signed Morrissey, W. M. Cobb to George B. Tullidge, April 16, 1923, and related material, CPR-George B. Tullidge.

CHAPTER 10. Coolidge, Common Cause, and the Politics of Scandal

1. Coolidge quote: *NYT*, August 3, 1923, 1; special report from San Francisco: *NYT*, August 3, 1923, 1; Sawyer breakdown: Ray Lyman Wilbur, *Memoirs* (Stanford, CA: Stanford University Press, 1960), 382; Christian quote: *NYT*, August 3, 1923, 6; reporters weeping: *NYT*, August 4, 1923, 2; Mark Sullivan, *Our Times*, vol. 6, *The Twenties* (New York: Scribner, 1946), 251–53, for Harding's expression, 251.

2. LOC, Theodore Roosevelt Jr. Manuscript Collection, Box 1, Diary 3, August 7, 1923, 530–31.

3. Oxygen and related questions: Sullivan Papers, Folder June 17–August 15, 1923, for August 8, also Folder November 7, 1923–January 20, 1924, for November 7; classic analysis of stories seeking to explain Harding's death: Robert H. Ferrell, *The Strange Deaths of President Harding* (Columbia: University of Missouri Press, 1996); Hoover comment: Ferrell, *Strange Deaths*, 111.

4. Description of Coolidge: Cameron Rogers, *The Legend of Calvin Coolidge* (Garden City, NY: Doubleday Dorn, 1928), 1, 4.

5. Coolidge quote (made in November 1923): Howard H. Quint and Robert H. Ferrell, eds., *The Talkative President: The Off-the-Record Press Conferences of Calvin Coolidge* (Amherst: University of Massachusetts Press, 1964), 57 (November 6, 1923);

Lindsay Rogers, "American Government and Politics: First and Second Session of the Sixty-Eighth Congress," *American Political Science Review* 13, 761–72.

6. Material on the burnings: Carl Sferrazza Anthony, *Florence Harding: The First Lady, the Jazz Age, and the Death of America's Most Scandalous President* (New York: W. Morrow, 1998), 486–89; on Harding: H. F. Alderfer, "The Personality and Politics of Warren G. Harding" (PhD diss., Syracuse University, 1928); for a critique of the Harding myth among academics in the 1920s and on: Robert K. Murray, *The Harding Era: Warren G. Harding and His Administration* (Minneapolis: University of Minnesota Press, 1969), 523–37.

7. *Outlook*, August 15, 1923, 134, 13; Ferrell, *The Presidency of Calvin Coolidge*, 43ff.

8. Dorothy G. Wayman, *David I. Walsh, Citizen Patriot* (Milwaukee, WI: Bruce Publishing, 1952).

9. George Wharton Pepper, *Philadelphia Lawyer: An Autobiography* (Philadelphia: Lippincott, 1944), 156. The Johnson-Reed Immigration Act of 1924 (PL 68-139) was approved May 16, 1924. The other sponsor was Congressman Albert Johnson.

10. Loren B. Chan, *Sagebrush Statesman: Tasker L. Oddie of Nevada* (Reno: University of Nevada Press, 1973), 9.

11. Robert Lee Bullard, *Fighting Generals: Illustrated Biographical Sketches of Seven Major Generals in World War I* (Ann Arbor, MI: J. W. Edwards, 1944), quotes, 290, 292; John F. O'Ryan and W. D. A. Anderson, *The Modern Army in Action: An Exposition of the Conduct of War* (New York: McBride, Nast, 1914).

12. O'Ryan quote: SH, 1750–52.

13. Samuel Bolles, National Adjutant, to John F. O'Ryan, April 16, 1923; John Thomas Taylor to John F. O'Ryan, telegram, May 15, 1923; Asa Bacon to David I Reed, March 29, 1923. NARA I, RG 46, Entry, Sen 68A-F22, Boxes 1 and 37, O'Ryan Investigative Files, Committee Working Files; O'Ryan Report, U.S. Senate, Committee on Investigation of United States Veterans Bureau, Second Preliminary Report (pursuant to S. Res. 466, 67th Cong., 4th sess.) 68th Cong., 1st sess. Report No. 103, Part 2, February 7, 1924, 1, 2, 4–8.

14. *NYT*, March 9, 1923, 14; *NYT*, April 11, 1923.

15. SH, 8, 9; O'Ryan to Walsh, October 4, 1923, NARA I, RG 46, Entry: Sen 68A-F22, Box 37 (O'Ryan Investigative Files, Committee Working Files).

16. "unavoidable": SH, 1416–17.

17. About Sawyer: *WP*, June 19, 1923, 13; *NYT*, August 26, 1923, 4; *WP*, September 18, 1923, 3; *NYT*, September 19, 1923, 1. Milton F. Heller, *The President's Doctor: An Insider's View of Three First Families* (New York: Vantage Press, 2000), 73–74, 123–34.

18. SH, 620–24, 1750–52, and for the Drain report, 1753–63.

19. Report of A. E. Graupner, Special Counsel US Senate Select Committee on Investigation of Veterans' Bureau Upon Conditions Surrounding the Purchase of the Hospital Site Near Livermore, Alameda County, California, October 20, 1923,

Typescript, Graupner Family Papers, Bancroft Library, University of California, Berkeley, California. Sawyer to Graupner, November 20, 1923, ibid. Miscellaneous papers, Carton 1, American Legion (Graupner report), quotes, 24–25; "I am perfectly frank...": SH, 91, and see SH, 1076–77, 1084–85.

20. Digest of Testimony, 38, 39; Mortimer: SH, 1391, 1406.

21. CRF, "Notable Personages," *Leavenworth New Era*, August 1926, 2; *WP*, September 16, 1923, 1.

22. In the Superior Court of the State of Washington for King County, Kate Forbes v. Charles Forbes, Case No. 169705, October 6, 1923, October 11, 1923. The divorce became final on August 13, 1924.

23. Quote: *WP*, October 27, 1923, 2; Walter B. Beals to John F. O'Ryan, October 27, 1923, Central Files for 225387, Enclosures, Box 205, F: Exhibit 76; SH, 1084–85, 1098–1102.

24. Telegrams courtesy of Russell's son, the late Richard Forbes, who rescued them from what was left of a cache of papers that had deteriorated over the years in a barn.

25. Wadsworth quote: *The Reminiscences of James W. Wadsworth* (New York: Oral History Collection of Columbia University, 1950), 293–94.

26. Burl Noggle, *Teapot Dome: Oil and Politics in the 1920's* (New York: W. W. Norton, 1962), 65. A classic.

27. Thomas Lunsford Stokes, *Chip Off My Shoulder* (Princeton, NJ: Princeton University Press, 1940), 141, 144.

CHAPTER 11. Rush to Judgment

1. *NYT*, October 23, 1923, 1; Henry Fountain Ashurst, *A Many-Colored Toga* (Tucson: University of Arizona Press, 1962), 205, cites diary for October 22, 1923.

2. The hearings were printed in two volumes with a combined total of 1,791 pages, which include 279 marked exhibits, ranging from committee reports and other business documents to hotel bills, coded telegrams, and personal letters. US Senate, 67th Cong., 4th sess., *Select Committee on Investigation of Veterans' Bureau. Hearings... pursuant to S. Res. 466* (Washington, DC: Government Printing Office, 1923), two volumes. Referred to here as SH. Forbes: SH, 2; O'Ryan: *NYT*, October 23, 1923, 1; also *BDG*, October 23, 1923, 5.

3. Hines: SH, 83–90; on Lindars: SH, 105.

4. *NYT*, October 23, 1923, 1; SH, 259.

5. *Atlanta Constitution*, October 26, 1923, 8.

6. "Forbes Allowed Fee...": *BDG*, October 24, 1923, 8; "Forbes Grafted...": *CDT*, October 24, 1923, 15; "Accuses Forbes....": *BDG*, October 25, 1923, 1; "Drinking Parties ...": *Atlanta Constitution*, October 25, 1923, 1; SH, 251, 258–60.

7. Forbes: *Danville (VA) Bee*, October 26, 1923, 4; Thompson: *WP*, October 26, 1923, 1; Hurley: *NYT*, October 26, 1923, 15; Reed: *NYT*, October 27, 1923, 19; Coolidge: *BDG*, October 28, 1923, 15; White House: *NYT*, October 27, 1923, 15.

8. There is no published biography of Easby-Smith. My thanks to Marcia A. Wiss, Esq. (who is, as was Easby-Smith, an eminent Washingtonian with strong connections to Georgetown University), for her help, enthusiasm, and advice.

9. Code: SH, 226–27, 229, 239; burglaries: SH, 208, 228–29, 257, 1372, 1392; *Trial Digest*, 84–85.

10. Williams: SH, 288–300; Perryville: SH, 620–637, 727, 779–80; "went out the other side": SH, 672; on Forbes: *Atlanta Constitution*, October 30, 1923, 1.

11. Sawyer's appearance: *Atlanta Constitution*, November 8, 1923, 23; *NYT*, November 8, 1923, 1; "autocratic power . . .": SH, 760; other quotes: SH, 756, 763, 766, 757, 759, 981.

12. EHM to G. B. Tullidge, November 8, 1923, Forbes Exhibit 10, SH, 1237–8; EKT to EHM, October 22, 1923, LP-EKT; EHM to EKT, January 2, 1924, LF-EKT.

13. SH, 1593–94, 1750.

14. C.V.C. [*sic*], Memorandum for Major Arnold, November 7, and ibid., November 9, 1923, DOJ Central Files for 225387, Enclosures, Box 1205, F: Exhibit 76.

15. *Atlanta Constitution*, November 14, 1923, 2; SH, 912–14; Forbes's multiple criticisms of Sawyer harmed him and were noticed by the press, e.g.: "Time and again he attacked Brig-Gen [*sic*] Charles E. Sawyer, personal friend and physician of President Harding," *LAT*, November 14, 1923, 11.

16. SH, 929, quotes at 1000, 1001.

17. SH, 961–62, quote at 981; on insubordination: SH, 981.

18. SH, 1006 and 945, respectively.

19. SH, 1028, 1006, and 1008, respectively.

20. SH, 1003, 1032.

21. SH, 1010.

22. SH, 1022.

23. SH, 1020. McAdoo was to be knocked out of the Democratic nomination by the association of his law firm with the oil interests on legal matters (garnering huge fees), exposed during the Teapot Dome hearings.

24. SH, 1009.

25. SH, 1033, 1036.

26. SH, 969–70.

27. SH, 1037; Forbes: SH, 1039. No proof was actually made public. However, Williams was not asked to testify at the trial, suggesting that his evidence did not hold up.

28. SH, 1044, O'Ryan, Forbes; on seeking sympathy: "and it was hard, General, as you know, to be charged with the responsibilities and the great responsibilities that

were placed upon one man in that institution and be shy of harmony and support."
SH, 1046. No response.

29. SH, 1049.

30. SH, 1065.

31. Headlines: *NYT*, November 16, 1923, 1; *Atlanta Constitution*, November 16, 1, respectively; Forbes's birthplace: SH, 1066; income: SH, 1067.

32. SH, 1068–69, 1074, 1098–99.

33. SH, 1106.

34. SH, 1108, 1114, 1131.

35. SH, 1150, 1155–56; on Colombia: SH, 1161–62; "Yes; I did": SH, 1163–64.

36. SH, 1165–68.

37. SH, 1175–76, 1179, 1181.

38. SH, 1207, 1212.

39. O'Ryan's questions: SH, 1222–23; Forbes's condition: *NY Evening Journal*, November 19, 1923, 1.

40. SH, 1243. *Appleton (WS) Post-Crescent*, evening, November 16, 1923, 1.

41. SH, 1263–64, 1308–11, 1372.

42. SH, 1393–94.

43. O'Ryan: SH, 1416–17.

44. James S. Easby-Smith to Kate Forbes, at her mother's home in Indiana, December 14, 1923, courtesy of Robert A. Barry.

CHAPTER 12. Scandal Weavers

1. Daugherty: *NYT*, December 2, 1923, 1; CPR–John W. H. Crim; political context: Robert H. Ferrell, *The Presidency of Calvin Coolidge* (Lawrence: University Press of Kansas, 1998), chap. 3. Thomas W. Miller was convicted, imprisoned, and eventually pardoned, another item in the list of "Harding scandals."

2. Crim to Daugherty and response: JWHC to HMD, December 1, 1923; HMD to JWHC, December 3, 1923, CPR-Crim.

3. The Savannah group was the "largest and most widely operating bootleg ring known since the passage of the Volstead Act": *NYT*, August 17, 1923, 15; James H. Pope to HMD, July 11, 1921, CPR-MWW.

4. NARA-CP, RG 60, Case 225387, Box 3855, MWW to Burns, March 31, 1924; MWW to David H. Blair, March 15, 1924, NARA-CP, RG 60, DOJ Central Files, Box 2491, F: 5–1003.

5. Henning: *CDT*, January 18, 1924, 1; Sullivan, *NY Tribune*, February 17, 1924; clipping, Sullivan Papers, Box 40, Veterans, February 18, 1924.

6. U.S. Senate, Committee on Investigation of United States Veterans' Bureau,

Preliminary Report (pursuant to S. Res. 466, 67th Cong., 4th sess.), 68th Cong., 1st sess., Report No. 103, January 28, 1924, 1–3 [First Preliminary Report]; ibid., Third Preliminary Report, Report No. 103, Part 3, June 6, 1924, 1, 2. The act was Public Law 68–242, June 7, 1924.

7. Ibid., Second Preliminary Report, Report No. 103, Part 2, February 7, 1924, 5. [O'Ryan Report], District personnel, 58; pleasure: 5, 20–21; "defraud the government,": 42–45; Perryville quotes: 40, 60, 70; O'Ryan's editing: Improper Sale of Property, Draft, NARA DC, RG 46, Entry: Sen. 68A-F22, Box 26 (O'Ryan).

8. Will Irwin, *The Making of a Reporter* (New York: G. P. Putnam's Sons, 1942), 358.

9. Introduction, O'Ryan report, 2; on Reed: *NYT*, February 10, 1924, 1; *LAT*, February 10, 1924, 1; *NYT*, Editorial, February 11, 1924, 14.

10. See Robert V. Hudson, *The Writing Game: A Biography of Will Irwin* (Ames: Iowa State University Press, 1982), esp. 113, 135; for Pickering's approach: Irwin, *The Making of a Reporter*, 53; "This man . . .": Irwin, *Propaganda and the News: Or, What Makes You Think So?* (New York: McGraw-Hill, 1936), 73; telegram, O'Ryan to Reed, January 28, 1924, NARA DC, RG 46, Entry: Sen-68A-F22, Box 26 (O'Ryan).

11. Quotes: *Atlanta Constitution*, February 12, 1924, 1; Irwin, *Making of a Reporter*, 401; Samuel Hopkins Adams, *Incredible Era: The Life and Times of Warren Gamaliel Harding* (Boston: Houghton Mifflin, 1939), 423 [statement to the writer by Mr. Irwin].

12. Irwin's quote: *Atlanta Constitution*, February 11, 1924, 1. Mortimer quoted by Irwin, ibid., February 13, 1924, 1.

13. For the main points, see Irwin's article in the *Atlanta Constitution*, February 11, 1924, 1.

14. CRF to KMF, February 15, 21, and 15, 1924, courtesy Richard Barry. Kate's letters to Forbes have not survived.

15. Quotes: *NYT*, March 2, 1923, 3, and March 7, 1924, 4.

16. "Robbing Wounded Veterans," *Literary Digest*, March 1, 1924, 46; "One Raider Indicted," [Forbes, of course], editorial, *Reno (NV) Gazette*, March 1, 1924, 4; "Veterans' Scandal Approaching Climax," *NYT*, March 9, 1924, XX4; Carl C. Dickey, "Plundering the Wounded Men," *World's Work* 48, no. 2 (June 1924): 167–74; Charles Merz, "The Betrayal of Our War Veterans," *Century Magazine* 108, no. 4 (August 1924): 435. The most pointed are Bruce Bliven's series, "The Ohio Gang," in the *New Republic*, the first article on May 7, 1924, 276, the fifth and last on June 4, 1924, 40; Forbes's quotes: *CDT*, March 18, 1924, 3.

17. Quotes: *Billings (MT) Gazette*, March 6, 1924, 21.

18. On Zihlman: *Frederick (MD) Post*, March 14, 1924, 1, 5; *WP*, April 1, 1924, 4; on Langley: see *US House of Representatives, Committee on Standards of Official Conduct, Historical Summary of Conduct Cases* in the House of Representatives; and

Langley's book *I Was Crucified*. Langley was pardoned in 1928. A file intriguingly titled "Mortimer's Irregularities with Congressmen" comes down through the years but with little still in it. In a third case, which came to attention later, Mortimer testified that he used Republican Congressman George W. Edmonds of Philadelphia to intercede for the local Rising Sun Brewery in a "tax penalty matter" and that Edmonds had received a check for $2,500 from the brewery as payment. Edmonds said that he had forced Mortimer to return $2,500, which Mortimer had extorted from the brewery for getting them a legal permit for which no fee was needed. Edmonds said he felt responsible because he had introduced Mortimer to the attorney representing the brewery. This case went nowhere: DOJ Central Files for 225387, Box 1206, *Chicago Daily Journal*, Wednesday, November 26, 1924.

19. MWW to Hayward, August 1, and response, August 11, 1924; Hayward to Crim, September 14, 1924; statements also came from the other defendants that Mortimer had not participated in any conspiracy or in criminal activities: NARA-CP, RG 60, formerly classified sub.corr. Class 23-Liquor violation, Box 1059, F: 23-51-55.

20. Burton K. Wheeler, with Paul F. Healy, *Yankee from the West: The Candid, Turbulent Life Story of the Yankee-Born U.S. Senator from Montana* (Garden City, NY: Doubleday, 1962), Wheeler's quotes, 215 and 221; James N. Giglio, *H. M. Daugherty and the Politics of Expediency* (Kent, OH: Kent State University Press, 1978), 163–80; Ruhl, "At the Capital's Vaudeville," *Collier's*, April 19, 1924, 7, 24. The hearings investigating the DOJ were led by Senator Smith Brookhart (Republican, Iowa) and Senator Burton K. Wheeler (Democrat, Montana).

21. The Maryland indictment charged that the defendants had arranged to sell about $3 million worth of army surplus supplies stored at Perryville for a fifth of their invoice value: *NYT*, April 15, 1924, 2, and April 17, 1924, 21.

22. "How about Forbes?": Senator George Wharton Pepper (Pennsylvania) made such comments at the state Republican convention in Pennsylvania; *Frederick (MD) Saturday Morning*, April 5, 1924, 2; *NYT*, April 26, 1924, 8; *CDT*, August 15, 1924, 1.

23. Crim quoted: *BDG*, May 22, 1924, 15A; see also *NYT*, March 12, 1924, 2; US Senate, 68th Cong., 1st sess., *Hearings . . . Pursuant to S. Res. 157. Investigation of Hon. Harry M. Daugherty*, I, 995, 998.

24. Kenneth D. Ackerman, *Young J. Edgar: Hoover, the Red Scare, and the Assault on Civil Liberties* (New York: Carroll & Graf, 2007), 374; Stone to Crim (JWHC), September 11, 1924, JWHC-CPR; Douglas C. Waller, *Wild Bill Donovan: The Spymaster Who Created the OSS and Modern American Espionage* (New York: Free Press, 2011), 68.

25. JWHC to Stone (HFS), June 2, and HFS to JWHC (Telegram and letter), June 5, 1924, JWHC-CPR. Crim added a private attorney to his staff and had the services of Leo W. Morrissey, a DOJ agent, as special assistant attorney, plus other assigned DOJ

agents, and from time to time a DOJ secretary (clerk-stenographer), Grace E. Adams, who otherwise worked for J. Edgar Hoover.

26. FBI, DOJ Director File, 62-3552-20, 34, 48, 51; Hoover for Burns to Crim, January 5, 1924; FBI, DOJ Director File, 62-3552-25, unattributed and undated memo, NARA-CP, RG 60, Central Files for 225387, Enclosures, Box 1208, F: Mrs. Charles Cramer; Marguerite Sweet to Crim, February 9, statement by Mrs. Merle Sweet, February 18, Merle Sweet to Crim, June 2, and to Rollin R. Winslow, June 1, 1924, DOJ Central Files, Box 1202, F: Sweet, Merle L.

27. FBI, DOJ Director File, 62-3552-37 and 41.

28. FBI, DOJ Director File, 62-3552-84.

29. Young O. Wilson, Re Charles R. Forbes, Attention Mr. Cunningham No. 3, File 3015, FBI, DOJ Director File, 62-3552.

30. FBI, DOJ Director File, 62-3552-71.

31. Forbes: *NYT*, May 19, 1924, 14; Cauley, To Whom It May Concern, May 17; Cauley to Easby-Smith, June 13; John T. Bottomley, Opinion, June 13, 1924, LP-CRF; JWHC to HFS, July 1, 1924, JWHC-CPR.

32. EKT to Katherine Mortimer, March 7, LP-EKT; George B. Tullidge to EKT, March 9; Katherine O'Donnell Tullidge to EKT, March 16, 1924, LP-EKT.

33. I draw here from reports in the *New Castle (PA) News*, May 17, 1924, 1; *Gettysburg (PA) Times*, May 17, 1924, 2; *Kokomo (IN) Tribune*, May 17, 1924, 17; *NYT*, May 17, 1924, 15.

34. "Three Involved . . .": *Frederick (MD) News*, May 16, 1924, 1; JWHC to MWW, May 15; MWW to Allegra, May 19; MWW to EHM, May 19, 1924, NARA-CP, RG 60, Box 3916, F: 226746.

35. MWW to JWHC, May 19, 1924, NARA-CP, RG 60, Box 3916, F: 226746.

CHAPTER 13. The Trial of Charles R. Forbes

1. There is no single collection of records on the Forbes-Thompson (or Thompson-Forbes) case. This chapter draws on four official sources: (1) U.S. District Courts, Northern District of Illinois, Eastern Division at Chicago, NARA, RG 21, Criminal Case Files, Case Files Box 359, United States v. Charles R. Forbes and John W. Thompson, defendants, no. 12511 (and related indictments); (2) United States Circuit Court of Appeals for the Seventh Circuit, October Term A.D. 1924, no. 3615, Charles R. Forbes v. United States of America, Transcript of Record, filed July 3, 1925; (3) the much longer, 1,621-page related document, no. 3616, John W. Thompson v. United States of America Transcript of Record, filed July 3, 1925 (cited hereafter as Trialdoc); and (4) an invaluable summary of the evidence, cited here as Digest of Testimony (fully referenced in Abbreviations). For the quotes: *Chicago Evening Post*, November

24, 1924, n.p., and *Chicago American,* November 26, 1924, reproduced in Trialdoc, 160, 163.

2. UPI report, *Sheboygan (WI) Press-Telegram,* February 7, 1924, 8.

3. Trialdoc, 219, 264–69, 418–419, 423; also *CDT,* November 27, 1924.

4. Lewis: *CDT,* January 28, 1925, 19.

5. Jurors named by Kinsley: *CDT,* November 26, 1924, in Trialdoc, 162.

6. *NYT,* November 25, 1924, 25; *CDT,* November 27, 1924, 2, and December 2, 1924, 4.

7. Quote: Kinsley, *CDT,* November 27, 1924, 2; Digest of Testimony, 77–78.

8. Digest of Testimony, 86–97.

9. Digest of Testimony, 103–5, 117–19, 130–44.

10. Digest of Testimony, 84–85. The six-month around-the-world flight, a coup for America's international image, was completed in September 1924. Martin's plane crashed into a foggy mountain in Alaska early in the flight, but others succeeded, and he remained the expedition's leader.

11. Katherine Mortimer did not testify. Trialdoc, 528–29; *CDT,* December 20, 1924, 3. In one source, Mortimer stated that he would "swear my soul to hell to get Forbes": *WP,* December 20, 1924, 3.

12. *CDT,* November 29, 1924, 4, 7, and January 27, 1925, 2.

13. *LAT,* December 12, 1924, 7.

14. Darrow, *The Story of My Life* (New York: Charles Scribner's Sons, 1932). Quote is at p. 64 of 1996 reprinted version by Da Capo Press.

15. Quote: Trialdoc, 1369.

16. *CDT,* December 2, 1924, Trialdoc, 176; *WP,* December 2, 1924, 11; *Chicago Herald and Examiner,* December 2, 1924, Trialdoc, 172–73.

17. Trialdoc, 379, 381, 382. Apart from Mortimer's claims there was no evidence that Forbes knew of the code before the Senate hearings in the fall of 1923.

18. Trialdoc, 397, 404, 410, 415, 524–25.

19. Trialdoc, 365, 456, 460, 545.

20. Trialdoc, 402; *NYT,* January 24, 1925, 16.

21. *Atlanta Constitution,* December 12, 1924, 1; Trialdoc, 485; *CDT,* December 11, 1924, 3; Trialdoc, 354; *CDT,* January 1, 1925; *WP,* January 2, 1925.

22. *CDT,* November 5, 1924, 11; Trialdoc, 172–73.

23. UPI report as in *Lima (OH) News,* December 5, 1924, 6; on Votaw: *CDT,* January 1, 1925, 3.

24. *CDT,* December 19, 1924, 15; *Billings (MT) Gazette,* December 20, 1924, 1.

25. Trialdoc, 201–2; *LAT,* December 23, 1924, 5; *NYT,* December 28, 1924, X12, and December 29, 1924, 32.

26. Mortimer to Crim, December 23, 1924, NARA-CP, RG 60, DOJ Central Files for 225387, Box 1208.

27. A potentially more dramatic case against Gaston Means, Thomas Felder, and Elmer Jarnecke opened in Federal District Court, New York, on January 5, 1925. See *CDT*, January 4, 1925, 1.

28. *NYT*, January 22, 1925, 2; *CDT*, February 5, 1925, 3; *LAT*, March 6, 1925, 4; Trial-doc, 445; *NYT*, December 5, 1924, 11; *Chicago Herald and Examiner*, January 28, 1925, included in Trialdoc, 194–95.

29. Trialdoc, 1357; *NYT*, February 5, 1925, 1.

30. UPI, as reported in the *Oelwein (IA) Daily Register*, January 23, 1925, 4.

31. *CDT*, January 28, 1925, 19; January 27, 1925, 2; January 28, 1925, 3; January 29, 1925, 2; *WP*, January 28, 1925, 19.

32. Quote: Trialdoc, 1359; *CDT*, January 30, 1925, 5; *NYT*, January 30, 1925, 8.

33. Trialdoc, 1363, 1365–66.

34. Carpenter's instructions: Trialdoc, 1373–75.

35. See, e.g., UPI, in *Freeport (IL) Journal-Standard*, January 30, 1925, 11; *BDG*, January 30, 1925, 11.

36. On the verdict: Trialdoc, 1376, 1377, 1379; *BDG*, January 31, 1925, 1; *NYT*, January 25, 1925, 1; *CDT*, January 25, 1925, 1; reactions: UPI, *Sheboygan (WI) Press*, February 4, 1925, 1, and *Oelwein (IA) Daily Register*, February 4, 1925, 1; see also *NYT*, January 31, 1925, 5; *CDT*, January 31, 1925, 1.

37. *CDT*, January 31, 1925, 1; *NYT*, February 1, 1925, 2.

38. Carpenter: Trialdoc, 1503; *NYT*, February 5, 1924, 1; *LAT*, February 5, 1925, 1; *NYT*, February 5, 1925, 1; reactions: *CDT*, February 5, 1925, 3; *Nation*, 120, no. 3110, February 11, 1925, 131–32; *Literary Digest*, February 14, 1925, 11–12.

CHAPTER 14. Making the Best of It

1. On the appeals: *NYT*, July 11, 1925, 11; November 12, 1925, 2; January 3, 1926, 16; January 29, 1926, 1; February 2, 1926, 5; and March 15, 1926, 44. There was still a suspicion that Judge Carpenter had called a six-day recess in the trial to go hunting. In 1928, there was support for the story, when Chief Justice Taft asked the senior circuit judges whether Carpenter (whom Taft had appointed in 1909) "does his end of the work," and was told no—and that Carpenter had adjourned a trial and taken off on a shooting trip to New Orleans. From then on, Carpenter was watched. Peter Graham Fish, *The Politics of Federal Judicial Administration* (Princeton, NJ: Princeton University Press, 1973), 56, 58, quoted in ftp.resource.org/courts.gov/fjc/judges .pdf.

2. Telegrams: Case 22537, NARA-CP, RG 60, Box 3856; Forbes's quote: *CDT*, March 19, 1926, 17.

3. Completed entry forms for Charles R. Forbes, Reg. No. 25021, United States

Penitentiary, Leavenworth, Kansas, March 20, 1926. Forbes's Leavenworth file is a major source for this chapter. Herein noted as LF-CRF.

4. *NYT,* March 16, 1926, 44; *Atlanta Constitution,* May 4, 1926; United States Penitentiary, Leavenworth, Kansas, Annual Report, 1926, Leavenworth: U.S. Penitentiary Press, 1926, various pages.

5. ARVB for the Fiscal Year Ended June 30, 1925, p. 355, Table 114.

6. For Hines and Coolidge: *LAT,* May 8, 1925, 3; editorials: *WP,* December 10, 1925, 6, and September 11, 6. Hines reportedly turned back more than $69 million of the VB appropriation of almost $482 million in fiscal 1925. On hospital beds: William P. Dillingham, *Federal Aid to Veterans, 1917–1941* (Gainesville: University of Florida Press, 1952), 65. The Veterans Administration, established by PL 71-536, added additional federal services for veterans to the old Veterans Bureau, including pensions for veterans of wars earlier than World War I (previously run by the Bureau of Pensions), and the National Home for Disabled Volunteer Soldiers, set up for northern veterans of the Civil War.

7. George B. Tullidge obituary, *Philadelphia Inquirer,* March 10, 1925, 7, and *Philadelphia Public Ledger,* March 10, 1925, clipping (my thanks to Jack Gumbrecht); other sources: *NYT,* March 30, 1925, 1, and March 31, 1925, 9; *WP,* April 2, 1925, 3; H. G. Heckman to Edward K. Tullidge, September 28, 1925 and James M. Maher, Superintendent of Police, Milford, CT, to US Marshal or Warden, Fort Leavenworth, June 5, 1926, LF-EKT. Edward K. Tullidge died in 1950.

8. Judicial District of Pennsylvania, Court of Common Pleas for Philadelphia County, Decree, June 15, 1925, Katherine T. Mortimer v. Elias H. Mortimer, December term 1922, No. 105. My thanks to Warren Kauffman, Esq., of Philadelphia for explaining the uses of different grounds for divorce before 1980, when the Pennsylvania divorce code was changed.

9. Finding evidence of the marriage was no mean feat. Katherine Forbes noted the date in her federal employment file on a Veteran Preference Claim form in the 1950s, and this enabled discovery of the wedding through FamilySearch.org.

10. Thanks to Arlene Nicely, Staunton Military Institute Alumni Association, for information about the career of George B. Tullidge, Jr.

11. Kate Forbes fell off the dock at the house on Vashon Island seriously damaging her legs on the stones below. Joan Barry Marsh, personal communication.

12. Crim: *CDT,* January 31, 1925, 1; Stone to Crim, March 2, 1925, CPR-JWHC; J. Curt Gentry, *J. Edgar Hoover: The Man and the Secrets* (New York: Norton, 1991), 142.

13. J. Edgar Hoover to Edward J. Brennan, July 30, 1924; CPR: EHM to Mabel W. Willebrandt, March 12, 1926; MWW to EHM, March 17, 1926, NARA-CP, RG 60, Case 225387, Box 3856.

14. Crim's quote is in a letter attached to J. D. Harris, General Agent, DOJ, Memorandum for Colonel Donovan, April 18, 1925; Hoover, Memorandum for Dono-

van, June 29, 1925, with report from Agent Conroy dated June 25, 1925, quote at 9; Hoover, Memo for Donovan, July 7, 1925, and February 4, 1925; Mortimer to Donovan, February 24, 1925; Memo from Donovan for the (F)BI, March 10, 1925; and J. D. Harris, General Agent, DOJ, Memo for Donovan, April 18, 1925, RG 60, Case 225387, Boxes 4037, 3855, 3856, 4037, 3856, and 3855, respectively.

15. *Minneapolis Journal,* August 18, 1928, 1; *Minneapolis Sunday Tribune,* August 19, 1928, 4; *LAT,* August 19, 1928.

16. Dorothy M. Brown, *Mabel Walker Willebrandt: A Study of Power, Loyalty, and Law* (Knoxville: University of Tennessee Press, 1984), 96–97; Battier story: *CDT,* December 29, 1927, 10; Daugherty quote: *NYW,* December 4, 1927, 2; T. B. White to W. T. Hammack, DOJ, September 5, 1927, LF-CRF. The admiring letters referred to in the text are in Willebrandt's federal employment file. She died in April 1963 at age seventy-three.

17. For "his health": C. A. Bennett to T. B. White, Deputy Warden, November 15, 1926; comments on Forbes's work at Leavenworth: Warden to Elwood G. Godman (one of Forbes's lawyers), August 27, 1926; Major C. A. Meals to T. B. White, June 18, 1927; T. B. White to W. T. Hammack, DOJ, September 5, 1927, LF-CRF. Forbes's Trusty Prisoner Agreement was dated March 17, 1927.

18. For analysis of the North Pole claims, see Robert Bryce, *Cook & Peary: The Polar Controversy, Resolved* (Mechanicsburg, PA: Stackpole Books, 1997). Bryce concluded that neither Cook nor Peary reached the Pole (669–673, 689). Cook was the most famous editor of the *New Era.* On his somewhat eccentric editorship, see James McGrath Morris, *Jailhouse Journalism: The Fourth Estate behind Bars* (Jefferson, NC: McFarland, 1998), 86–88.

19. Forbes's Hawaii pieces appeared on page 1 of the *New Era* for April, May, June, and July 1926. Quote on Harding: *New Era,* August 1926, 1. Forbes discussed the condition for probation in December, drug addicts in January. Further articles by Forbes on crime and punishment appeared in May and June 1927. On the self-supporting penitentiary: May 1927. CRF, "Validity of the Polar Claims," April 1927, and "Did Life Begin at the Pole?," July 1927.

20. Hoover, *The Memoirs of Herbert Hoover,* vol. 2, *The Cabinet and the Presidency, 1920–1933* (London: Hollis & Carter, 1953), 55.

21. James N. Giglio, *H. M. Daugherty and the Politics of Expediency* (Kent, OH: Kent State University Press, 1978), 192; *Time,* July 27, 1931; David H. Stratton, *Tempest over Teapot Dome: The Story of Albert B. Fall* (Norman: University of Oklahoma Press, 1998), 344–48.

22. "Forbes seeking Parole, Report," unattributed newspaper clipping under the UP byline, June 27, 1926, 3A; Day letter, CRF to Mrs. Harry Judkins, January 21, 1927; draft telegram, denied by Leavenworth censors, from "Uncle Bob" to G. K. Perkins, Union Trust Building DC, January 23, 1927; draft telegram, "Bob Forbes" to Charles

W. S [*sic*], City Editor, *El Paso Herald,* January 24, 1927; MF Judkins to Warden, February 2, 1927; Professor Ralph H. Major, MD, to Dr. C. A. Bennett, February 5, 1927, LF-CRF.

23. Clarence W. Barron, Arthur Pound, and Samuel Taylor Moore, *They Told Barron* (New York: Harper & Brothers, 1930), 234; quotes on the press by Silas Bent, *Ballyhoo: The Voice of the Press* (New York: Boni & Liveright), 1927, 197–98; and see Bent, *Strange Bedfellows: A Review of Politics, Personalities, and the Press* (New York: H. Liveright, 1928), 210, 212; William Allen White, *Masks in a Pageant* (New York: Macmillan, 1928), 424–36.

24. Samuel Hopkins Adams, *Revelry* (New York: Boni & Liveright, 1926), for quotes, 111, 222–249. On asking prospective jurors at the Fall-Doheny trial: *NYT,* November 23, 1926, 1.

25. Forbes comments: *NYT,* November 30, 1927, 26; Arnold Mulder, "A Novelist's Problem" *Appleton (WS) Post-Crescent,* January 26, 1927, 6; Editorial, *Williamsburg (IA) Journal-Tribune,* November 25, 1926, 4; *NYT,* November 30, 1927, 26; Adams, *Revelry,* 252, 37, 318, respectively.

26. *NYT,* February 8, 1927, Section: Amusements, 25; Harry M. Daugherty and Thomas Dixon, *The Inside Story of the Harding Tragedy* (New York: Churchill, 1932), 198; *Time,* November 29, 1926.

27. CRF to Russell M. Forbes, May 12, June 2, and June 12, 1927, courtesy of the late Richard M. Forbes.

28. Department of Justice Release, July 7, 1927, "Report to Collect Fine Imposed on Charles R. Forbes," NARA-CP, RG 60, Case 225387, Box 3856. See George E. Q. Johnson, US Attorney, DOJ, Northern District of Illinois to Warden, about a civil suit against CRF and the Hartford Accident Company on the matter of his appeal bond, charging that the agreement between the defendant and the court was violated, February 9, 1928. The certificate is included in Forbes's Leavenworth record, as is the signed statement of his debts.

29. An undated [November 1927], torn fragment from a newspaper, which I have been unable to identify, prints Forbes's statement, apparently in full: DOJ FOIA, Charles R. Forbes, 62–3552. The reporter cited is Irwin I. Femrite, *Daily Northwestern,* November 26, 1927, 9; Cook, *Leavenworth New Era,* vol. 14, December 1927, 1; mother's greeting: *NYT,* November 30, 1927, Section: Lost and Found, 26.

CHAPTER 15. Charlie and Bob, Masks and Mirrors

1. "Tells of Prison Dope," *Lancaster Daily Eagle,* December 22, 1927, 8; *WP,* December 17, 1927, 3; *Evening State Journal* and *Lincoln (NB) Daily News,* December 16, 1927, 1 (UP).

2. I use the version of Forbes's article that appeared in the *NYW,* December 4, 1927, 1–3.

3. Re Jeff Sims: *NYW,* December 4, 1927, 2.

4. For headlines: *CDT,* December 4, 1927, 1; *LAT,* December 4, 1927, 1; Daugherty quote: *NYW,* December 5, 1927, 2.

5. "when he was drunk": William Allen White, *Masks in a Pageant* (New York: Macmillan, 1928), 430; Reily: *NYT,* October 25, 1928, 11; Gaston B. Means, as told to May Dixon Thacker, *The Strange Death of President Harding* (New York: Guild Publishing, 1930), 259, 262–64; Nan Britton, *The President's Daughter* (New York: Elizabeth Ann Guild, 1928), frontispiece; Capone quote: *CDT,* December 6, 1927, 1. For major studies on the peculiar history of Harding's reputation: Robert H. Ferrell, *The Strange Deaths of President Harding* (Columbia: University of Missouri Press, 1996); and Phillip G. Payne, *Dead Last: The Public Memory of Warren G. Harding's Scandalous Legacy* (Athens: Ohio University Press, 2009).

6. "devil god": White, *Masks in a Pageant,* 420; *LAT,* February 4, 1928, 1; *NYW,* November 28, 1927, 1.

7. *Sheboygan (WI) Press,* March 20, 1928, 1; *NYT,* March 19, 1928, 9; *NYT,* March 2, 1928, 21; *NYT,* March 15, 1928, 1; *WP,* February 7, 1928, 3. Miller spent eighteen months in prison, was paroled in 1929 and pardoned by President Hoover in 1933.

8. Robert H. Ferrell, *The Presidency of Calvin Coolidge* (Lawrence: University Press of Kansas, 1998), 191, 205, 207. Arthur M. Schlesinger, *The Age of Roosevelt,* vol. 1, *The Crisis of the Old Order, 1919–1933* (Boston: Houghton Mifflin, 1957), 155, 165, Reed quoted (in 1932) at 268.

9. *Pasadena Star-News,* Part 2, March 28, 1929, 11; *Pasadena Post,* March 27 and 28, 1929, both p. 1; *LAT,* March 28, 1929, A12. Thanks to the Pasadena Public Library for introducing me to Pasadena Digital History and, for assistance, especially Wei Zhang and Dan McLaughlin. Obituary of Christina N. Forbes: *Pasadena Star-News,* February 23, 1931, 2.

10. Fall quotes: *LAT,* July 15, 19, 21, 22, 24, 25, 27, 1931; Burl Noggle's book is a classic account: *Teapot Dome: Oil and Politics in the 1920s* (Baton Rouge: Louisiana State University Press, 1962), see esp. 214. Fall's biographer, David H. Stratton, estimated that Fall received more than $400,000 in total value from Doheny and Sinclair, but if he had wanted a real bribe, he would have gone for $4 million: Stratton, *Tempest over Teapot Dome* (Norman: University of Oklahoma Press, 1998), 305, 348.

11. Daugherty and Dixon, *The Inside Story of the Harding Tragedy* (New York: Churchill, 1932), 179–85; James N. Giglio, *H. M. Daugherty and the Politics of Expediency* (Kent, OH: Kent State University Press, 1978), 155–57; Fanny Butcher, review: *CDT,* January 30, 1932, 12.

12. *WP,* August 2, 1933, 1; *WSJ,* August 17, 1933, 3.

13. Katherine's career: CPR-KTF.

14. Richard F. Barry, personal communications, 2010, 2013; Joan Barry Marsh, personal communication, 2010. Richard and Joan were two of the three children of Marcia Forbes Barry, the daughter of Forbes's second marriage. The third sibling, Robert, was a toddler at the time. Forbes's third wife, Katherine, had no children, and his first family was estranged. Forbes's grave is at Section 3, Site 1847-E. For this and confirmation about the funeral: Records of Arlington National Cemetery. Biffle as "helpful pal . . .": Roger Butterfield, *Life Magazine*, June 6, 1946, 65.

15. Robert D. Leigh, *Federal Health Administration in the United States* (New York: Harper & Brothers, 1927), 210–11; Preston William Slosson, *The Great Crusade and After, 1914–1928* (New York: Macmillan, 1930), 77; Frederick Lewis Allen, *Only Yesterday: An Informal History of the Nineteen Twenties* (New York: Harper & Row, 1931), 124, 105, 112, respectively; M. R. Werner, *Privileged Characters* (New York: Robert M. McBride, 1935), 201, 210; William Allen White, *A Puritan in Babylon: The Story of Calvin Coolidge* (New York: Macmillan, 1938), 239.

16. Hoover, *The Memoirs of Herbert Hoover*, vol. 2, *The Cabinet and the Presidency, 1920–1933* (London: Hollis & Carter, 1953), 54; *LAT*, June 17, 1931, 4. On partisan criticism of his speech, see Editorial, *CDT*, July 11, 1931.

17. *WP*, March 1, 1934, 8.

18. E. S. McPherson to US Veterans Bureau [*sic*], May 8, 1945; G. H. Sweet to E. S. McPherson, May 25, 1945, CPR-CRF.

19. Harding-Forbes correspondence records: JWH Crim to Wm. J. Donovan, October 9, 1924, NARA-CP, RG 60, Case 225387, Box 3855. Crim went to the White House to look for papers that might be helpful in protecting Harding, as well as important in the Forbes case, because it was Forbes's practice to write to the president when he needed specific authority, with a draft letter from WGH that would give him that authority. Crim: "There is a very large file consisting of papers of this sort, of discussions concerning the sites, of the political considerations involved, directions from the President to Forbes, letters of criticism of Forbes which were sent to him by the President, and of memoranda made by the President of criticisms of Forbes made to the President personally." He did not find the file. Merle Sweet said that the letters Forbes took with him when he left office were of a "strictly personal nature" (SH, 1334). On Forbes's papers: Thomas H. Tullidge, personal communication, 2007; Mark Sullivan quote: *Our Times*, vol. 6, *The Twenties* (New York: Scribner, 1946), 365.

20. D. A. Reed to Mark Sullivan, July 1, 1935, Sullivan Papers, Box 15. Another respondent, Charles G. Dawes, supported his old friend, the late Dr. Sawyer, and praised his "initiative and consequent discovery of Forbes's dishonesty." Dawes to Sullivan, July 1, 1935, Sullivan Papers, Box 6. See also Sullivan, *Our Times*, 6:143–44.

21. Samuel Hopkins Adams, *Incredible Era: The Life and Times of Warren Gamaliel Harding* (Cambridge, MA: Riverside Press, 1939), dust jacket, preface, and, respectively, 234, 108, 233, 238, 290–91, 335, 441; H. F. Alderfer, "The Personality and

Politics of Warren G. Harding" (PhD diss., School of Citizenship and Public Affairs, Syracuse University, 1928), 248–50. See also Samuel V. Kennedy III, *Samuel Hopkins Adams and the Business of Writing* (Syracuse, NY: Syracuse University Press, 1999), 187–189.

22. Karl Schriftgiesser, *This Was Normalcy: An Account of Party Politics during Twelve Republican Years: 1920–1932* (Boston: Little, Brown, 1948), 81–82, 110–13; Henry J. Taylor, "Was Corruption as Bad under Harding?," *Reader's Digest*, August 1952, 59–60.

23. Robert K. Murray, *The Harding Era: Warren G. Harding and His Administration* (Minneapolis: University of Minnesota Press, 1969); John W. Dean, *Warren G. Harding* (New York: Times Books, 2004). Internet examples: "dashing playboy," Wikipedia; $200 million, Britannica.com; both accessed 7/11/2015.

24. 1931–1932 figure: A. A. Friedrich, *Encyclopaedia of the Social Sciences*, vol. 15, "Veterans" (New York: Macmillan, 1935), 245; *Memoirs of Herbert Hoover*, 285. In the early 1930s, there were almost twice as many veterans hospitalized for non-service-connected than for service-connected conditions: Gustavus A. Weber and Laurence F. Schmeckebier, *The Veterans' Administration, Its History, Activities and Organization* (Washington, DC: Brookings Institution, 1934), 477.

25. Bonus Army: see esp. Paul Dickson and Thomas B. Allen, *The Bonus Army: An American Epic* (Walker, 2004), 30; Stephen R. Ortiz, *Beyond the Bonus March and GI Bill: How Veteran Politics Shaped the New Deal Era* (New York: New York University Press, 2010), 1; quote: "I can see . . .": Thomas Lunsford Stokes, *Chip Off My Shoulder* (Princeton, NJ: Princeton University Press, 1940), 303. Another future general, George S. Patton, was also in the military team.

26. For a detailed treatment of Forbes's role as initiator of the Veterans Health System, see Jessica L. Adler, "A Solemn Obligation: Soldiers, Veterans, and Health Policy in the United States 1917–1924." Submitted in partial fulfillment of the requirements for the PhD in the Graduate School of Arts and Sciences, Columbia University, 2012, 407–12. And, Jessica L. Adler, *Burdens of War: Politics, Necessity, and the Birth of the Veterans Hospital System* (Baltimore: Johns Hopkins University Press, forthcoming). Current information on veterans' services: www.va.gov.

Coda

1. Philip Kinsley, *CDT*, various dates November–December 1924.

2. The characteristics are drawn from Roger A. McKinnon, Robert Michels, and Peter J. Buckley, *The Psychiatric Interview in Clinical Practice*, 2nd ed. (Arlington, VA: American Psychiatric Publishing, 2006), 353–83.

3. Clinton W. Gilbert, *Behind the Mirrors: The Psychology of Disintegration at Washington* (New York: G. P. Putnam's Sons, 1922), 114.

4. In 1947, James V. Forrestal, previously US secretary of the navy, became the first US secretary of defense, responsible for coordinating the formerly independent departments for the army, navy, and air force against substantial resistance from within—and with insufficient authority to insist on their cooperation. Legislation in 1949 remedied some of the problems, but by then Forrestal had resigned. Suffering from severe depression and in danger of suicide, he entered psychiatric treatment. His body was found on a low roof below the window of his sixteenth-floor room of the National Naval Medical Center in Bethesda, Maryland, and though his mental illness cannot be ascribed solely to his job, the exhaustion, conflicts, and frustrations he faced cannot have helped. The inscription on his gravestone at the Arlington National Cemetery, carved in capital letters, reads: "In the Great Cause of Good Government."

In 2003, Tom Ridge, a Republican with an esteemed reputation—possible future president, former governor of Pennsylvania, and before that a longtime congressman—took on the grueling job of creating the Department of Homeland Security during the administration of George W. Bush, which involved the regrouping of 180,000 employees from twenty-two different agencies. Following two years of never-ending work, tensions among disparate cultures, inevitable mistakes, widespread criticism and barbs, and on occasion ridicule from the media, Secretary Ridge resigned with his political capital spent and abandoned full-time service in the public sector.

Index